THE AYMARA

Strategies in Human Adaptation to a Rigorous Environment

Studies in Human Biology

VOLUME 2

Series Editor

KENNETH M. WEISS

Department of Anthropology and Graduate Program in Genetics,
The Pennsylvania State University

The titles published in this series are listed at the end of this volume.

THE AYMARA

Strategies in Human Adaptation to a Rigorous Environment

edited by

WILLIAM J. SCHULL

The University of Texas at Houston,
The Genetics Centers,
Graduate School of Biomedical Sciences

and

FRANCISCO ROTHHAMMER

University of Chile,
Department of Cellular Biology and Genetics,
Medical School, Santiago

With collaborating editor

SARA A. BARTON

The University of Texas at Houston,
The Genetics Centers,
Graduate School of Biomedical Sciences

KLUWER ACADEMIC PUBLISHERS

DORDRECHT / BOSTON / LONDON

Library of Congress Cataloging in Publication Data

The Aymara : strategies in human adaptation to a rigorous environment / edited by William J. Schull, Francisco Rothhammer, with collaborating editor, Sara A. Barton.
p. cm. -- (Studies in human biology ; v. 2)
Includes bibliographical references (p.) and index.
ISBN 0-7923-0969-3 (acid free paper)
1. Aymara Indians--Anthropometry. 2. Aymara Indians--Health and hygiene. 3. Altitude, Influence of. 4. Anoxemia. I. Schull, William J. II. Rothhammer, Francisco. III. Barton, Sara A. IV. Series.
F2230.2.A9A89 1990
612'.098--dc20 90-5335

ISBN 0-7923-0969-3

Published by Kluwer Academic Publishers,
P.O. Box 17, 3300 AA Dordrecht, The Netherlands.

Kluwer Academic Publishers incorporates
the publishing programmes of
D. Reidel, Martinus Nijhoff, Dr W. Junk and MTP Press.

Sold and distributed in the U.S.A. and Canada
by Kluwer Academic Publishers,
101 Philip Drive, Norwell, MA 02061, U.S.A.

In all other countries, sold and distributed
by Kluwer Academic Publishers Group,
P.O. Box 322, 3300 AH Dordrecht, The Netherlands.

This book was produced in camera-ready form with an IBM PC compatible computer, using Quicksoft's *PC-Write* word processor and a Hewlett-Packard LaserJet Series II printer, with "Tms Rmn" and "Prestige Elite" soft fonts. Robert Schwartz customized the printer driver and developed the formatting codes to obtain the desired layout.

Printed on acid-free paper

Printed in the Netherlands

TABLE OF CONTENTS

FOREWORD

South America's Andean highlands have seen the rise and decline of several impressive, indigenous civilizations. Separated somewhat in time and place, each developed its distinctive socio-cultural accouterments but all shared a need to adjust to the individual, societal and environmental limitations imposed by life at high altitude. Partial oxygen pressure, temperature and humidity fall systematically as altitude rises, but there are other changes as well. Darwin, Forbes, von Humboldt, von Tschudi and other naturalists of the eighteenth and nineteenth centuries who weaved their way through South America commented repeatedly on the tolerance or apparent indifference of the indigenes to the rigors of life at altitudes above 3000 meters but its impact upon lowlanders. Von Tschudi (1847), for example, observed 'in the cordillera the effect of the diminished atmospheric pressure on the human frame shows itself in intolerable symptoms of weariness and an extreme difficulty of breathing. . . . The first symptoms are usually felt at the elevation of 12,600 feet (3800 m) above the sea. These symptoms are vertigo, dimness of sight and hearing, pains in the head and nausea. . . . Inhabitants of the coast and Europeans, who for the first time visit the lofty regions of the cordillera, are usually attacked with this disorder.' But von Tschudi's description of acute mountain sickness was hardly the first; his Spanish predecessors had known and commented upon it too. The earliest account is probably that of the Spanish Jesuit, Father Joseph de Acosta although it has recently been argued that acute gastroenteritis was either a more likely cause of the symptoms he described than acute mountain sickness or at least a complicating factor in his experiences (Bonavia et al., 1985). Be this as it may, Acosta wrote (1590, see also Purchas, 1628; in particular the 1905 reprinting, volume 15, pp. 27-29):

> 'There is in Peru, a high mountaine which they call Pariacaca, and having heard spoke of the alteration it bred, I went as well prepared as I could, according to the instructions which was given me, by such as they call Vaguianos, or expert men: but not withstanding all my provision, when I came to mount the degrees, as they called them, which is the top of the mountaine, I was suddenly surprized with so mortall and so strange a pang, that I was ready to fall from the top to the ground: and although we were many in company, yet every one made haste (without tarrying for his companion,) to free himselfe speedily from this ill passage. Being then alone with one Indian, whom I entreated to helpe to stay me, I was surprized with such pangs of straining and casting, as I thought to cast up my heart too; for having cast up meate, flegme, and coller, both yellow and green; in the end I cast up blood, with the straining of my stomacke. To conclude, if this continued, I should undoubtedly have dyed; but this lasted not above three or foure houres, that wee were come into a more convenient and naturall temperature, where all our companions (being fourteene or fifteene) were much wearied. .... But commonly it doth no important harme, onely this paine and troublesome distates while it endures: and not onely the passage of Pariacaca hath this propertie, but also all this ridge of the Mountaine, which

> runnes above five hundred leagues long, and in what place soever you passe, you shall finde strange intemperatures .... I therefore perswade my selfe, that the element of the ayre is there so subtile and delicate, as it is not proportionable with the breathing of man, which requires a more grosse and temperate ayre, and I beleeve it is the cause that doth so much alter the stomacke, and trouble all the disposition.'

Two features of Acosta's early description warrant special attention as testimonies to the astuteness of his observations. First, he correctly deduced that it was the 'thinness' of the air that induced the symptoms, and second, that these effects occurred throughout the Andes if the altitude was high enough, but were generally transitory and harmless.

These chroniclers also noted that the indigenous peoples differed one from another but had in common disproportionately large chests which they ascribed to the demands of the altitude. They were intrigued too by the changes in body dimensions of highland peoples who colonized low altitudes. Most of these early observations were limited in scope and number, and frequently bordered on the anecdotal. Systematic study of the processes of acclimatization and adaptation to the hypoxia of altitude did not begin until roughly a century ago with the studies of the great French physiologist, Paul Bert (1878). Much of the earliest work was in the Alps. This century has seen an expansion of interest to Africa, the Himalayas, the Andes and their peoples, and the search for commonalities in adaptation in these different geographic areas. Of particular relevance have been studies in the Andean area and the contributions of the Peruvian high altitude physiologists and the Pennsylvania State University anthropologists, including their students.

The Aymará who are the objects of the present volume were first studied, at least in recent times by Ricardo Cruz-Coke, a physician and geneticist, who became interested in high altitude research some years ago during a stay in Lima where his father was the Chilean ambassador. Cruz-Coke promoted the interest of other health scientists, who joined him in various field visits organized between 1962 and 1968. During a post-doctoral training period at the University of Michigan, in 1971, one of us analyzed most of the data collected by Cruz-Coke and his colleagues under the guidance of the other, who was then a member of the faculty of the Medical School of the University of Michigan. From this scientific collaboration emerged the multidisciplinary research to be set forth in subsequent pages. Although the main body of information was collected and analyzed between 1973 and 1978, additional data collection and evaluation continue.

Our interest in the Aymará and thus our perspectives are essentially biomedical but in an anthropological and genetic context. Broadly stated, our aims in this monograph are to describe changes in function, in healthy and diseased states, of the pulmonary and cardiovascular systems and in cardiopulmonary relationships in anthropologically defined, biologically homogeneous groups, living in adjacent but sharply different environmental niches. Furthermore, we are interested in assessing, if possible, the genetic contribution to man's adaptation to hypoxia, more specifically, to quantify changes in genetic variability with increasing oxygen pressure. Finally, we wish to understand the ethnogenesis and the evolutionary relationships of the Aymará and of Andean populations in general to other indigenous groups in South America as they are revealed by a series of genetic markers. We are under no illusion that the study to be described achieved the stated ends in all of its particulars. It patently has shortcomings. Some of these were apparent at its initiation, but represent the inevitable compromises forced upon a study of its nature; others have become so as analysis of the data has progressed. One of the explicit aims of this monograph is to expose these limitations in order that subsequent investigators will profit.

Although each of the essays that comprise this book is intended to be self-contained, we have attempted to depict the Aymará as they reside in environments of different physiological and socioeconomic stress so that some of the environmental interactions, interactions that characterize all societies, can be seen in their complexity. It is these interactions that must be identified and understood if progress is to continue in studies of human adaptability. Finally, as the literature readily reveals, there are numerous different transliterations of the names of the various Andean cultures; for consistency we have fixed on one, possibly not always the best, but where alternatives exist, these will be found in the Glossary.

The Editors

ACKNOWLEDGEMENTS

Studies of this magnitude and complexity, carried out under circumstances alien to most of the investigators involved, clearly owe whatever measure of success they achieve to numerous people and many local and national institutions, but we are especially beholden to the now defunct Junta de Adelanto de Arica and its then president, Luis Beretta. Without the unqualified endorsement of this body, as well as the enthusiastic support of all members of the Department of Community Development and Andean Plan – particularly its chief, Carlos Solari – this study would have not been possible. We owe much to the National Health Service of Chile, the Servicio Nacional de Salud, the practicantes of the Chilean police, and the teachers who gave selflessly of their time and energies to make our examinations a success. We are also indebted to numerous persons and institutions at the local and national levels in Bolivia, but especially to Coronel Antonio Ovando of the Corporación de Desarrollo de Oruro, Padres Emery Mulaire and Santiago Monaste, Gilberto Pauwels, and Srs. Juan Capurate and Teófilo Ayma. Finally, we wish to express our gratitude too to the numerous members of our field teams and the residents of the study locales who in patience and good humor tolerated our questions, pokings and proddings.

This work was supported by grants from the National Heart, Lung and Blood Institute (HL-15614, HL-05266), the Institute of General Medical Sciences (GM-28574) of the National Institutes of Health, the Wenner-Gren Foundation and the John S. Guggenheim Foundation of the United States; from the Special Program for Research and Training in Tropical Diseases of the World Health Organization; from MAB/UNESCO; from the Fondo Nacional de Desarrollo Cientifico y Tecnologico (FONDECYT); and the Universidad de Chile. We are grateful to all of these institutions and agencies for without their help this study would never have been undertaken, and if undertaken, could certainly not have been adequately implemented.

LIST OF CONTRIBUTORS

Allison, Marvin J.
Professor of Pathology
Virginia Commonwealth University
Medical College of Virginia
Department of Pathlogy
PO Box 662
Richmond, Virginia 23237

Bailey, Julia K.
Graduate Student
2312 Suffolk Dr.
Houston, Texas 77027

Barja, Ita
Nutritionist
Perseo 577
Santiago, Chile

Barton, Sara Ann
Research Instructor
The University of Texas
Graduate School of Biomedical Sciences
Center for Demographic and Population Genetics
PO Box 20334
Houston, Texas 77225

Castro Williams, Nélida
Nutritionist
15427 Linkshire
Houston, Texas 77062

Chakraborty, Ranajit
Professor
The University of Texas
Graduate School of Biomedical Sciences
Center for Demographic and Population Genetics
PO Box 20334
Houston, Texas 77225

Díaz, Biffret
Pediatrician
Velasquez 1320, # 303
Arica, Chile

Ferrell, Robert E.
Professor
Department of Human Genetics
University of Pittsburgh
Graduate School of Public Health
Pittsburgh, Pennsylvania 15261

Figueroa Tagle, Leonardo
Associate Professor of Applied Analytical Chemistry
Universidad de Tarapacá
Casilla 7-D
Arica, Chile

Gallegos, Daniel
Physician
PO Box 693
Quito, Ecuador

Goldsmith, Robert I.
Ophthalmologist
1708 Shadford Road
Ann Arbor, Michigan 48104

González Ureta, Mariluz
Analytical Chemist
Universidad de Tarapacá
Casilla 7-D
Arica, Chile

Lunny Lenart, Vivian
Cardiologist
36 Manor View
Stevenage Herts
SG2 8PF, England

McFarlane, Judith
Professor
College of Nursing
Texas Woman's University
1130 M.D. Anderson Blvd.
Houston, Texas 77030

Mueller, William H.
Professor
The University of Texas
School of Public Health
PO Box 20186
Houston, Texas 77225

Murillo, Federico
Physician
Sucursal de Correos Miraflores
PO Box 110097
La Paz, Bolivia

Palomino, Hernán
Associate Professor
Universidad de Chile
Facultad de Medicina
Departamento Biología Celular y Genética
Casilla 70061
Santiago 7, Chile

Razmilíc Bonilla, Blago
Professor Analytical Chemistry and Instrumental Analysis
Universidad de La Serena
Facultad de Ciencias
Departamento de Biología y Química
Casilla 599
La Serena, Chile

Rothhammer, Francisco
Professor
Universidad de Chile
Facultad de Medicina
Departamento Biología Celular y Genética
Casilla 70061
Santiago 7, Chile

Schull, Victoria
1400 Hermann Drive, #16E
Houston, Texas 77004

Schull, William J.
Director and Ashbel Smith Professor
The University of Texas
Graduate School of Biomedical Sciences
Center for Demographic and Population Genetics
PO Box 20334
Houston, Texas 77225

Soto-Heim, Patricia
Anthropologist
Museé National D'Histoire Naturelle
Anthropologie
Museé de L'Homme - 17
Place du Trocadéro
75116 Paris, France

Spotorno, Angel E.
Associate Professor
Universidad de Chile
Facultad de Medicina
Departamento Biología Celular y Genética
Casilla 70061
Santiago 7, Chile

Veloso, Alberto
Director
Facultad de Ciencias
Universidad de Chile
Departamento de Ecologia
Las Palmeras
Santiago, Chile

Weidman, Betsy
Audiologist
Mayo Clinic
Rochester, Minnesota 55905

Weidman, William H.
Cardiologist
Professor of Pediatrics
Mayo Clinic
Department of Pediatric Cardiology
Rochester, Minnesota 55905

WILLIAM J. SCHULL

Chapter 1
INTRODUCTION: THE PLACE AND THE STUDY

Northern Chile is a land of contrasts – verdant coastal valleys and soaring, perpetually snow-capped mountains separated by the formidable, rainless expanse of the Atacama desert. The shore is a striated, pink-brown cliff face rising in some places to a height of 1000 meters, pierced here and there by modest rivers that arise in the cordilleras to the east. At the bottom of this cliff are sea-eroded terraces, on which are built the towns. Beyond the coastal escarpment, at an elevation of 600 meters or so, and somewhat to the south, are the Pampas de Chaco and Camarones, a series of old lake floors of varying widths – the northern limits of the Atacama desert. Eastward the land rises rapidly into the Sierra de Huaylillas and the Cordillera Central to fall briefly to the altiplano and rise again to the Cordillera Oriental – the boundary between Bolivia and Chile; the crest of these mountains has an average elevation of 5000 meters with occasional peaks over 6000 meters high. This latter barrier is broken at about 4000 meters by a mountain pass, the Portazuela de Tambo Quemado, some 80 kilometers from the sea.

This is an area of frequent natural calamities and has undoubtedly been so for millennia; it is the interface of two active tectonic plates. Earthquakes and tidal waves – frequent sequela of an earthquake – occur with disturbing regularity. In post-Columbian times southern Perú, including parts of what is now northern Chile has been visited by major quakes in 1586, 1604, 1615, 1681, 1746, 1831, 1833, 1868, 1877 and 1895 (Keller, 1946; Urzua, 1969) as well as others more recent. Squier (1878; see also Urzua, 1969, pp. 54-56), a onetime U. S. Commissioner to Perú, wrote tellingly of the havoc a tidal wave can visit on these valleys, specifically at Arica. He said, 'The water rose till it reached a height of thirty-four feet (10 m) above high-water-mark, and overflowed the town, and rushed through the streets, and threw down what the earthquake had left. And all this rise and overflow of the waters took only about five minutes. The water rushed back into the ocean more suddenly than it had advanced upon the land. This awful spectacle of destruction by the receding flood had hardly been realized when the sea rose again, and now the vessels in port began dragging. The water rose to the same height as before, and on rushing back it brought not only the debris of the ruined city with it, but even a locomotive and tender and a train of four cars were seen carried away by the fearful force of the waves. During this advance of the sea inland, another terrific shock, lasting about eight minutes, was felt. At this time all around the city the dust formed into clouds, and, obscuring the sky, made things on land quite invisible. It was then that the thundering approach of a heavy sea-wave was noticed, and a minute afterwards a seawall of perpendicular height to the extent of from forty-two to forty-five feet

William J. Schull and Francisco Rothhammer (eds.), The Aymará: Strategies in Human Adaptation to a Rigorous Environment, 1-18. ©1990 *by Kluwer Academic Publishers.*

(13 to 14 m), capped with a fringe of bright, glistening foam, swept over the land, stranding far inshore the United States steamer Wateree, the America, a Peruvian frigate, and the Chanarcillo, an English merchant-vessel.' The ill-fated Wateree settled some three kilometers from the coast, and since it was obviously impossible to refloat it from this distance, it ended its existence, ignominiously for a man-of-war, as a hotel (Urzua, 1969).

The coastal valleys and the high intermontane plain we have described have been settled for millennia. Social intercourse, as archaeological evidence attests, and gene flow between the peoples of these regions have long occurred. But some five centuries ago the dimensions of their cultural, economic and biological interdependence were altered. The rise of Incan hegemony and the arrival of the Spanish conquistadors brought decimation and ultimately loss or absorption to the coastal peoples and enslavement to the Andean indigenes. A rapacious search for noble metals led to the displacement of populations and eclipsed agricultural and pastoral pursuits. The cultural syncretism prompted by the competing autochthonous and Spanish ways of life compromised values and the traditional awareness of the fragility of the ecology of the sierra and western altiplano.

THE ECOLOGICAL NICHES

Broadly speaking, the area of which we write is divisible into three sharply differentiable but geographically adjacent ecological zones – the costa, the sierra, and the altiplano – that differ strikingly in temperature, rainfall, and oxygen pressure; associated with changes in these are biotic changes that limit the types of economies that can be practiced, and thus lifestyles. A brief characterization of these different environments follows (see also Keller, 1946; Cruz-Coke, Cristoffanini, Aspillaga and Biancani, 1966; Santolaya, Donoso, Apud and Sanudo, 1973; Cruz-Coke, 1977).

The coastal valleys

The northern coastal zone (the costa) of Chile embraces four valleys, the Lluta, the Azapa, the Codpa and the Camarones, and the terrace on which the city of Arica sits. While portions of these valleys are lush, as a result of irrigation and the rivers that arise in the mountains to the east, rainfall is sparse, and this appears to have been true throughout their human occupation (Bird, 1963). Many coastal areas habitually see less than one millimeter of rain a year. Temperatures are moderate. The annual average maximum in Arica is 21.8°C and the annual average minimum is only 14.9°C; the diurnal cycle is small, normally less than 10°C. Seasonal differences are limited to a five-month cloudy period (June-October) when each morning the sky is possessed by fog or low clouds that dissipate during the day; most afternoons are sunny. It is a salubrious climate, moderated by the Pacific high pressure center to the west, swept by the southeast trade winds.

These are conditions conducive to crop diversity; grains, olives, grapes, melons, sugar cane, vegetables and a variety of citrus fruits are or have been grown. Even cotton was raised commercially at one time (Squier, 1878, p. 219). Most of these crops are not indigenous; they as well as the cattle that is husbanded have been introduced at one time or another since the arrival of the Spanish. Agricultural enterprises, which can be initiated at any time of the year, now depend either upon labor imported from other areas in Chile or from the west of Bolivia. Malaria was either already prevalent in the area, or more likely, given the rapid decimation of the indigenous population, became so shortly after the Spanish arrived, possibly introduced through the slaves they imported. It persisted until 1945 (Wormald, 1968). Interestingly, given its importance as a staple at higher altitudes, the potato is not generally cultivated here, nor was it in the recent historic past. Von Tschudi (1847, p. 178) too had noted: 'Potatoes are not planted on the coast, where, it appears, the climate and soil are unfavourable to them. In those parts they are small and watery. On the higher ridges which intersect the coast at short distances from the sea, the potato grows wild. I am inclined to believe that the root is indigenous in these parts, as well as in Chiloe and Chile, and that the ancient Peruvians did not obtain this root from the south but that they removed it from their own high lands in order to cultivate it on a more favourable soil.'

The city of Arica, the economic and administrative focus of the northernmost zone of the Province of Tarapaca, dominated by its Morro, the scene of one of the decisive battles of the Pacific War, has a population in excess of 100,000 persons and sprawls over the flatlands at the mouth of the Quebrada Azapa. The area it presently occupies has been inhabited for thousands of years, as numerous indigenous burial sites witness. Arica's importance as a port in post-Columbian times followed the discovery in 1545 of silver at Potosi in Bolivia. Soon thereafter, Sir Francis Drake (in 1579) and Thomas Cavendish (1587), and subsequently, Bartholomew Sharp and John Watling (1681) and other freebooters of the time, attracted by the promise of wealth, exercised their sails and guns off Arica's coast; sometimes as in John Watling's case, their efforts cost them their lives (Urzua, 1969). Arica and the other coastal communities of the north, such as Iquique, were parts of a flourishing coastal trade that extended at least as far south as Chiloe. Von Tschudi (1847) noted that boats from the latter island regularly plied as far northwards as Callao, the port of Lima, carrying wood, brooms, hams and potatoes and returning with linen, woolen and cotton cloths, ironware, tobacco and spirits. Although Arica is the coastal terminus of a rail line to La Paz, and serves as one of Bolivia's outlets to the sea, its importance as a port waned as mining declined, revived briefly when the area was a free-trade zone, and it is not now as great as formerly. It does not compete significantly with Antofagasta, Valparaiso or San Antonio, Chile's major ports to the south. Most of Arica's present inhabitants are relatively recent immigrants, drawn to it primarily within the last five decades or so.

The sierra

In the sierra to the east of the Atacama desert, the terrain is rugged and highly irregular. It is a xeric zone of columnar cacti and ephemeral plants, a chaparral-like region of xerophytic scrub. Villages, largely of indigenous peoples, either squat on tablelands or commingle with highland valleys; most are at elevations of 3000 to 3500 meters and are generally situated near springs or mountain streams. The majority of these villages are old, and have been recorded on maps of the area for centuries. However, virtually all have fewer than several hundred inhabitants. At these heights, partial oxygen pressure is approximately 100 mm (as contrasted with 149 mm at sea level). Cosmic and ultraviolet activity are much more intense. Rain, though markedly seasonal, occurs with increasing intensity from 2500 meters upwards. Temperatures, particularly the daily and annual minima, are substantially lower than those of the coast, and the diurnal temperature cycle often exceeds 30°C. In the dry season the humidity rarely reaches 20 per cent, and the more fragile plants, such as the phlox-like flowers that brighten the mountainsides in the rainy season, literally dessicate in situ.

The soil is generally poor, and crops are less diverse than on the coast; economically, the most important one is alfalfa, grown as fodder for the cattle and sheep. Oregano, which has been introduced as a cash crop, and some corn, potatoes, quinoa and other vegetables are cultivated for home use. Llama and alpaca, contrary to common thought, are not particularly numerous, and some wild guanaco persist. Trees are few, and then mostly imported conifers or eucalyptus. Irrigation is primitive but effective. Cultivation is generally by hand, or with the aid of an occasional burro or horse. Equatorially (north) facing slopes are more productive; presumably the difference of a few degrees in soil temperature is significant.

The altiplano

Over 40 per cent of the Departamento de Arica lies above 4000 meters; much of this is a rolling high plain, the so-called altiplano, delimited on the east and west by mountains that occasionally exceed 6000 meters. It is an austere land, alternately wet (December-March) and dry (April-November), punctuated in the north by salt flats and intimidated in the south by an active volcano, Guallatiri, the highest in the world. Temperatures commonly oscillate as much as 30°C in the course of 24 hours and even greater changes have been recorded (Keller, 1946). Snowfall is slight, except in the high mountains, and is confined almost exclusively to the rainy season. Little shelter exists from the chilling, parching winds, creators of 'dust devils' and rachitic plants, that blow through much of the year; there are virtually no trees, save the tortuous queñua (*Polylepis incana*) and the coarse grass (ichu). The scrubby growth that does occur rarely attains a meter's height. Here and there are marshy oases of green peat bogs, the bofedales, stepchildren of the melting snows or erratic meanderings of small streams, that support herds of alpaca and llama and a few domesticated burros or the occasional feral one. Vicuña, the graceful kin of the alpaca and llama; viscacha, a shy rock-loving rabbit-like rodent; nandu, the South American rhea; condors and perdiz, a partridge of a kind, are commonplace, and the lakes, Chungará, and Cotacotani, are graced with pink flamingos, the parina, that rarely stray (Hernández, 1970).

Potatoes are staples; other crops are few. Corn will not thrive, and quinoa, that does well in Bolivia, does poorly here. A large cauliflower-like woody plant, called llareta (*Laretia compacta*), provides one of the few combustibles with which to cook or relieve the cold in the simple thatched adobe dwellings. This is a remarkable place and its inhabitants, a remarkable people. Deeply etched in their faces and social fabric is a durability that belies an often dour countenance, and the hardships that fashion their lives. However, skin weathered to an elephantine abrasiveness, cheeks often unnaturally rosy, and eyes etched with an actinic patchwork of capillaries speak eloquently to the physical hardships of their life.

The peripatetic nineteenth century chronicler, von Tschudi (1847, pp. 303-305) described this land as follows: 'Between the Cordillera and the Andes, at the height of 12,000 feet (3600 m) above the sea, there are vast tracts of uninhabited table-lands. These are called in the Quichua language the Puna; and the Spaniards give them the name of the Despoblado (the uninhabited). These table-lands form the upper mountain regions of the South American Highlands. They spread over the whole extent of Perú, from north-west to south-east, a distance of 350 Spanish miles, continuing through Bolivia, and gradually running eastward into the Argentine Republic. .... The climate of these regions is not less rigorous than that of the high mountain ridges. Cold winds, from the west and south-west, blow nearly all the year round from the ice-topped Cordillera; and for the space of four months these winds are daily accompanied by thunder, lightening, and snow-storms.' He continued, 'The aspect of the Puna is singularly monotonous and dreary. The expansive levels are scantily covered with grasses of a yellowish-brown hue, and are never enlivened by fresh-looking verdure. Here and there, at distant intervals, may be seen a few stunted Queñua trees (*Polylepis racemosa*, R.P.), or large patches of ground covered with the Ratanhia shrub (*Krameria triandria*, R.P.). Both are used by the Indians as fuel, and for roofing their huts.' He further observed, 'In the heights of the Cordillera the effect of diminished atmospheric pressure on the human frame shows itself in intolerable symptoms of weariness and an extreme difficulty of breathing. The natives call this malady the Puna or Soroche; and the Spanish Creoles give it the names of Mareo or Veta. ..... The first symptoms of the veta are usually felt at the elevation of 12,600 feet (3800 m) above the sea. These symptoms are vertigo, dimness of sight and hearing, pains in the head and nausea. Blood flows from the eyes, nose and lips. Fainting fits, spitting of blood, and other dangerous symptoms, usually attend severe attacks of veta.' To this litany of threats to well-being, Forbes added 'Another scourge of the traveller in the Cordillera, is the disease called the Surumpe. It is a violent inflammation of the eyes, caused by the sudden reflection of the bright rays of the sun on the snow. By the rarefied air and the

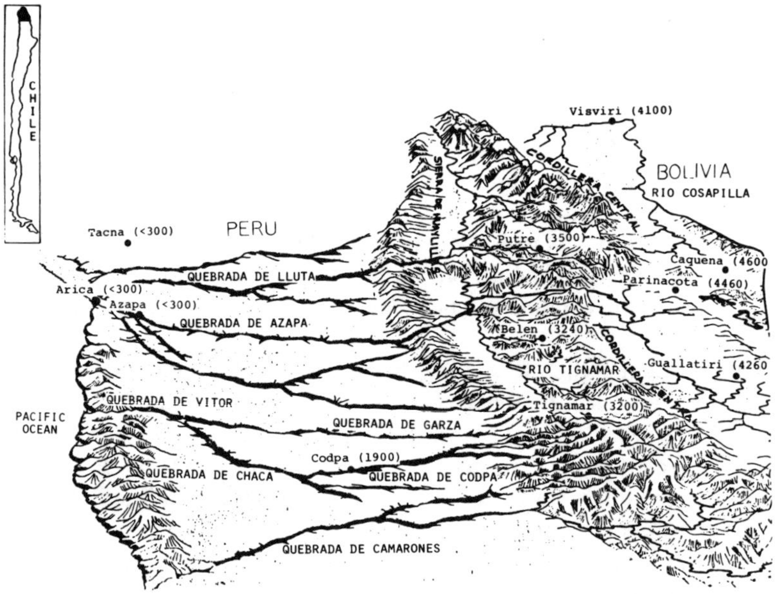

FIGURE 1. A physiographic sketch of the Departamento de Arica with some of the village locations and altitude

Clench et al. (1981), Figure 1, p. 749. Reprinted with permission of Alan R. Liss, NY.

cutting wind, the eyes, being kept in a constant state of irritation, are thereby rendered very susceptible to the effects of the glaring light.'

THE PEOPLE

Scattered across the altiplano and through the quebrada of the Sierra de Huaylillas and the Cordillera Central are villages of Aymará (see Figure 1). Several thousands live in the area (many more are in Western Bolivia). Their villages and caserios range from tens of individuals to a few hundred. Until recently they have been primarily peasant pastoralists deriving their livelihood from herds of alpaca and llama, or subsistence agriculturalists, the former in the altiplano and the latter in the sierras. Little is known with certainty of their social structure in pre-Columbian times, but to the extent that this structure persisted into the years of early European contact, they were not tribally organized, but existed as loose, more-or-less autonomous villages or hamlets within which some social hierarchical levels occurred.

THE STUDY

Scientific characterization of the differences between Andean and non-Andean peoples began over a century ago; efforts to understand the anatomical, biochemical and physiological bases of their adaptation have mounted in the last half century. Speculation colors observation, but the latter adaptation could occur, as Frisancho (1975) has noted, through modifications in pulmonary ventilation, lung volume and pulmonary diffusing capacity, transportation of oxygen in the blood, diffusion of oxygen from blood to tissues, utilization of oxygen at the tissue level or some combination of these. All of these alternatives may be operative but differentially, and the genetic contributions to these diverse adaptive pathways too may differ. Environmental modulation of growth and development could loom large in some instances and small in others.

The Multinational Andean Genetic and Health Program was organized in 1972 in the Departamento de Arica in close cooperation with the Departamento Desarrollo Comunal y Plan Andino of the Junta de Adelanto de Arica and has involved professionals from Bolivia (Universidad de San Andres), Chile (Universidad de Chile, Santiago; Universidad del Norte, Arica; Servicio Nacional de Salud), Ecuador (Universidad Central), Perú (Universidad de San Marcos) and the United States (Universities of Michigan and Texas, and the Mayo Clinic). Broadly stated, the objectives of this program were to appraise the impact of differences in ambient oxygen tension, temperature and humidity upon disease and disability among the Aymará, and to assess the role of genetic variation in their adaptation to the hypoxia of altitude. Another, less immediately scientific but no less important objective from the public health perspective was the assessment of the health problems and needs of these people. To these ends, some 2525 individuals, inhabitants of 14 villages and locales in northern Chile and western Bolivia, were examined in the years 1973-75.

Traditional adaptive and health parameters were studied, but special attention was focused upon the estimation of the frequencies of a number of biochemical markers to ascertain the extent, if any, of non-indigenous contribution to the present gene pool and to identify simply inherited biochemical variants which appear to be responding directly, in frequency, to changes in oxygen tension. Of particular interest were those enzymic and non-enzymic proteins associated with red cell glycolysis and oxygen transport or the regulation of the latter. An effort was also made to measure a number of the intermediates involved in the regulation of glycolysis including adenosine triphosphate (ATP), the energy currency of the body.

The examination or observations on each individual include: a complete medical history, including the Rose and Blackburn (1968) cardiovascular questionnaire, and a general physical examination, embracing pulmonary function tests, resting electrocardiogram and cardiac function as evaluated clinically, and an ophthalmoscopic examination involving, in addition to the clinical assessment of the health of the eye and its adnexa, visual acuity, color vision tests and tensiometry. Oral and dental appraisals were routinely conducted, and craniofacial measurements, dental casts and anthropometric measurements obtained on virtually all participants. Auditory acuity was assessed on all individuals old enough to understand the testing procedure. Simple neuromuscular performance tests, such as tapping, were also conducted and nutritional, reproductive and residential histories were collected. Finally, either an ACD-preserved specimen of venous blood, or a perchloric or trichloracetic acid precipitated specimen, or both was collected. Other measurements, obtained on specific subsets of examinees include serum lithium concentrations, dark adaptation tests, and continuous cardiac monitoring. Aspects of the village environs were also measured, such as the concentrations of common and trace metals in water and foodstuffs, in an effort to appraise, albeit not comprehensively, environmental differences that could impinge on biological ones.

ACD-preserved blood specimens were separated through centrifugation into cells and sera on a daily basis, and the resulting aliquots stored in transportable liquid nitrogen containers for subsequent movement and study. Although hemoglobin and hematocrit were measured in the field, using, in the first instance, an AO colorimeter or, in Bolivia, a spectrophotometer, and, in the second, an hematocrit microcentrifuge, all other laboratory determinations, except the immunoglobulin tests that were conducted at the University of Michigan, occurred in the Genetics Marker Laboratory of the Graduate School of Biomedical Sciences at the University of Texas Health Science Center.

To achieve as much standardization of the various procedures as possible with a multi-membered, multi-national investigative team, manuals in English and Spanish were prepared that described in detail how each measurement was to be made, observations obtained and recorded, and the intent of each question on the various questionnaires. Every examiner was provided with one of these manuals, in his or her language of choice, to serve as a reference when need arose. Each examination sheet or questionnaire was bilingual, English and Spanish, and color-coded to facilitate prompt recognition. Insofar as practical, all entries of measurements and responses to questions were self-coding. The various records on a participant were contained in a heavy manila envelope that could be tied. To track the flow of participants through the numerous different examinations and to ensure that no examination was missed, the face of this envelope provided a brief record of the examinations, including the time and examiner, that each examination had been completed, and a summary of pertinent health findings to aid the exit interview. One person was routinely assigned to ensure that participants were moved through the examinations expeditiously without undue waiting.

A diary was maintained in which to document changes in the initial protocol that proved necessary and the reasons, to record daily temperature and humidity, and the results of the standardization of those machines where this was required.

For example, the lung function machine was standardized twice daily, at the beginning of the morning examinations and again in the afternoon. A small hand-held dictating machine was available to supplement entries in the diary. Training sessions and periodic discussions and evaluations of performance occurred in the field.

ENLISTMENT OF PARTICIPANTS

Clearly, the success of this study hinged entirely upon our ability to involve the individual villager and to satisfy his or her expectations wherever feasible. Chary of outsiders, rapport with the Aymará is not easily established, but can be won if they are candidly apprised of what their participation in a study entails, and perceive some benefit to themselves. Obviously they are concerned about their health and that of their children. They could, therefore, see benefit to the health examinations that comprised an integral part of our study. Most, however, are unfamiliar with such devices as a lung function machine, an electrocardiograph, or an audiometer. To allay their concerns and to explain fully to them what the examinations entailed, the following routinely occurred:

(1) Before our appearance in a particular village, representatives of the Junta de Adelanto de Arica, familiar to the villagers, called upon the village authorities to explain our study and its objectives, and to obtain their concurrence in participation.

(2) Upon our arrival, before the initiation of actual examinations, the villagers were invited to a public meeting at which the program was carefully explained, and a film in Spanish illustrating each of the successive steps in the investigation was shown. Initially, the film that we used had been prepared in Houston, but in the course of the first year's activities, a second was made in Chile in surroundings familiar to the participants utilizing Aymará volunteers. Questions prompted by either the film or the explanation of the program were welcomed. The most frequent questions concerned the time that would be involved and the amount of blood to be drawn.

(3) Before an individual was examined, the steps in the examination were again explained, and the individual was given an opportunity to refuse any part of the examination without prejudice to participation in the remainder, or to treatment or referral for treatment of their health problems where such treatment could be extended. All treatments were prescribed and initiated by physicians licensed in Chile, and with the approval of the Servicio Nacional de Salud.

(4) Finally, upon completion of the examination, a physician explained to each participant any significant health findings on his or her health, responded to queries, dispensed any medication deemed necessary, and presented the individual with a written summary of the findings, and certain normative values, e.g. blood pressure, height, weight, etc. Although this exit interview was usually in Spanish, staff physicians were available who could explain the findings in Aymará, Quechua or Uro-Chipaya. Where medical follow-up was indicated, or

more extensive treatment required, arrangements were made with the Servicio Nacional de Salud hospital in Arica to have the person accepted for treatment.

THE STUDY SITES

Fourteen different examination sites were used, one each in the Azapa and Lluta valleys, six in the sierra (Belén, Chapiquiña, Murmuntani, Putre, Socoroma, and Tignamar), four in the Chilean altiplano (Caquena, Guallatiri, Parinacota and Visviri), and two in the Bolivian altiplano (Toledo and Turco). Most of the villages involved were accessible at the time of these examinations only by four-wheel drive vehicles over unimproved roads. Accordingly, all of the examinations occurred either in October or November of 1973 or 1974, or March of 1975. At this time of the year, normally the areas involved are dry, roads are passable, and the temperatures more tolerable. Examinations were made either in schools, a social hall, a village meeting place, or a governmentally maintained policlinic if one existed in the village. In the coastal valleys, public transportation was available, but in addition, through the courtesy of the Junta de Adelanto de Arica, there were vehicles to transport examinees from the outlying villages to the examination location. Transport was also provided in the sierra and altiplano, where walking is the normal means of movement.

As would be anticipated, these sites, although similar in many ways, differed in a number of particulars such as the presence of a policlinic, which assured access to a higher level of emergency medical care, schools, and a carabinero post with radio connections with the coast. Save in the coastal valleys none of the villages has a closed sewage system. Water is generally obtained either from wells or more commonly springs, and it is the presence of the latter that has largely determined the situating of the various villages.

None of the sierran or altiplano churches in this region of Chile has a resident priest, and religious services occur on an indifferent schedule, usually at the time of the annual feast day of the village's patron saint or at church celebrations such as Easter.

A brief description of each of the villages or areas of study follows:

Azapa Valley: This 25 kilometer long, green subtropical valley, known as the Quebrada Azapa, extends eastwards from the city of Arica along the course of the San José River. It embraces the principal agricultural zone in the Departamento, and is particularly famous for its olives. Examinations were conducted in a school at Las Maitas, some 15 kilometers from the city. Most of the participants came from the immediate area, and were predominantly of mixed racial ancestry, so-called mestizos, or Spanish.

Belén is located 140 kilometers from Arica at an elevation of 3240 meters. It is one of the older continuously inhabited sierran villages, having come into existence in 1625 in the early colonial period, and was once the principal center of the Spanish administrators of the highland interior. In its vicinity are a number of substantial springs that serve as sources of water for the community, and the area is relatively rich in eucalyptus trees. Herding and agriculture, largely cultivation of oregano, occur. The village has an elementary and intermediate school, and a church of some historical importance established in the seventeenth century.

Caquena is in the altiplano at an elevation of 4600 meters adjacent to the Río Caquena and surrounded by grazing lands that support some of the largest herds of alpaca and vicuña to be found in the northern Chilean puna. It is 195 kilometers from Arica, and the location of a school, a church (established in 1690, restored in 1891), an experimental station of the Corporación de Fomento de la Producción (CORFO), largely concerned with the biology and breeding of the indigenous camelids, a policlinic, and a small carabinero post (a retén).

Chapiquiña is situated in the sierra to the south of Putre at an elevation of 3180 meters. It is approximately 115 kilometers from Arica on the dirt road from Putre to Belén. It has an elementary school, a small facility of Empresa Nacional de Electricidad (ENDESA), but no church nor a policlinic. Communicants attend the church at Pachama, six kilometers away. Alfalfa and oregano have been introduced as cash crops, and there is herding, particularly of sheep.

Guallatiri is in the altiplano at a distance of about 180 kilometers from Arica. It sets at an elevation of 4,260 meters in the shadow of one of the few continuously active volcanoes, Guallatiri (6060 m), along this stretch of the cordilleras. There is an elementary school, a church (constructed in the seventeenth century), and a small carabinero post within the village. One of the tributaries of the Lauca River, arising on the flank of the volcano, borders the community immediately to the east. No significant cash crops are grown, and herding involves llama and alpaca that graze along the green belt adjacent to the tributary.

Lluta Valley: All of the examinations were conducted in the governmentally maintained policlinic in Poconchile, a small community astride the highway from Arica to the interior, some 28 kilometers from the delta of the Lluta River. Participants were drawn, however, from all of the communities within the valley extending as far to the interior as Molinos (57 kilometers from Arica). Poconchile, itself, is approximately 38 kilometers to the north and slightly east of the city of Arica. Most of the settlers in this valley are either agriculturalists or raisers of cattle or goats. Some are self-employed but many work at the larger estates.

Murmuntani is primarily an altitude acclimatization base for the Rancagua Regiment which is normally stationed in Arica. It is approximately 80 kilometers from the latter city at an elevation of 3400 meters. Participants were drawn not only from this community but from another small village, Zapahuira, some eight kilometers distant. Alfalfa, garlic, and oregano are commercially cultivated, and there is herding, confined largely to goats and cattle. There is no church, nor school, nor policlinic. Examinations were conducted at the military base which had only a maintenance garrison at the time.

Parinacota is located 160 kilometers from Arica at an elevation of 4480 meters. It has an elementary school and a church (originally constructed in 1699 and reconstructed in 1789); there is a small carabinero post and policlinic located at Chucuyo about four kilometers away where the examinations were conducted. Some 17 kilometers to the east of Parinacota are the Lakes Chungará and Cotacotani, and still further eastward are the presently dormant volcanoes, Pomerape (6240 m) and Parinacota (6330 m), known collectively and more commonly as the Payachata, that is, the twins, because of their similarity in heighth and appearance.

Putre was established in 1580, is the largest and principal community in the sierra, and is the seat of administrative authority for the sierra and altiplano. It is situated on a tableland at an elevation of 3500 meters, 145 kilometers from Arica. There is an elementary and intermediate school, a policlinic, two churches (one Catholic, constructed in 1600, and one Protestant), a forest nursery, a carabinero commissary, and radio service located in the community. The area, if not the present town, has long seen human habitation, and in its vicinity in the Quebrada Chilcacahue are a number of indigenous artifacts, mostly rock paintings (at Villacaurani). Alfalfa and oregano are the main cash crops, but lettuce, asparagus, celery, broad beans, artichokes, and potatoes are cultivated, and substantial herding of cattle, goats, llama, and sheep occur in the area. At the time of our studies there was also a small military detachment present as well as an internment camp for political prisoners.

Socoroma is a sierran community at an elevation of 3000 meters about 92 kilometers from Arica. It sets five kilometers off the present main road from Arica to the Bolivian border, but in the colonial period was astride the silver route from the mines at Potosi to Arica. There is an elementary school and one of the largest churches in the north (originally constructed in 1560), a social hall, but no policlinic. Alfalfa and oregano are cultivated; herding is largely of sheep.

Tignamar, and its sister village, Saxamar, are sited at 3200 meters about 145 kilometers from Arica. Tignamar is on the Río Tignamar, one of the tributaries of the Río San José. Although this river is normally small, it has been known to flood, and in 1959 did extensive damage to the village. Tignamar has an elementary and intermediate school, a church (dating from the late seventeenth or early eighteenth century), and a forest nursery. Oregano is the principal cash crop in the vicinity; herding is largely confined to cattle and sheep.

Toledo is at an elevation of 3752 meters in the western Bolivian altiplano some 40 kilometers southwest from Oruro, across the flood plains of the Río Desaguadero which empties into Lake Poopó to the south of Toledo. It is a community of about 7,000 inhabitants, a provincial (Saucari) administrative and commercial center. It has a primary, secondary, and high school, a church established in the eighteenth century with a resident priest, regular mail, truck and telegraph services, and a clinic staffed by two practicantes.

Turco, elevation 3980 meters, lies at the southern foot of the Cerros de Turaquiri, in the western Bolivian altiplano. It is approximately 240 kilometers west from Oruro, and 100 from Tambo Quemado on the Chilean border. It is a quiet, undistinguished village with a primary and intermediate school, a church dating from the late sixteenth century again with a resident priest, and a small clinic with a live-in nurse. There is no regular mail nor transportation service, but there is a shortwave radio connection with the outside. This village like most of the others in the Bolivian altiplano is more sharply defined than its Chilean counterparts. There is the customary village square onto which faces the church, the schools, and the governmental buildings. Much more farming occurs in the area than is characteristic of the Chilean altiplano; the principal crops are potatoes and quinoa. Weaving of textiles and clothing from wool derived locally provides a source of cash income.

Visviri: This village, whose Aymará name translates as the 'origin of the winds', is the largest in the Chilean altiplano and is the border checkpoint for the railroad connecting Arica with La Paz. It is at an elevation of 4100 meters some 255 kilometers from Arica, and near the Bolivian-Chilean-Peruvian junction. Immediately across the Bolivian border is the town of Charaña. Visviri has a policlinic, an elementary and intermediate school, offices of the Registro Civil, and the headquarters (the tenencia) of the carabineros in the altiplano, but no church. There is regular, twice-weekly mail service, and provisions can be brought by rail.

THE EXAMINEES: THEIR NUMBER AND LOCATIONS

Table 1 sets out the village of residence and the village of examination for the 2525 individuals who were examined; their ages ranged from 15 days to over 90 years (Table 2). The numbers examined within a given village or locale reflect the population densities and the ease or difficulty of travel. Censuses were conducted in each of the villages of the coast, sierra and altiplano before the initiation of examinations by employees of the Junta de Adelanto de Arica or village school teachers. Comparison of the census findings with the rosters of the individuals actually examined reveals our study population to represent 70 to 93 per cent of any given village in the sierra and altiplano; no effort was made to study the coastal communities exhaustively. Our resources were inadequate for the latter, and moreover the bulk of the inhabitants of these communities were not Aymará. Most of the individuals who were not examined were elsewhere with their flocks and herds, or lived too far from the village of census to make an appearance at the examination site practical. We are not aware of any systematic bias that this may have introduced, nor is a bias suggested by the sex and age characteristics of the 'not-examined' group as indicated in the census areas. Some notion of the extensiveness of the family data available in Chile and Bolivia can be gleaned from Table 3 where we distribute nuclear families as a function of the number of parents and offspring examined.

ANCESTRY AND RESIDENCE

Two matters of moment, basic to the study, are the algorithm by which an individual is designated, first, to be Aymará, and second, a coastal, sierran or altiplano resident. Their ethnic origins have been assessed socio-culturally through the 'Aymaraness' of their maternal and paternal surnames, and

TABLE 1
Distribution of examinees by place of residence and place of examination

Place of residence[1]	Altitude niche of examination			
	Coast	Sierra	Altiplano	Total
COAST				
Arica	33	30	3	66
Valle Azapa	286	0	0	286
Valle Lluta	279	0	0	279
Other	1	0	0	1
SIERRA				
Belén	0	88	0	88
Chapiquiña	0	113	1	114
Murmuntani	0	30	0	30
Putre	0	381	0	381
Socoroma	0	58	0	58
Tignamar	0	135	0	135
ALTIPLANO				
Caquena	0	3	146	149
Charaña	0	0	3	3
Guallatiri	0	0	89	89
Parinacota	0	0	96	96
Visviri	0	0	315	315
Turco	0	0	300	300
Toledo	0	0	129	129
UNKNOWN	4	1	1	6
TOTAL	603	839	1083	2525

[1] Residence here implies presently living in the stated village or its immediate environs; boarding students are assigned to the village in which their school is located and not to the village of their parents, if the two are different.

Adapted from Schull and Rothhammer (1977), Table 2, p. 153.

biologically through the use of genetic markers. Aymará names are recognizably different from Spanish ones, and thus presumably individuals with such names are readily classifiable (see Schull and Rothhammer, 1977, for a listing of these names), providing admixture, if it had occurred, was sufficiently recent. Most Aymará in the Departamento de Arica are Catholics, at least nominally, and substantial numbers have taken or more frequently been given Spanish surnames at baptism. Such persons pose classification problems if the surname is the sole criterion of Aymará origin. Wormald (1969; p. 46) states that the census of 1871 reveals 39 to 57 per cent of the Aymará inhabitants of the precordilleran villages of Belén, Chapiquiña, Putre and Socoroma had Spanish surnames, whereas 25 to 56 per cent of the Aymará inhabitants of the altiplano villages of Caquena, Guallatiri and Parinacota were so named. The origins of some of these names are known, and frequently their advent in a village can be dated (Urzua, 1969).

TABLE 2
Distribution of the ages of the Bolivian and Chilean examinees by sex and region of examination

	Village of examination							
	Coast		Sierra		Altiplano		Total	
Age (yrs)	Males	Females	Males	Females	Males	Females	Males	Females
<1	12	13	14	15	23	23	49	51
1-4	29	27	17	39	76	65	122	131
5-9	38	46	79	70	93	91	210	207
10-14	54	59	81	59	89	90	224	208
15-19	30	16*	40	18*	26	31	96	65*
20-29	32	46	37	44	56	74	125	164
30-39	38	41	42	28	64	54	144	123
40-49	35	25	40	41	51	53	126	119
50-59	12	12	35	34	33	31	80	77
60-69	14	14	33	30	22	12	69	56
≥70	5	5	20	23	15	11	40	39
Total	299	304	438	401	548	535	1285	1240

* Note the differences in these classes. We presume this reflects the commonly encountered reluctance of young women of these ages to disrobe for the physical examination and anthropometric measurements.

Adapted from Schull and Rothhammer (1977), Table 3, p. 154.

Customarily in Spanish-speaking countries, an individual has two surnames, his or her father's family name and the name of his or her mother's father's family. The scheme of classification that evolved was based upon the four names of an individual's parents, and the completeness of that information. Nine alternatives were recognized; these ranged from the case where all four parental surnames were known and were conspicuously Aymará to the case where only two names were known and these were both Spanish, that is, not traditional Aymará or Quechua surnames. Both the socio-cultural assessment and the genetic one suggest the sample is approximately equally divided among Aymará, mestizo and non-Aymará individuals. It should be noted, perhaps, that the surname algorithm is a conservative one in the sense that many Aymará were undoubtedly classified as mestizo.

As more roads have penetrated the sierra and altiplano, and as the economic attractions of the city of Arica have grown, largely in the last four decades, the population of the interior has become more mobile. Many individuals have moved permanently to the city; others visit the coast for days, weeks, or even years but consider their residence to be in the interior. No fully satisfactory method for the assignment of such individuals to residential groups exists. If one insists that an individual who is to be designated a resident of the altiplano must have been born at that altitude, and never lived at any other altitude even for a day, too few individuals will qualify. Similarly, if the strictures on residence are too loose, real differences provoked by a lifetime at different oxygen pressures

TABLE 3
The distribution of nuclear families examined in Chile and Bolivia as a function of the number of parents and offspring examined

Number of siblings examined	Number of parents examined			
	0	1	2	Total
1	993	167	50	1210
2	95	63	43	201
3	28	35	58	121
4	12	22	33	67
5	2	10	21	33
6	0	6	6	12
7	0	2	1	3
8	0	1	1	2
Total	1130	306	213	1649

Adapted from Schull and Rothhammer (1977), Table 4a, p. 155 and Murillo et al. (1980), Table 2, p. 57.

may be obscured. We have selected a middle road. Residence is here defined on the basis of place of birth, and proportion of life lived at a given altitude. Thus, an individual born in an altiplano village who has spent at least 90 per cent of his or her subsequent life in an altiplano village, although not necessarily the one of birth, was considered an altiplano resident and assigned to his current village of residence. If, however, he or she had resided mostly at some lower altitude, assignment was to his or her current village in that altitude. This procedure is conservative in that those effects, genetic or otherwise, secondary to one altitude will be assigned to a lower altitude and thus lessen the 'true' differences that would prevail if no residential ambiguities existed. The effects of this definition are illustrated in Table 4 where the numbers of individuals born in the coastal, sierran and altiplano communities in Chile who asserted that they had lived either their entire lives at their present elevation (possibly in a different village, however) or for other amounts of time, are given.

ACQUISITION AND MANAGEMENT OF DATA

Studies of this size and complexity require substantial preliminary preparation, not the least of which concerns the management of the data that are collected. The traditional field notebook hardly suffices as a means of recording observations. More than 300 measurements (exclusive of laboratory determinations) were made on or questions asked of each participant, the average day saw 35 or more individuals examined, and never less than 12 examiners or interviewers were involved in the collection of the observations. To achieve the implied rate of data acquisition and the requisite uniformity among examiners and interviewers all questionnaires or observational records had to be self-coding, as far as possible. As earlier noted, to manage conveniently the array

TABLE 4
Residential permanence as a function of residential niche. (Data restricted to Chi

Residential niche	Percentage of life lived in stated niche						
	100	>90	>80	>70	>60	<50	Total
Coast	391*	396	411	430	486	145	631
Sierra	410	463	522	549	619	193	812
Altiplano	483	524	550	566	591	62	653
Total	1284	1383	1483	1545	1696	400	2096

* The entries 100 through >60 inclusive, represent the cumulative number of individuals within the percentage of life lived in stated niche.
Adapted from Schull and Rothhammer (1977), Table 6, p. 160.

of measurement or observational domains the records associated with each were color-coded, and all forms were bilingual, Spanish and English. Most Chilean Aymará understand and can speak Spanish; for those who could not, one of the examiners was also fluent in Aymará, Quechua and Uro-Chipaya, collectively the major languages of the altiplano of Bolivia, northern Chile and southern Perú. All forms were completed in duplicate, one copy to be stored in Chile and the other in the United States.

Once the records were machine-retrievable, a 'logical' verification of each entry occurred – all coded values were examined to see whether they lay within the alternatives specified in the code itself, singly and as a logical group. Many questions, for example, were contingent upon the answer to a prior question; the logic of such concatenations was verified. All quantitative observations were screened singly and pairwise. In the first instance, means, variances, maxima and minima were determined to ascertain whether these accorded with experience or reason. In the second instance, bivariate arrays were plotted by machine to search for 'outliers' or discrepant observations. This search occurred within age class, altitude group, or for a specific measurement when multiple observations of a particular kind were made, e.g., in the case of lung function analysis. All seemingly atypical measurements were reexamined (with the aid of the original form), and ultimately either the discrepancy was reconciled, or the measurement was assigned to an 'unknown' category.

Of great importance to us were those data relevant to gene segregation, for a surprisingly small number of family studies have been done on the attributes associated with adjustments to altitude. Control of the quality of this information was not, however, straightforward. Many of these people are illiterate; moreover, there is no clearly established convention for the written forms of their surnames, if the latter are Aymará. Each interviewer could, therefore, transliterate a particular name differently. Families frequently did not appear at the examination location as a group, and even had this been so, it was likely that they would have been interviewed by different persons. Accordingly, it was necessary, once the data were machine-retrievable, to standardize names – to verify that a given name was always transliterated in the same manner (see Schull and Rothhammer, 1977). This does not, of course, imply that our transliteration was phonetically the best, but merely that we were consistent in its use. Consistency was necessary, for we proposed to link (and have linked) family units on the basis of their names (as well as ancillary evidence, such as a woman's reproductive history). Linking of families through names is unquestionably more accurate in countries where an individual bears two surnames, a patrinym and a matrinym, as is commonly the case in South America.

Finally, all atypical biochemical genotypes have been contrasted with as many 'standards' as available or practicable. All biochemical and serological genotypes have been examined, of course, in the context of the family in which they occur. Our aim was to establish non-paternity or non-maternity, and to isolate discrepant genotypes.

Chapter 2
FLORA AND FAUNA

The various rises of the Andes from Miocene to Pleistocene times have isolated a substantial portion of the South American continent, producing conditions that resulted in the emergence of two new high altitude life zones: the northern Paramos and the southern altiplano. We examine here the conditions prevailing in the altiplano now, and how they can be related to the present distributional patterns of its flora and fauna. We also describe how such conditions might have influenced the development of permanent human settlements, particularly through the emergence of agriculture and the domestication of the region's animals, either as beasts of burden, or sources of food, or both.

Any explanation for the origin and differentiation of a local biota should consider the geological and climatic aspects of the specific region. The high mountains that presently comprise the Andean chain are the result of two major kinds of geologic events (Ramos, 1989). First, there has been magmatic activity, the eruption and accumulation of thick piles of rock, primarily andesite, poured out by the volcanoes such as Guallatiri dispersed along the chain. The magma itself stems from the partial melting of the oceanic crust subducted to depths of hundreds of kilometers beneath the continental plates as the latter collide with the oceanic ones. This subduction generates considerable friction and deformation, and the strains of this deformation result in earthquakes that represent fractures in the brittle lithosphere, the outer crust, reaching the surface. And, second, the volcanic and interbedded sedimentary rocks have been compressed through the tectonic activity with the convergence of an oceanic and a continental plate. Much of modern Chile is thought to have once been an independent terrane, known as Chilenia, that drifted into Gondwanaland, as the ancient continent of South America and Africa has been termed, from the west in the late Paleozoic era. Its arrival shifted the volcanic belt westward from its previous location in present Argentina. The uplift of the Andes began in the Middle Cretaceous after the separation of Africa from South America and the formation of the South Atlantic Ocean. These processes have extended over hundreds of millions of years, and continue.

Prior to Miocene times, there was a well-established biota which was drastically changed by new ecological conditions produced by the Andes themselves. First, the uplifting of the land acted as a new barrier to moisture-laden Pacific winds, and many of the savanna woodland forms, animal and plant, previously existing in the area retreated northward (Patterson and Pascual, 1972; Webb, 1978). Second, Plio-Pleistocene volcanic activity strongly modified the altiplano relief (González, 1974), with volcanic effusions contributing to alter water regimes and subsequent formation of rivers and lakes, particularly in the

William J. Schull and Francisco Rothhammer (eds.), The Aymará: Strategies in Human Adaptation to a Rigorous Environment, 19-32. ©1990 *by Kluwer Academic Publishers.*

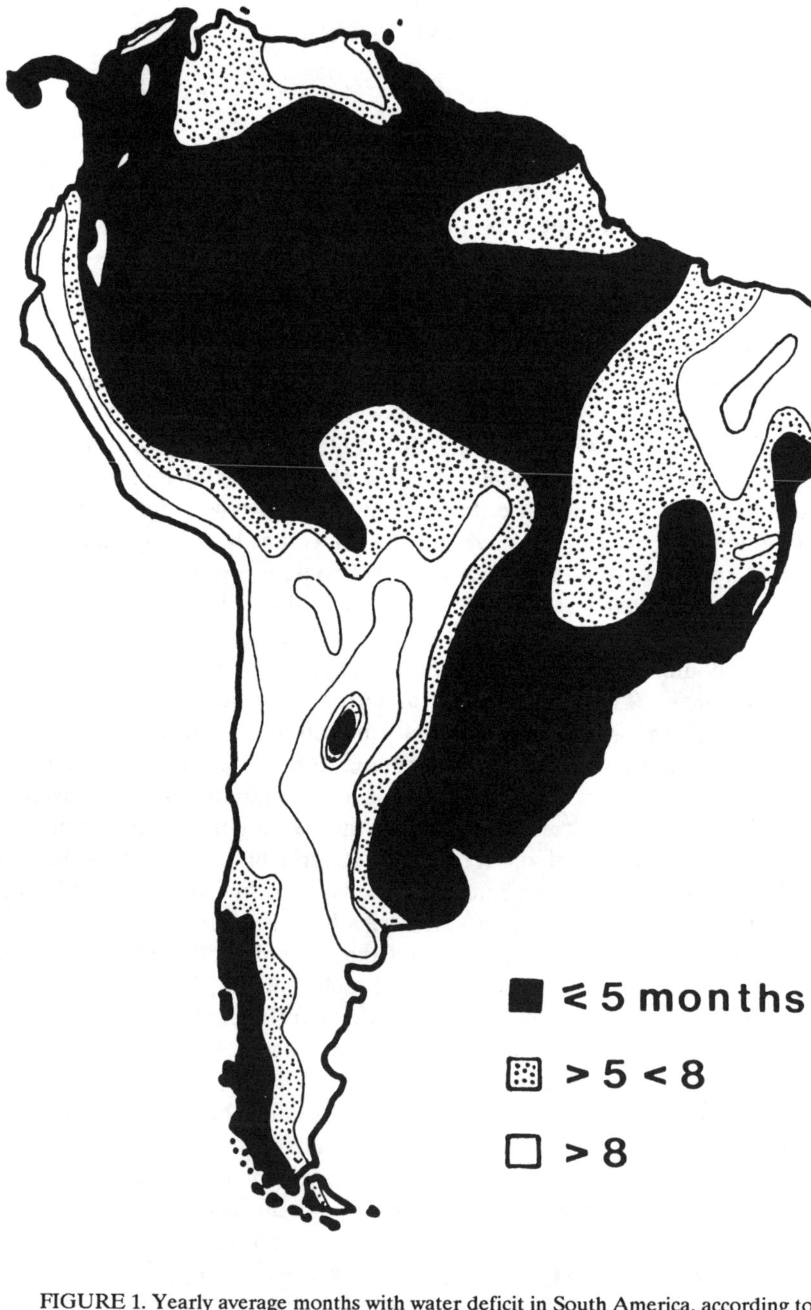

FIGURE 1. Yearly average months with water deficit in South America, according to Thornthwaite's balance (figure slightly modified from Burgos, 1979)

southern altiplano. Finally, one major consequence of the uplift was colder conditions that enhanced the effects of glaciation. These factors, briefly introduced in Chapter 1, will be further considered more extensively here in relation to their specific biological effects.

As previously stated, the altiplano can be characterized as a cold, arid and barren plateau formed between the two cordilleras, a part of the large northwest-southeast dry diagonal crossing South America (see Figure 1) and having more than eight yearly months of water deficit (Burgos, 1979). This precipitation regime has produced most of the dry plant formations all over the continent (Sarmiento, 1975; see Figure 2), among which three are found within or around the altiplano: the Puna formation (in the altitudes between 3000 and 4300 meters), the High Andean formation (from 4300 up to the limit of vegetation at about 5000 meters), and the Sierra formation, in the western cordillera of Perú.

The Puna itself can be subdivided into three vegetational belts: (a) the humid or moist zone to the north of the altiplano, (b) the dry or 'tola' belt, both running parallel to the dry diagonal previously mentioned, and (c) the thorn or desert Puna, often termed the 'Puna de Atacama,' in the south of the altiplano (Cabrera, 1968; for maps and descriptions see Molina and Little, 1981; and Cabrera and Willink, 1973). The latter is the coldest and most arid environment of the central Andes. Within these formations and belts, there are many minor localized biotic communities, shaped by particular combinations of soils, temperature, exposure, water or rainfall (Table 1). This mosaic is more frequent in both cordilleras; beyond them, the driest of the earth's deserts to the west and the tropical forest to the east complete the striking features of these landscapes.

The origins and relationships of the Puna formations can be estimated by similarity indices calculated from the number of plant genera shared by the dry formations in South America. The most dissimilar formations are the Caatinga and the High Andean ones; in between lie the rest, usually in geographic contiguity with two exceptions, namely, the high similarities of the High Andean (and Puna) to the distant Patagonia and of the sierra to central Chile. The first of these exceptions can be partly explained by the cold conditions they share. To understand the second, the changes in the permanent snow line and the limits of the belts during glacial times can be invoked (Vuilleumier, 1971). In fact, during the glaciation, the central Chilean scrub thorn formation was 330 kilometers north of its present position (see Figure 7.6 in Simpson, 1979). Analogous arguments have been advanced to explain the similarities of the High Andean and Patagonian formations.

The average number of yearly months with a rainfall deficit rises with altitude along the western slope of the central Andes (Figure 1), producing a gradient from the dry and warm desert on the Pacific coast to the moist and cold Puna. As would be expected, in a coast to altiplano transect, a corresponding gradient in the total plant cover can be observed, with values from 0.1% at the limit of the Atacama desert to 70% at about 4000 meters. This gradient diminishes at greater altitudes (Villagrán et al., 1982; see Figure 3a). It is clear that dryness

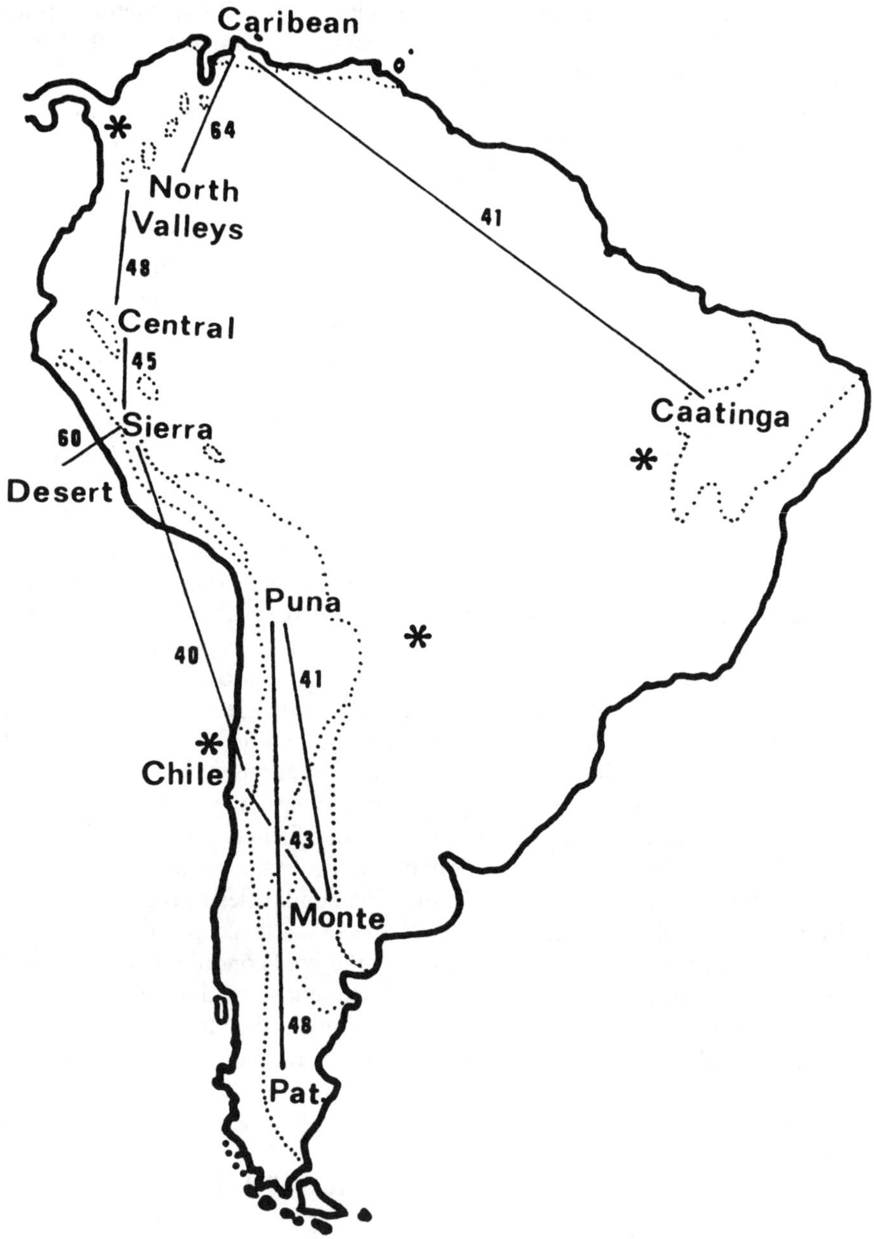

FIGURE 2. Distribution of dried plant formations in South America.
High Andean formation within the Puna not shown. Numbers are Sorensen coefficients of similarities based on the number of shared plant genera. (Data from Sarmiento, 1975)

TABLE 1
Vegetational units, number of species and characteristic species of plant associations in the southwest altiplano

Vegetational Unit (Local name) Characteristics	No. of Species Arica[1]/ Toconce	Plant association Characteristic species with vernacular names
PRE-PUNA BELT ("Pampa") Desertic plateau with sparse shrub cover From 1540 to 2800 m.	21/18	*Atriplex microphyllium,* tola blanca *Franseria meyeniana*, pega - pega *Tarasa operculata*, quella hembra *Browningia candelaris*, cardón, ure
PUNA BELT ("Tolar") Woody shrubs From 3,000 to 4,000 m.	138/41	*Fabiana densa*, tola quipa *Baccharis boliviensis*, chack'a tola *Diphlostephium meyenii*, tola mazanillón
HIGH ANDEAN BELT ("Pajonal") Cold zone w/ "icchu predominance Higher than 3,700 m	68/23	a) *Parastrephia lepodiphylla*, K'jaña tola *Baccharis santelices*, ñacatola *Stipa leptostachya*, paja sikuya b) *Parastrephia lucida*, k'oa tola b.1) *Festuca orthophylla*, wicho b.2) *Azorella compacta*, llareta b.3) *Polylepis tarapacana*, queñoa c) *Festuca orthophylla* c.1) *Valeriana nivalis*, k'jata *Perezia ciliosa*, aicha-aicha *Senecio* sp. c.2) *Pycnophyllum* sp., K'jota
BOFEDAL ("Vega")	22/6	*Oxichloe andina*, orko pak'o *Distichia muscoides*, k'achu pak'o *Werneria heteroloba*, takerere

1 Transect Arica - Lake Chungará. Data from Castro et al., 1982 and Aldunate et al., 1981.

and cold are the limiting factors producing the antimodes at both ends in such a curve. The influence of cold is further shown by the increasing predominance of tufted grasses and cushion mats over scrubby plants and cacti (see Figure 3b). The number of plant species also increases with altitude up to 3000 meters in the western Cordillera (Figure 3c). Over 60% of these species from 2000 meters up are of punean origin (Kalin Arroyo et al., 1982).

If we follow the sampling to the south, we would find that these particular species become rarer, and are more and more replaced by other species of southern origins, particularly at 23° south. Only 25% of the original species remain at the southern limit of the altiplano, the site of the largest penetration of the Atacama Desert into the continent. There is also a north to south decrease in the total number of species, from 394 at 18°S to 223 species at about 32°S (Villagrán et al., 1983). By contrast, the hard cushion plant community, called

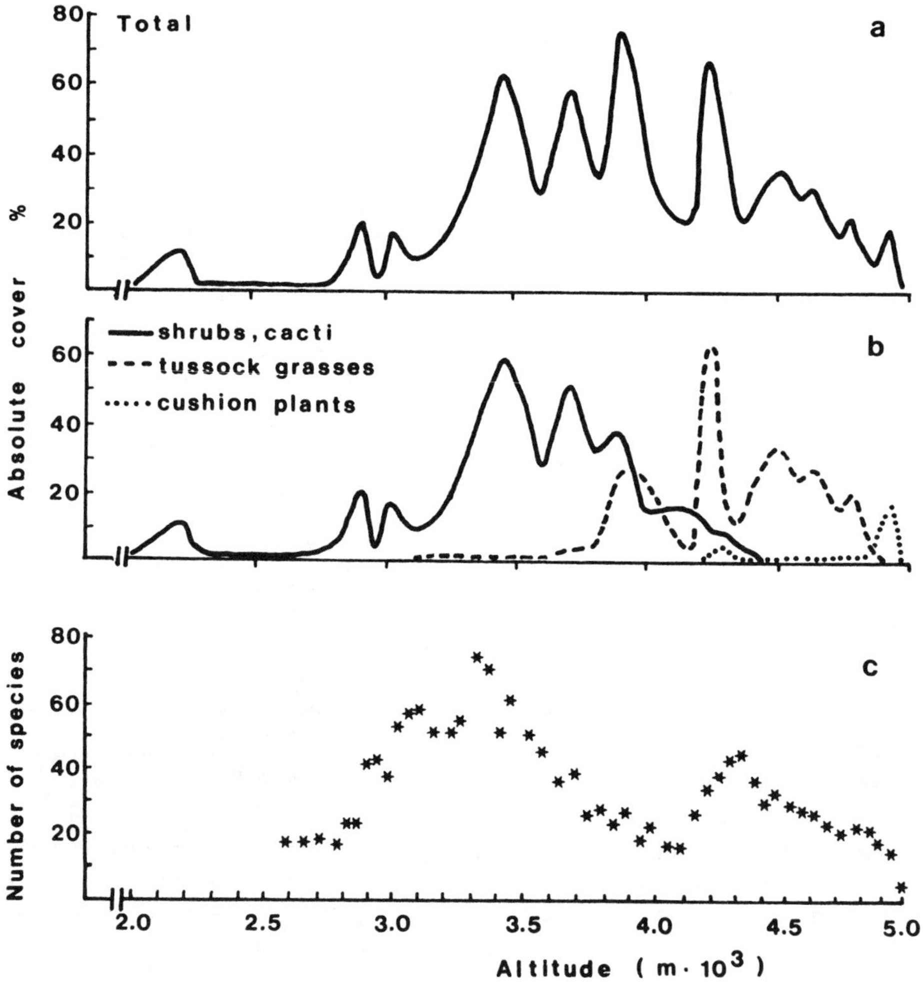

FIGURE 3.
Plant coverage and diversity according to altitude in a transect studied in Northern Chile. a) Total cover. b) Cover provided by shrubs and cacti, tussock grasses and cushion plants. c) Absolute number of species found at different sites of the transect. (From Kalin Arroyo et al., 1982 and Villagrán et al., 1982)

TABLE 2
Mammalian diversity in different regions of the world[1]

Region	Surface area ($10^6 km^2$)	No. of genera	No. of Species	Genera-species ratio
Africa	30.4	231	744	3.2
Australia	7.7	117	364	3.1
Neotropica	17.8	278	810	2.9
West N. America	2.6	114	360	3.2
South S. America	3.7	105	238	2.3
Altiplano	2.0	30	46	1.5

[1] Data drawn from Keast, 1972; Eisenberg and Redford, 1982; and Hershkovitz, 1972.

'bofedal,' shows a much more uniform floristic composition through all of the southern altiplano and the central-south Andes sites, a fact explained by the homogeneity of the microclimatic conditions required by this community (Villagrán et al., 1983) and the efficient mechanisms of dispersion of its components (Kalin Arroyo et al., 1982).

Animal life is abundant in South America; almost a fifth of the extant species of mammals live there (Hershkovitz, 1972) and the continent has been called 'the paradise of birds.' By contrast, all over the altiplano only 46 species of mammals (Hershkovitz, 1972; see also Reig, 1983) and 91 species of birds (Vuilleumier and Simberloff, 1980) are to be found; these are small numbers in relation to the size of the altiplano (see Table 2 for comparisons using mammalian data). There is only a small amount of diversification, judging by the small ratio of species number over genera number. All this seems to contradict the statement that the 'rate of speciation is directly proportional to the evolutionary history of lithospheric complexity for a given interval of space and time' (Cracraft, 1982; page 361), which is the main hypothesis of the most recent development of evolutionary theory. Such theory also claims, however, that 'the likelihood of extinction is inversely proportional to the degree of environmental favorableness to which a species is subjected' (Cracraft, 1982; page 362). A highly favorable environment is characterized 'by a high mean annual temperature (23-28°C), low mean annual range of temperature (less than 10°C) and high annual rainfall (generally 200-250 centimeters or more) dispersed evenly throughout the year.' It is clear that the conditions predominating in the altiplano are precisely the opposite. This suggests that the rate of species extinction in the altiplano as well as the speciation rate was very high. For some of the tetrapod vertebrates for which observations are available, the species number found in several sites in the central Andes are shown in Figure 4.

Some trends emerge from these data. First, there is a tendency for species number to be high in the western cordillera, particularly in all transects for rodents and lizards. Second, there is a tendency for species number of all groups to be high at the center of the altiplano, near the Titicaca region, with figures

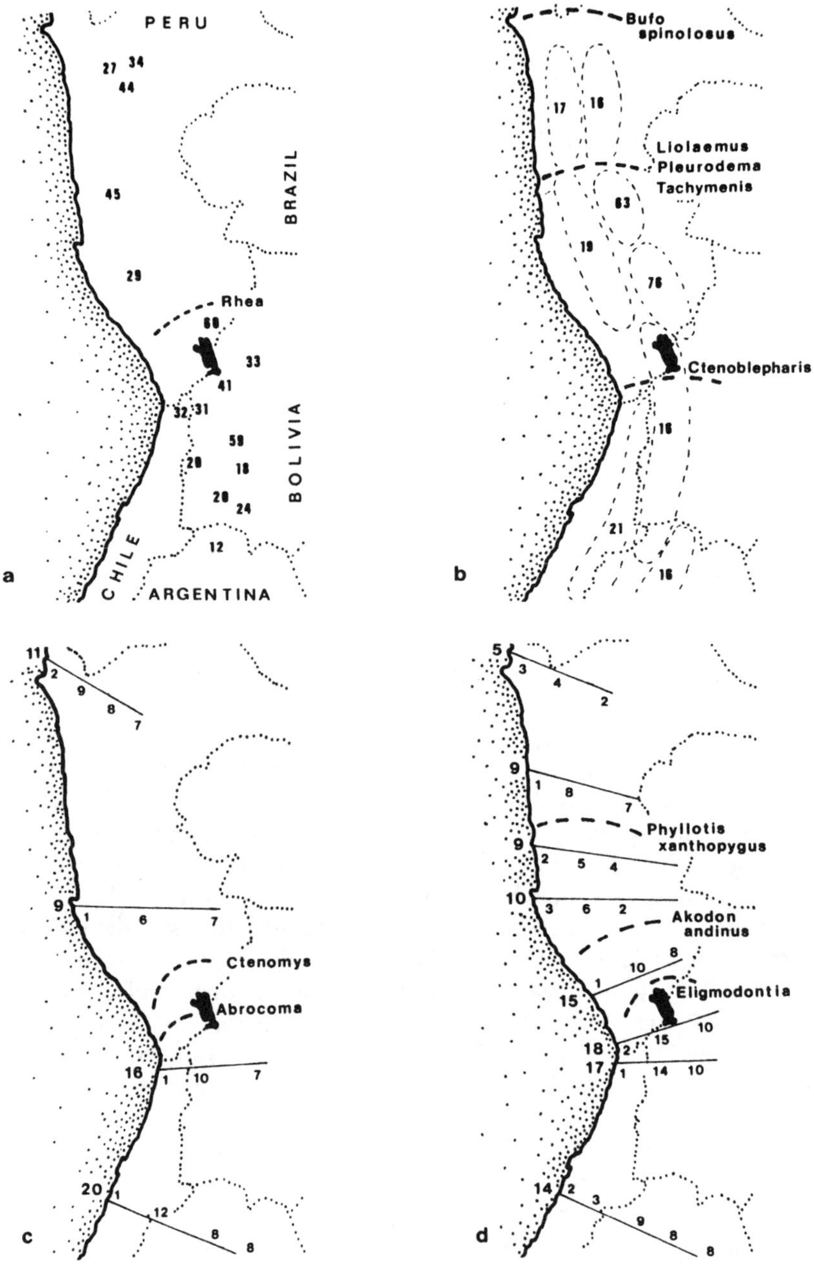

FIGURE 4. Number of species found at different sites or regions in the Central Andes. a) Birds (data from Vuilleumier and Simberloff, 1980). b) Reptiles and amphibians (data from Duellman, 1979). c) Caviomorph rodents (data from Mares and Ojeda, 1982). d) Phyllotine and Akodontine cricetid rodents (data from Pearson, 1982; Mares, Ojeda and Kosco, 1979; and unpublished observations). Broken lines refer to geographic limits of taxa. Large numbers to the left in c and d refer to the total number of species found in a particular transect.

decreasing north and south along the main axis of the altiplano. The first trend is concordant with absolute plant cover and diversity just discussed (unfortunately, there are no quantitative data on plants for the oriental cordillera, but the high species numbers of birds, reptiles and frogs are also concordant with the seemingly high plant coverage and high precipitation). The rugged topography also produces patchiness conditions promoting isolation, divergence and eventually, speciation.

In their study of Puna birds, Vuilleumier and Simberloff found a significant correlation between number of species and number of different biotypes estimated from a knowledge of the ecology of different species, but not for altitude (op. cit.). Pearson and Ralph (1978) also found a correlation in the number of bird species with foliage height diversity and percentage of ground cover, but not for mammalian species in a transect in southern Perú. This might be connected with the second trend. The richness of species in the vicinity of Lake Titicaca can be ascribed to the history of the region as well as to the ecology of the species involved. Simpson (1975) observed that 'if we look at distribution patterns across [along in this case] the altiplano, we find genus after genus with several sympatric species or taxa which shows distributional boundaries at specific localities.' One such locality is around Lake Titicaca where plant taxa like *Cremobolus peruvianus* (Crucifera), *Baccharis tricuneata var. ruitana* (Compositae) and *Mutisia cochabambensis* (Compositae) reach their southern limits, and some related forms, *Cremobolus subscandens*, *Baccharis tricuneata var. pulverulenta* and *Mutisia lanigera*, respectively, reach their northern limits (Simpson, 1975; see Figures 14, 15 and 16). Similar cases can be presented for cricetid rodents (the family of small rodents including the hamsters) of the puna, where *Auliscomys pictus* of the northern puna (part) meets its sister species *Auliscomys sublimis* around Lake Titicaca; they are well differentiated morphologically and they have the same karyotype, an unusual condition for the genus (Pearson and Patton, 1976). Another example is the encounter and probable crossing of *Phyllotis xanthopygus chilensis* and *Phyllotis xanthopygus rupestris* (maps of distribution in Pearson, 1958). Such patterns can be explained by the Pleistocene glaciations where 'the combination of the extended [Titicaca] lake and mountain glacier seemed to have prevented north-south migrations during glacial periods along the eastern side of the lake. The glacial lake Minchin, which included Lago Poopó and the Salares de Coipasa and Uyuni, probably isolated populations of plants [and animals] to the north and south of it' (Simpson, 1975; legend of Figure 20).

It is obvious from these cases that isolation sometimes resulted in speciation, when there are no crosses in sympatry, and in some others, hybrid zones are formed when speciation was not completed. It has been observed that in southern Perú, the following genera reach the Tambo Valley which is to the north of Lake Titicaca: the rodents Galenomys, Ctenomys, Eligomodontia and the bird Pternocnemia (the rhea) (Figure 4), (Pearson, 1982). These facts suggest that the removal of the glacial barrier allowed the passage of these and other taxa to the north and to the south (further examples are in Simpson, 1975, and Vuilleumier and Simberloff, 1980). It should also be noted that of the five most strikingly aberrant sites detected in a multiple regression study of 17 puna bird sites, three are in the Lake Titicaca region; moreover, from a total of four sites where many more species are observed than predicted, three are located in this same region. In other words, there is something anomalous in this portion of the altiplano where more species occur than would be expected for the altiplano as a whole. This species richness may be a temporal event; we may be seeing the contemporary inter-glacial mixing of two differentiated biota produced by the removal of a glacial barrier.

Environmental constraints, natural and recently man-made, seem to be acting on the distribution of altiplano animals. As more of the interior has become accessible through roads and with the planned diversion of water for hydroelectric purposes or to irrigate the farms of the coastal valleys, many of the species of birds tetter precariously on the brink of extinction (see McFarlane 1975a, b), and still others have had their habitats sharply curtailed. Among herpetozoans, amphibian species are restricted to water streams, abundant at the 'bofedal,' while lizards are found within shrubby vegetation. For amphibians, a severe constraint for dispersal is imposed by their dependence on water for their reproductive processes and the discontinuity of suitable 'bofedal' sites, and now the diversion of water. This is not the case for reptiles, all of them viviparous. Constraints for their distribution are probably associated with food availability in terrestrial environments (Veloso et al., 1982).

Overall, the altiplano is the land of the wild vicuña and guanaco, and of the domesticated alpaca and llama. Despite the ecological, cultural and economic importance of the only extant American camelids, their taxonomy and relationships are not well-established as yet (Walker, 1975). The greatest similarities are between the guanaco and the llama when contrasted with the alpaca and vicuña, because the former pair are large at birth and at adulthood, have the longest gestational periods, close-rooted incisors, browser and grazer habits, low elevation habitats, largest geographic distribution and short and coarse hair (Franklin, 1982). It is usually stated (i.e., Leon, 1939) that crosses in pairs of all combinations give fertile descendants, despite the fact that all four species have maintained their biological distinctiveness over time. The vicuña is the most dissimilar form, but some of its characteristics are shared by the alpaca. This has led some investigators to suggest that the latter species may have had a vicuña ancestor.

Such issues cannot be settled as yet, however, due to the absence of strong evidence, particularly data from careful reproductive and genetic analyses, including contemporary DNA techniques. At present, the origin of the alpaca is the most obscure of all. The different alternatives are, in the order of their general acceptance, that it was domesticated from (a) the guanaco, together with the domestication of the llama, (b) from the vicuña, and (c) from a wild guanacoid species now extinct. What follows is an attempt to argue against the first of these alternatives.

TABLE 3
Convergent characters in two phyletic lines of altiplano mammals[1]

	Llama	Alpaca	*Auliscomys*	
	(guanaco)	(vicuña)	*pictus*	*sublimis*
Distribution (altiplano)	W. North (West)	Central (South)	North	South
Elevation	2300-4000 (0-4250)	4400-4800 (3700-4800)	3350-4500	4000-5500
Size	large	small	large	small
Fur	short-coarse	long-fine	long fur	unusually long, soft
Hair color		(white undersides)	darker	lighter
Feeding habits	browser grazer	grazer		
Diet	less succulents	more succulents	8% insects 66% vegetation	27% insects 42% vegetation
Incisors	close roots	open roots	wide	narrow
Other			diurnal nocturnal	nocturnal gregarious
			long tail	short tail

[1]Data from Pearson, 1951, 1958; Franklin, 1982; Pizzimenti and de Salle, 1980; and unpublished observations.

Our reasoning begins with two facts. First, the wild vicuña and guanaco are geographically disjunct species now, and probably in the past, although the evidence in this respect is limited. Second, despite domestication, alpaca herds tend to be concentrated in the same geographic distribution as the vicuña, that is, in the altiplano proper. In contrast, the llama tends to have the wide distribution of the guanaco (see maps and comments in Franklin, 1982). It is reasonable to assume that a domesticated form would tend to adopt a similar geographic (the optimal) distribution to that of its wild ancestor, and this is the case for the guanaco and llama. The observation that the alpaca does not tend to follow either the guanaco or the llama distribution operates against the first alternative. Additional indirect evidence of an eco-morphologic nature can be obtained through the comparison of the characters also observed in another pair of altiplanic mammalian species mentioned previously, that is, *Auliscomys pictus* and *A. sublimis*. The latter also deserves a close look because it 'lives at the highest altitude [type locality at 5500 meters] from which mammalian life has been recorded in the New World, and in the Old is only surpassed in this respect by a few of the Himalayan species' (Thomas, 1900).

A biometric comparison between all Auliscomys using principal component analysis (Spotorno, unpublished results) showed that the southern sublimis is smaller than the northern pictus. From such analysis and data from the available reports, Table 3 was constructed. Based on the first five characters (the rest are not clearly cohesive but included for completeness), it is apparent that the morphological and ecological relationships of the alpaca-llama pair are paralleled by the ones of the sublimis-pictus pair. This might be called ecological convergence of two unrelated taxa when one considers that the southern altiplano is drier than the northern part (Figure 1), the former with most of the desert and dry, cold puna belt (Winterhalder and Thomas, 1978) and the latter with the main moist, warm Puna belt. These particular conditions would explain the long, fine and lighter colored furs of sublimis and its analogues, the alpaca and vicuña, in contrast with those qualities shown by the northern pictus and its guanaco and llama analogues. On these grounds, the view that the alpaca has some characters associated with the desert puna suggests that it was domesticated from a species that is or was living there, the vicuña or another one. Since the vicuña is so divergent from the rest, the plausibility of the third alternative seems less remote.

How might the variety of climatological and biological conditions here presented have influenced the establishment of permanent human settlements which later evolved into a mature culture? Patently, the development of agriculture and the domestication of animals are central to this issue. Two factors that can limit these latter developments are the leaching of soils by high precipitations and the availability of a sufficiently large and adequate genetic variability for a successful crop. The first one refers to the fact that, in addition to the removal of nutrients from soils, the tillage of land destroys the vegetal soil layer and increases soil leaching by rain. If there is a rainy season, planting schedules can be adjusted to limited and predictable rain with supplementary water given by irrigation. The dramatic sequence of forest clearing, fast planting and cropping, and leaving the field, practiced by many tropical forest aborigines (Meggers, 1971) would not favor a permanent settlement. In fact, the dark areas of Figure 1 are those where a high degree of soil leaching occurs every year and where intense supplementary feeding of the soil and herds is required. The second factor is based on the knowledge that artificial selection cannot create new variability; thus we can only use and accumulate that which is naturally provided at a slow rate, particularly those variants that are already adapted or pre-adapted to an unusual and harsh environment. The relative richness of the zone around Lake Titicaca would increase the feasibility of obtaining enough genetic diversity to start and sustain long-term attempts to adapt plants to agricultural practices.

The present diversity of cultivated plants in the Andes was the result of domestication processes started almost 8,000 years ago (Kaplan et al., 1973), although a primarily agricultural strategy was not adopted until 4,000 years ago

(Hammond, 1976). High altitude crops include the chenopods qanahua or cañihua (*Chenopodium pallidicaule*) and hupa or quinoa (*Ch. quinua*), normally cultivated in the cold puna, between 3000 and 4000 meters (Frere et al., 1978), and with a yield far larger than any other grain in the highlands (Sauer, 1963). From material collected in Ecuador, Perú and Bolivia, three varieties were found in Cuzco, four around Titicaca Lake, three in the southern altiplano and two in Potosi. The southern altiplano varieties (Real de Puno, Salinas and Sajama) were found to be more resistant to hail than the northern ones (Frere et al., 1978). Compared to other crops, the two chenopods are more resistant to freezing and to salty soils, and they produce grains with a high protein content and high quality amino acids, making them comparable to animal food. The qanahua, found exclusively in the Andes, is the only diploid species among cultivated and wild chenopods (Heiser and Nelson, 1974), suggesting a probable altiplano origin for the crop (Heiser, 1979).

The presently widely raised potato, a tetraploid plant, also arose in the Andes as a cultivated species (Heiser, 1979). For those accustomed to a few clones of the so-called 'Irish' potato (*Solanum tuberosum*), Andean potatoes show a striking diversity of color, shape and taste. The main Andean groups are the tetraploid *andigena*, followed by the diploid *stenotomum*, cultivated up to 4000 meters; there are other diploids, triploids and pentaploids. 'The richest zone in clones in Bolivia and Perú is between 3600 and 3900 meters. The number of clones diminish markedly to the North, Colombia - Venezuela, and to the south, Chile - Argentina ....' (Frere et al., 1978). Other domesticated Solanum species are cultivated in South America for the fruits rather than for the tubers: naranjilla (*S. quitoense*), topiro (*S. topiro*) and kachuma or melonpear (*S. muricatum*) (Heiser, 1979).

One of the prominent characteristics of Andean agriculture is the domestication of tubers. In addition to potatoes, oqa or oca (*Oxalis tuberosa*), a carrot-like tuber of many colors, and colluku or ulluco (*Ulluco tuberosis*), a waxy skinned, nutty tasting root, as well as yakuma or yakon (*Polymnia sonchifolia*), rakacha or arracache (*Arracia xanthorhiza*), a white, yellow or purple root, ajipa (*Pachyrhizus* sp.) and the butterscotch scented maca (*Lepidium mejenii*) were domesticated (see Sauer, 1963; Heiser, 1979 and Brush, 1982 for reviews). Oca is the second most widely cultivated tuber in the Andes, in rotation with potatoes (Frere et al., 1978). All these tubers were the main dietary items before the introduction of maize from Mesoamerica 4,000 years ago (Hammond, 1976); however, maize is a poorly cold adapted species cultivated only in the warm valleys of the Andes.

The places or precise dates where the domestication of animals occurred are obscure (Spotorno, 1982). In the best documented study of altiplanic preceramic faunal remains (Wheeler Pires-Ferreira et al., 1976), it is striking that there is not a single camelid bone at the oldest level (10000 to 7000 BC), where cervid and horse remains predominate. The next level (7000 to 5500 BC) shows the sudden appearance of camelids whose bones account for 54.9% of the 175 identifiable pieces found, a figure which increases to 82.3% at level 5 (5500 to

TABLE 4
Number of vernacular names (Quechua and Aymará) for plant and animal species

Plants[1]		Animals[2]	
Compositae	22	Insects	12
Solanaceae	5	Other arthropods	2
Cactaceae	5	Pisces	2
Umbelliferae	3	Birds	16
Charyophyllaceae	3	Herpetozoa	6
Papilionaceae	2	Mammals	17
Geraniaceae	2	TOTAL	55
Cruciferae	2		
Juncaceae	2		
Malvaceae	2	Mammals[3]	25
Other	24		
TOTAL	72		

[1] Only for the Chilean altiplano; for a complete list, see Castro et al., 1982.
[2] From Ebbing, 1965 *Gramática y diccionario Aimará*. La Paz, Bolivia: Editorial Don Bosco.
[3] From Murphy, 1976.

4200 BC) and to 84.8% at level 4 (4200 to 2500 BC). More recent sites in southern Perú also show a continued predominance of camelids over cervids (Miller, 1979). Since the camelids are territorial and presumably easier to hunt than the fast and gracile cervids and horses, it is difficult to explain the absence of camelid remains at the Junin puna (central Perú) if these species were, in fact, living there. This suggests again the southern altiplano as the probable place of camelid domestication.

Andean peoples have developed a detailed knowledge about the flora and fauna of the altiplano in centuries of permanent residence. Individuals from Putre, Parinacota and Zapahuira in northern Chile recognized and gave vernacular names to 74% of 225 local plant species (Castro et al., 1982); of these 68% were used as food, fuel, medicine, building materials or for religious purposes. People from Toconce, at the extreme south of the altiplano, recognized 91% of a sample of 154 local plant species and 119 were used in some manner for themselves or their herds (Aldunate et al., 1981). Andean men and women have coined names for many plant and animal species (Table 4). They have been successful too in the selection and adaptation to culture of dozens of plant species (Brush, 1982) and in the use and domestication of enough species to make a living (Gilmore, 1950), becoming aware of the particular ecological constraints imposed by a complex mosaic of diverse environments (see Aldunate et al., 1981, for a description of the environment as perceived by Toconce inhabitants). Consequently, they have been able to invent successfully socio-ecological ties to circumvent low local production (Murra, 1975) partly derived from restricted crop diversity at any particular site. And it seems that they have done all of this with the few resources a rigorous Nature gave them here and there, no single one sufficient by itself but enough when such diversity is summed up and combined.

WILLIAM J. SCHULL, BLAGO RAZMILIC,
LEONARDO FIGUEROA, AND MARILUZ GONZALEZ

Chapter 3
TRACE METALS

The waters that nurture the lands we describe arise largely in the mountains to the east and are replenished in their ceaseless efforts to reach the sea through the rains and snows of the altiplano. Six riverine systems are involved, four along the coast and two in the altiplano. Among the former are the Lluta, San José (Azapa), Vitor and Camarones systems, all of which originate in the sierra; among the latter are the Río Lauca and the Río Uchusuma. Originally the Río Lauca, and its major tributaries, the Río Quiburana and Río Sajama, drained into the Lago de Coipasa in Bolivia; however, several decades ago, with the consent of Bolivia, to meet the increased water needs of the Azapa Valley agricultural enterprises and the growing electrical requirements of Arica, some of the waters of the Lauca were diverted into the Río San José that sustains the Azapa Valley.

Europeans who early reached these areas commented frequently on the toxicity of some of these waters for beast and man, especially notorious was the 'agua de verruga' alleged to produce a serious disease, manifesting itself in great bleeding, boils or carbuncles, and often death (von Tschudi, 1847; Squier, 1878). Some of these observers suggested that minerals might be a factor in the occurrence of disease in these areas. Von Tschudi, for example, observed (1847, p. 265): 'Every valley has its own peculiar disease, which frequently does not extend beyond the boundary of a few square miles, and is quite unknown in neighbouring districts. The origin of these disorders is, doubtless, to be traced to certain mineral or vegetable influences as yet unknown. It is remarkable how unequally these baneful visitations affect the different races of the inhabitants.' Similarly, Forbes (1870, p. 224) noted that 'In some districts, particularly in the provinces of Larecaja and Munecas, the Indians suffer from wens or goitre, which often attain a great size. Amongst the inhabitants of Quiabaya and Sorata it is so common that they have received from their neighbours, not so affected, the nickname of 'Ccotosos,' from Ccoto, the Aymará word for goitre. ... In Bolivia, dried seaweed from the shores of the Pacific is employed in the cure of goitre. ... The employment of this substance in medicine is remarkable, as showing how similar results may be arrived at in far distant parts of the globe; for it is quite evident that the curative properties of the seaweed are due to the iodine contained in it; yet in Europe the discovery and employment of preparations of iodine in the cure of goitre are comparatively of very recent date.' This description of the simple effects of iodine deficiency would have been apt until the introduction of iodized salt and is still true in many of the remote areas of the altiplano.

William J. Schull and Francisco Rothhammer (eds.), The Aymará: Strategies in Human Adaptation to a Rigorous Environment, 33-44.

As these rivers and streams of the interior of the north to which we have alluded flow coastward, it is now known that they accumulate a heavy burden of metals, many noxious. Arsenic, boron, copper, lithium, sodium, and potassium are common constituents and may themselves contribute to ill-health in this region. Thus, for example, the concentration of arsenic in the Río Camarones near the village of Camarones is 1.1 ppm or over 20 times the U.S. Public Health Service recommended value of 0.05 ppm. Similarly, inhabitants of the Lluta valley have significantly higher serum burdens of lithium. This would be merely a curious but possibly unimportant finding were it not for the recognized toxic and adverse responses of individuals to therapeutic doses of lithium. Nitrates and sulfates as well as other cations or elements too are conspicuously elevated by world standards.

But it is difficult to generalize about the burdens of these rivers for each is more-or-less unique, and their natural burdens have often been altered by the spoil from mining activities in the sierra and altiplano. At various times in the past, and to a lesser extent now these mines have produced antimony, arsenic, bismuth, copper, gold, lead, manganese, molybdenum, silver, sulfur, and zinc (Salas, Kast, Montecinos, and Salas, 1966). The San José River, for example, until the diversion of a portion of the Lauca, had very few feeder streams originating in the altiplano and was not connected to any thermal area. Thus the quality of its water was far better than most of the other rivers, but the quantity it carried was very much less, and rarely, save in years of exceptionally heavy rain in the sierra, did its waters actually reach the Pacific. The Lluta, on the other hand, is the strongest flowing and has the largest catchment area in the region. However, it is highly acidic at its point of origin near Mount Tacora, remains so as far westward as Poconchile, and often reaches the Pacific still acidic. Its tributaries, the Azufre and Tacora Rivers, arise in a sulfur rich area, and are also acidic (pH hovers around 2-3), as are the waters it derives from thermal springs, some of which are exceptionally rich in borax (Wright et al., 1961 and Wright and Meléndez, 1963). Both the Azufre and Tacora Rivers are highly toxic to livestock and travellers. Near Humalpaca these rivers are joined by the Caracarani, and the further addition of the waters of the Putre and Socoroma Rivers, which are alkaline and apparently serve well the terrace gardens of the farmers in the vicinity of Putre, does not significantly alter the acidity of the main river but does apparently lessen its toxicity. The result of this confluence of small rivers of quite different character is the anomaly of highly alkaline agricultural soils being irrigated by strongly acid water. And this concatenation may be responsible for the periodic crop failures that occur. However, archaeological remains are common in the Lluta valley, suggesting that the indigenous pre-Columbian population was able to utilize the water.

The pathways of ingestion of noxious or potentially noxious constituents of these waters are numerous, for they not only support the people, but the crops they cultivate and the animals they husband. Little is known about the concentrations of most metals in these components of the local food chains, but we can surmise that they too must be high. Even less is known about the effects of these metals, at these concentrations on human growth and development, and health. Some are known to be prejudicial, indeed toxic at still higher concentrations, but others may actually be beneficial, for example, selenium. A measured review of the evidence to support these contentions for all of the metals these waters contain, or the potential complexity of the cellular interactions that may occur lies outside our purpose; however, a brief consideration of one metal, lithium, will serve to illustrate our concern.

BIOLOGY OF LITHIUM

We select lithium for a variety of reasons of which three are especially prominent. First, few other areas of the world appear to exhibit concentrations of lithium in surface waters the equal of those encountered in northern Chile. Second, lithium, although nominally a member of the alkali metals group (sodium, potassium, rubidium and cesium), exhibits some properties analogous to those of the alkaline earths (barium, calcium, magnesium, strontium). Finally, while much is known about the absorption, distribution and excretion of calcium, magnesium, potassium and sodium, all elements essential to man, it is not known how their cellular kinetics may be altered in the presence of substantial but non-therapeutic amounts of lithium, an element which actively competes with the others.

Lithium is widely, albeit not abundantly distributed throughout the earth's crust. It is concentrated in the silicates and alumino-silicates of acidic igneous rocks, in pegmatite dikes, in evaporites and lake clays of volcanic origin, as well as in waters from hot springs, oil-field brines, highly mineralized waters, salt lagoons, and hydrologically closed basins. These are conditions which characterize northern Chile to greater or lesser extent. Lithium is easily removed from rocks and sediments in weathering and tends to remain in solution because of the high solubility of its most common salts.

Lithium can affect plant growth and development, sometimes adversely and sometimes beneficially. It stimulates growth of members of the family Solanaceae, for example, but apparently retards the growth of citrus. While plants differ in their tolerance, generally their lithium content correlates well with that of the soils in which they are rooted. Lithium accumulates first in the root and then moves into the older leaves where it becomes immobilized. Some plants can tolerate large amounts of lithium; prominent among these are members of the families Chenopodiaceae and Solanaceae. The latter family includes potatoes and the former quinoa (also spelled quinua), both widely cultivated staples of the middle and higher Andean altitudes.

A recent estimate of daily intestinal absorption of lithium in human beings suggests a value of 20 micrograms; this is substantially less than the average total daily human intake and implies that not all lithium in foods is absorbed by the intestine. Intake itself can, of course, vary widely. It is generally believed that medicinal lithium salts in drinking water are completely absorbed, and thus water may constitute the major source of lithium for man and animals. The absorbed lithium is largely excreted within 24 hours, save for a small portion that is retained intracellularly. It is for this reason that under equilibrium conditions, daily urinary excretion of lithium is held to be a reliable measure of daily intestinal absorption. Geographical differences in the lithium content of human urine are known to exist which suggest the influence of geographical differences in the lithium concentrations of food and water.

A. Human body burdens of lithium

An extensive literature relates therapeutic dosages of lithium to amounts to be seen in plasma, erythrocytes and other tissues. Some tissues concentrate lithium relative to plasma; others do not. Whole brain, for example, exhibits concentrations of lithium roughly comparable to those seen in plasma; whereas bone and thyroid tissue exhibit amounts severalfold greater. Surprisingly sparse, however, are data that describe human body burdens as functions of the concentrations of lithium in non-medicinal sources, that is, in water and foodstuffs. Presumably some, possibly all of the observations made at therapeutic concentrations are also applicable at lesser exposures, for lithium is not metabolized and its pharmacokinetics are dependent solely upon absorption, distribution and excretion. Maternal and fetal plasma concentrations in lithium treated women, for example, never differ by more than the analytical error, and thus there appears to be full equilibration across the placenta. Lithium concentrations in the milk of lithium-treated nursing mothers is about half that seen in the plasma of the women themselves. It seems reasonable to presume, given the latter observations in particular, that cow's and goat's milk may also be an important source of lithium in areas where they are extensively used. Cattle and goats find potable water that humans do not, and their ruminations should serve to release plant-bound lithium that could then be concentrated in milk. Indeed, in the Camarones and Lluta valleys, lithium levels in milk are often two-fold or more higher than those in the water (Razmilíc, unpublished observations).

B. Toxic and adverse response to therapeutic doses of lithium

Currently the most common medicinal use of lithium salts is in the control of manic-depressive psychosis (Lazarus, 1986) although historically it has also been used in the treatment of gout, as a hypnotic, a salt substitute, and in other ways, specifically to treat some hematologic disorders (Barr and Galbraith, 1983). Its use in the latter instances stemmed from the presumption that lithium enhances granulopoiesis while inhibiting erythropoiesis (Chan, Saunders, and Freedman, 1980), but as Barr and his colleagues have shown this does not appear to be the case (Barr, Koekebakker, Brown, and Falbo, 1987). Stimulated growth is not cell lineage specific; growth is enhanced in all clones, whether erythroid or granulocytic, until toxic levels are reached. Effective therapy in manic-depressive psychosis appears to rest upon the maintenance of satisfactory plasma concentrations of lithium. Experience suggests plasma concentrations of 1.0 to 1.5 milliequivalents per liter (mEq/liter) or so are sufficient to attain these ends, and are normally achievable at daily doses of approximately 3 mg of ionic lithium per kilogram of body weight. Doses of this amount can, however, if maintained over appreciable periods of time, give rise to a variety of adverse responses. We identify here only a few of the more striking of these; an account of all of the purported adverse reactions will be found in Jefferson and Greist (1977).

Polyuria and polydipsia occur in over 40% of individuals receiving lithium therapy. Less common is a more severe diabetes insipidus-like syndrome in which urine volumes as high as 9 liters per day have been reported. It appears the polyuria stems from a lithum-induced inhibition of antidiuretic hormone-sensitive renal adenyl cyclase. The polydipsia may be merely a secondary consequence of the polyuria, but some animal experimental evidence suggests lithium has a direct effect on thirst.

Lithium has complex effects on thyroid function and carbohydrate metabolism. It may induce a diffuse, nontender goiter; hypothyroidism with or without a goiter, or merely abnormal laboratory tests of thyroid function without conspicuous clinical effects. Although normally lithium's effect on the thyroid is a suppressive one, occasionally thyrotoxicosis occurs. Interestingly, lithium concentrations in thyroid tissue commonly exceed plasma concentrations two to five-fold.

Insofar as carbohydrate metabolism is concerned, animal studies reveal no less than five separate stages of metabolism which lithium may affect; the net result is, however, increased glycogen synthesis. The nephrogenic diabetes insipidus that develops in about one-third of lithium treated patients is probably accounted for by impairment of cyclic-AMP-induced water flow responses in the kidney. In the gastrointestinal tract, the uptake and transport of sugars (glucose, xylose, etc.) and water is partially dependent on a sodium transport system, and the substitution of lithium for sodium decreases intestinal absorption of both glucose and water. Parenthetically, lithium is also known to stimulate the sodium pump in the red blood cell, but the efflux it provides depends upon the amount of potassium that is present. At the organismal level the actions of lithium on carbohydrate metabolism appear to be quite similar to insulin. Since carbohydrate metabolism at this level is largely hormonally controlled and appears to be mediated by stimulation or inhibition of adenylate cyclase to produce cyclic-AMP, the effects of lithium can be explained if lithium blocks activation of adenyl cyclase by hormones such as glucagon and adrenocorticotropic hormone. It does not appear that lithium itself is diabetogenic and the evidence that it may alter the frequency of diabetes is confusing and unpersuasive.

Lithium may also impinge on any enzymatic process requiring magnesium or calcium. Much attention has focused on the effect of lithium on the well characterized ten major enzymes of glycolysis, six of which have been shown to be magnesium-dependent. It can be argued that any enzyme that is involved in the utilization or generation of ATP, the major energy currency of metabolism, is potentially liable to lithium action because the active form of ATP is the ATP-Mg complex, and lithium is able to compete with magnesium in the formation of this complex. Specifically, lithium has been shown to inhibit enolase, pyruvate kinase and hexokinase, but to have no inhibitory effect on phosphoglycerate kinase or magnesium dependent ATPase.

Finally, leukocytosis, specifically a neutrophilia, is the most frequently encountered hematopoietic side effect of lithium; white cell counts frequently reach 14-15,000 cells per cubic millimeter, and values as high as 24,000 have been reported. This expansion of the total blood granulocyte pool apparently reflects an increased production of neutrophils in the bone marrow. Barr and his colleagues (Barr, Koekebakker, Brown and Falbo, 1987) have shown that ultratrace levels of lithium, in the nanomolar range, will stimulate clonal proliferation of granulocyte precursors in vitro, and suggest that lithium and its elemental relatives may play a role in the control of human blood cell production. They further suggest that boron may also play an essential role in human physiology (Clarke, Webber, Koekebakker and Barr, 1987). This is of particular interest insofar as the Lluta Valley is concerned, for the waters of the Río Lluta carry especially high concentrations of the salts of boron. Although elemental boron is thought not to be toxic, accumulation of its salts is. Boracic acid occurs in nature as the mineral sassolite; it is soluble in water, and protracted exposure can presumably produce borism with its dry skin, eruptions and gastric disturbances (Merck Index, 1976).

Given the possible essential role of lithium in hematopoiesis, it is tempting to speculate upon the prevalence of infectious disease in areas of relatively high exposure to this metal if, indeed, the leukocytosis is linearly related to plasma lithium concentrations. However, bacterial localization such as that seen in infective endocarditis appears to involve platelet aggregation, and lithium inhibits ADP-induced aggregation. Epidemiological efforts to identify untoward effects of lithium at those concentrations naturally and commonly encountered have not been compelling. It is important to note, however, that in all of these studies the range in lithium concentrations was modest, from 0 to 160 parts per billion. These are concentrations very much less than those associated with the riverine valleys of which we write.

C. Genetic control of lithium transport

Several lines of evidence suggest that the cellular transport of lithium is under genetic control. First, Dorus et al. (1974; see also Dorus et al., 1975) have shown that both in vivo and in vitro the intrapair difference in red blood cell uptake of lithium is smaller, on the average, in identical than in non-identical twins. Indeed, they estimate that some 76% of the inter-individual variability in in vitro lithium ion uptake in erythrocytes is due to genetic factors. An even higher heritability appears to hold in plasma concentrations of lithium. Their findings are reinforced by studies of Schless et al. (1975) who have demonstrated that in sheep with genetically determined differences in potassium concentrations,

TABLE 1
Lithium content in potable surface waters by river system, from highest to lowest altitude, and year of collection

Site	Altitude (m)	Lithium (ugm/l) 1977	1978	1979	1980
RIO LLUTA					
Putre	3640		138	210	
Ancolacaye			180		
Larancagua			722		
Socoroma	3000			50	
Zapahuira	3400		19	30	
7 km. above Molino (km 69)	750		800		
Molinos (km 62)			800	830	
10 km below Molino (km 52)			800		
Bocanegra				870	
Poconchile (km 39)	500		1000	940	
Km 36				1650	
Rosario (km 25)			1170	1490	
Km 20				1800	
Parcela 17	150		1100		
Diez y seis (school) (km 16)				850	
Sta. Lucia bridge (km 13)				1900	
Chacalluta bridge (km 10)	50		1300	2300	
River entry to ocean	0		1300		
RIO SAN JOSE					
Rio Lauca					148
Chapiquiña	3181			39	
Belén	3240			30	
Lupica	2900			21	
Saxamar	3100			19	
Tignamar	3160			22	
5 lowland valley sites	< 200			104-152	99-123
RIO CAMARONES					
Rio Caritaya					4000
Illapata	2200	1200	1500	2300	
Esquiña	2200			450	
Taltape	1500	1600	2000		
Cuartel Viejo				2710	
Umallane				2800	
Camarones	1500			2960	
Conanoxa	300	2000	2600	4480	
Cuya	150	2100	2700		
Baden		2600	3300		
Cuya Bridge	50	3000	4000	6150	6398
River entry to ocean	0	3500	4600		7600

differences also exist in lithium ion concentration. Animals with low red cell potassium ion concentrations had greater lithium concentrations than high potassium sheep. They speculate that lithium ion distribution may be controlled by the same genetic factors that regulate potassium ion distribution.

TABLE 2
Lithium concentration in surface waters and the association with plasma levels

Ecological niche		No.	Mean (mEq/l)	s.d.
Altiplano	(0.00072)	5	0.00319	0.00042
Sierra	(0.01983)	14	0.00462	0.00070
Coast	(0.21494)	12	0.01239	0.00762

Second, Pandey and his colleagues (1977) have described a manic patient and some members of this family whose red blood cells revealed little or no evidence of the phloretin-sensitive $Li+/Na+$ counterflow system that characterizes normal erythryocytes. The latter cells exhibit at least three operationally distinct transport pathways; one of these is inhibited by ouabain (a glycoside derived from the wood of *Acocanthera ouabaio* or from the seeds of *Strophantus gratus* and used as an African arrow poison), one by phloretin (an aglucon of phlorizin derived from the bark or roots of a variety of rosaceous trees, e.g., apple, pear, plum), and one by furosemide (a furfuryl-sulfamoylanthranilic acid). Under physiological conditions, the distribution of lithium between erythyrocytes and plasma depends mainly upon the lithium-sodium counterflow system (the phloretin-sensitive pathway to which reference has been made) and the furosemide pathway. Pandey and his colleagues argue that the similarity in lithium transport defect seen in the patient and several of his siblings makes it probable that this defect is inherited.

Third, although lithium therapy produces dramatic improvement in those individuals whom it helps, failures to respond do occur in the treatment of bipolar patients (those who have episodes both of mania and depression), and lithium's role in the treatment of unipolar (depressed only) patients is still poorly defined. Mendlewicz and his associates (1972) have presented the results of a family study of all patients admitted to a double-blind trial of lithium prophylaxis which suggest that lithium responsiveness can be predicted from the patient's family history. Specifically, they found that response to lithium was significantly correlated with the presence of bipolar illness in the proband's first degree relatives, and argue from this that responsiveness is inherited.

D. Lithium concentrations in this region and the associated body burdens

Analysis of water samples obtained over several years reveal, first, that in the three broad ecological niches that obtain in the north of Chile, lithium concentrations are lowest in the altiplano, intermediate in the sierra and highest in the coastal valleys (see Table 1). Second, this general gradient suggests that within the coastal valleys, where the population is densest, exposure to lithium increases as the streams and rivers flow coastward, and finally, to the extent that body burdens are proportional to concentrations of lithium in the waters that sustain a population, these burdens should increase coastwardly. Of these

TABLE 3
Analysis of variance of variability within and between families within niches

Source	Sum of Squares	df	Mean Square	F
Between sibships within niche	0.0025700	6	0.0004283	8.32**
Within sibships within niches	0.0005146	10	0.0000515	
Total	0.0030846	16		

** $P < 0.01$

speculations, only the latter is testable with the materials at hand.

Tables 2 and 3 present the body burdens of a haphazardly drawn sample of individuals from the designated areas as reflected in their plasmas, and the statistical significance of the correspondence between burden and concentration in water. We note the following: 1) average body burdens may be curvilinearly related to the concentrations of lithium observed in surface water, 2) variation in body burdens changes from village to village; the villages exposed to the highest water concentrations also exhibit the greatest variation in plasma concentrations, and 3) variation within families is significantly smaller than that between families (Table 3).

Plasma concentrations are not significantly different in males as contrasted with females and do not vary with age over the range of ages studied (7-66 years). The values recorded in Table 2 are amazingly similar to those described by Zaldivar in samples taken in 1971 (Zaldivar, 1980). It should be noted that our venous blood specimens were collected in a 15 ml vacutainer to which had been added 3 ml of acid-citrate-dextrose solution as a cell preservative; as a consequence, the values presented in Table 2 underestimate the 'true' plasma concentrations by approximately 20%. This does not compromise our conclusions for all are derived from comparisons within similarly obtained specimens; it does mean, though, that if absolute measures are desired, the values here presented must be increased by 20% or so.

While the numbers in Table 2 are admittedly small, and warrant no more than speculation at the moment, at least two different events could account for the seeming curvilinearity. First, at lower lithium concentrations in water, the contribution of foodstuffs to the body burden may loom larger. Second, at low concentrations of lithium gastrointestinal absorption may be enhanced whereas at higher concentrations absorption may be dampened. Obviously much more needs to be done to characterize not only the variation of lithium concentrations in this area, but the associated body burdens.

OTHER TRACE METALS

Data on other water-borne metals with toxic effects in these rivers, such as arsenic, cadmium, copper, lead, manganese, and zinc, are generally more limited

TABLE 4
Variation in selected metals in surface rivers of northern Chile[1]

Site	Elevation above sea level (m)	Li (mg/l)	Na (meq/l)	K (meq/l)	As (mg/l)	B (mg/l)
RIO LLUTA						
7 km above Molino	750	.8	7.8	.54	.5	9.5
Molino		.8	7.8	.54	.25	8.8
10 km below Molino		.8	7.8	.64	.19	8.8
Poconchile	500	1.0	10.9	.78	.12	11.3
Parcela 17	150	1.1	12.2	.87	.12	13.0
Chacalluta Bridge	50	1.3	13.5	1.0	.10	14.5
River entry to ocean	0	1.3	13.5	1.0	.09	14.3
RIO SAN JOSE						
Bocatoma	250	.1	2.9	.5	*	.5
San Miguel	200	.1	2.9	.5	*	.6
Alto Ramirez	150	.1	3.5	.4	*	.6
RIO CAMARONES						
Taltape	1500	2.1	11.7	.64	.83	9.8
Conanoxa	300	2.6	14.3	.82	.73	12.3
Cuya	150	2.7	14.3	.78	.70	12.8
Baden		3.4	21.3	.97	.54	16.5
Cuya Bridge	50	4.5	26.1	1.15	.54	21.3
River entry to ocean	0	4.8	32.6	1.15	.80	23.8
USPHS mandatory limit					.05[3]	5.0[3]
Recommended limit			10.0[2]		.05[2]	1.0[3]

* imperceptible
[1] Source: Unpublished data, O. Zumaeta, B. Razmilíc
[2] Koning, 1987
[3] USPHS, 1970

than those on lithium (see Table 4). However, sufficient information has accumulated on some, arsenic for example, to limn the potential magnitude of the environmental hazards. The acute toxicity of inorganic arsenic has been repeatedly documented, and recent studies have established its probable carcinogenicity. It is apparently associated with an increased risk of cancers of the skin, lung, liver, kidney and bladder as well as vascular disease (see, e.g., Wu, Kuo, Hwang, and Chen, 1989). Arsenic is known to have a high affinity for sulfhydryl groups, and it is generally presumed that the protean nature of its biological effects reflect the number of enzymes whose activity depends upon the sulfhydryl group (Reeves, 1976). Given this affinity, arsenic tends to accumulate in those organs of the body rich in sulfhydryl groups, such as the skin, hair, fingernails, arteries and kidney. The most common route of absorption is through ingestion, but arsenic can also enter the body through inhalation or through the skin, and thus even bathing in contaminated waters could increase absorption.

Insofar as these valleys are concerned, Razmilíc and his colleagues (unpublished recent observations) have reported the annual mean concentration of arsenic in the Río Camarones to be 0.91 mg/L; more strikingly the concentration of arsenic in cultivated soils is 206.2 mg/Kg and values in the alfalfa grown in the valley are three to eight times higher than those seen in the Lluta or Azapa valleys. The 'edible' shrimps (*Cryphiops caementarius*) captured in the Camarones River have exceptionally high burdens of arsenic; values in the viscera as high as 468 mg/Kg (on a dry weight basis) have been recorded. Exposure of the human inhabitants of the Camarones Valley to these levels of arsenic has persisted for centuries as analysis of the remains of some 15 mummies, dating from 570 to 630 years prior to the present, reveals. Figueroa et al. (1987) found average arsenic levels in the skin to be 20 mg/kg, and varied in the internal organs from 3.8 mg/kg in the lungs to as high as 41.4 mg/kg in the liver (the kidney exhibited an intermediate value – 21.8 mg/kg). Measurements of the concentrations of arsenic in the fingernails and hair disclosed values of 49 and 143 mg/kg, respectively (for comparison, the average fingernail value in Valdivia, a non-arsenical area of southern Chile, is 4.82 mg/kg (see Borgoño et al., 1980)). Elimination of arsenic is either through vomiting, in the case of acute intoxication, or more slowly through urinary excretion and desquamation of the skin when exposure is chronic. Presumably the concentrations seen in the soft tissues – skin, liver and kidney – reflect these known pathways of elimination of arsenic, and the substantially lower levels in the lung, the fact that the metal was ingested not inhaled. The biological half-life of arsenic in humans appears to be fairly short, a matter of a few days, but the time depends upon the nature of the arsenic or arsenical compound to which one is exposed. About 70% of 'fish arsenic,' for example, is eliminated in the urine within a week, but the remainder seems to be eliminated much more slowly (Vahter, 1983). To the extent that the paleoindian inhabitants of this valley supplemented their diets with riverine fish or crustaceans this slower elimination could have contributed to the body burdens we have cited.

Although we know little about the prevalence of cancer among these early indigenes, it is interesting that the tissues with high concentrations of arsenic are those associated with arsenic-related malignancies. It is important to bear in mind, however, that the toxicity of arsenic and its in vivo metabolism appear influenced by other trace metals, such as selenium, and in Chile, high concentrations of arsenic are usually accompanied by high concentrations of selenium, molybdenum and borax. This association speaks again to the need for studies that examine the environmental pathways through which exposure occurs and the biological effects of these potential water-borne toxicants simultaneously rather than singly. The riverine systems of northern Chile would appear to provide an unusual opportunity to achieve this end.

CONCLUSIONS

Until their collective roles can be better defined, we can merely identify some of the possible implications of exposure to the one element, lithium, that has been extensively studied. First, we call attention to the importance of glycolysis in acclimatization and adaptation to the hypoxia and hypocapnia of altitude and note that the enzymes involved in aerobic and anaerobic glycolysis are under genetic control. Second, lithium competes with magnesium in the formation of the Mg-ATPase complex essential to the proper functioning of many of the enzymes involved in glycolysis, and thus differences in concentrations of lithium in water could influence glycolysis and hence adaptation or acclimatization to diminished oxygen and carbon dioxide. Third, lithium is known to be preferentially accumulated in some plants. Among these are the families Chenopodiaceae and Solanaceae, that is, the families to which two of the major foodstuffs of the indigenes belong, the potato and quinoa.

Clearly one can speculate further about the probable impact of these ecologic differences upon health and disease, but such speculation seems unproductive at this juncture. Our aim has been solely to call attention to the complexity of possible gene-environment interactions even in a geographic setting that seems more homogeneous than many, and to suggest that these complexities must be understood before it will be practicable to define the role of either genes or environment or gene-environment interaction in the adaptation of the indigenous peoples to their environment as precisely as would be desired.

Such an understanding would contribute not only to our knowledge of trace metal metabolism but to adaptation to an hypoxic environment. As Iyengar and Gopal-Ayengar (1988; see also Iyengar, 1988) have argued, excesses (and deficiencies) of trace metals are sufficiently pervasive in the high altitude areas of the world that trace element research is essential to the delineation of the hypoxic effects of high altitude. They contend that living at higher elevations involves many stresses, not solely a lower ambient partial oxygen pressure. As an illustration of their concerns, they note (citing the work of Agostini and his colleagues, 1983) that Andean residents show significantly lower serum levels of selenium and glutathione peroxidase compared to subjects from low altitudes, and that selenium deficiency implies a suboptimal protection of cells against oxidant stress. Similarly, in a discussion of the origins of the reported differences in hemoglobin concentration between Himalayan and Andean populations, Frisancho (1988) notes that these concentrations are similar if the comparison is restricted to Andean values derived from non-mining areas and suggests that, since mining is associated with pollution that accentuates hypoxia, the Andean values in mining areas represent a response to not onlu altitude but to mining. Monge, León-Velarde, and Arregui (1989) have reported that the prevalence of excessive erythrocytosis increases with age among healthy, high altitude Peruvian miners but whether this is an effect of age or reflects protracted exposure to mining pollutants (which would be correlated with age) is not clear.

FRANCISCO ROTHHAMMER

Chapter 4

THE AYMARA: AN OUTLINE OF THEIR PRE AND POST-COLUMBIAN HISTORY

The first highland hunters that settled the area presently inhabited by the Aymará lived in small rock shelters some 10,000 years ago. In fact, the archaeological sites of Las Cuevas (7590 BC), Tojotojone (7900 BC), Hakenasa (6390 BC) and Patapatane (6210 BC) provide evidence that these Paleoindian hunters made projectile points from obsidian, basalt and quartz and hunted the American Camelidae, mainly vicuña (Dauelsberg, 1983).

Around 6000 BC, a small glacial advance took place in the highlands and most rock shelters in the area had to be abandoned. Approximately at the same period, the first fishermen and collectors of shellfish made their appearance on the coast near the outlet of the Azapa valley. To catch fish, they employed hooks made from the shell of the mussel mytilus (*Choromytilus choro*). Later these artifacts were replaced by cactus needle hooks, which were used with bait (Bird, 1963). These archaic fishermen lived on the shore protecting themselves from the fresh breeze using primitive wind shelters made from cattail.

It may be postulated that these fishermen and shellfish gatherers were descendants of highland Paleoindian hunters who gradually adapted their technology to the exploitation of marine resources. However, the finding of embalmed mummies, dated around 5000 BC, in the same geographic area seems not to fit entirely with this hypothesis. The embalming technique, which is characteristic of the so-called Chinchorro phase (ca. BC 6000-2000), was very elaborate. After removing the internal organs, including the brain, the embalmers cut away the skin and the hair, and removed the muscles. The body was then smoked and filled with wool, feathers, and rubble, and covered with clay, molding carefully the limbs and the face. Finally, the skin was put in place again and the embalmed body painted either red or black (Uhle, 1919; see also Schiappacasse and Niemeyer, 1984). Through time, over a lapse of 3000 years, the technique changed gradually becoming progressively less elaborate.

It is difficult to imagine that this highly sophisticated embalming method was the result of a local cultural development. Recently, we have suggested that the origin of the Chinchorro phase has to be found in the tropical forest and its presence on the Pacific coast of Chile was the result of a transandean migration that took place around 6000 BC (Rivera and Rothhammer, 1986, see also Chapter 15).

Between 2000 and 1000 BC, around Lake Titicaca, on the highlands, several human groups started a remarkable cultural elaboration that culminated in the cultures of Pukara, Wankarani, and Chiripa. This last one, in turn, gave rise later to the impressive Tiwanaku culture. Again, there are uncertainties as to whether

William J. Schull and Francisco Rothhammer (eds.), The Aymará: Strategies in Human Adaptation to a Rigorous Environment, 45-48.

these cultural developments were the result of local differentiation, of a diffusion process originating in the tropical forest, or a mixture of both. It is known, however, that Pukara exerted an important influence on the human groups that peopled the Azapa valley and contributed to the origin of the Alto Ramirez phase around 500 BC. Pukara is responsible for the introduction of semi-tropical cultivars, such as quinoa, yuca, sweet potato, and chili pepper, as well as novel burying practices, specifically the construction of funerary mounds. The Alto Ramirez people began, during this period, to manufacture rude pottery and basketry, and to cook and store their agricultural products. Remarkable, too, is the development of tinctured tapestry with representations of human heads, llamas, frogs, crosses and ladders (Muñoz and Focacci, 1983).

Tiwanaku's influence begins in the coastal valleys around 380 AD with the Cabuza phase and is present during the Maitas phase (ca. AD 750-1000). The San Miguel and Gentilar phases that followed (ca. AD 1000-1300) are characterized by some regional cultural differentiation. These different phases are primarily defined on the basis of pottery types, and represent, first, the influence of different stages of development of the Tiwanaku culture and, subsequently, the adaption of these to local conditions.

After the collapse of Tiwanaku, the Mollo culture evolved east of Lake Titicaca, giving thereafter origin to the regionalized post-Tiwanaku kingdoms (Browman, 1985). Shortly before the arrival of the Spanish, the Bolivian highlands and the valleys were markedly influenced by the Inca culture.

Meanwhile the cultural development of the valleys changed continuously under the influence of different highland cultures, the fishermen on the coast, however, remained relatively isolated, and were only indirectly influenced by these changes. The Changos, primitive fishermen described by the Spanish conquerors, at the beginning of the sixteenth century, may be considered the last descendants of the archaic shellfish gatherers that initially peopled the coast (Rothhammer et al., 1982).

According to Cuneo Vidal (1919; cited by Hidalgo, 1978) some 10,000 Aymará Indians lived in Tacna in 1535. The geographic origin of these Indians was, according to the same author, the highland area between Puno and the Desaguadero River, that is to say in the regionalized post-Tiwanaku kingdom of Chucuito. The Indian population of the Tacna valley belonged to two chieftainships, the 'hanansaya' and the 'urinsaya,' occupying the upper and lower portions of the valley, respectively. The population grew until land and water became scarce. As a consequence, the regulus of Chucuito decided to colonize the Lluta and Codpa valleys, and the area of Socoroma, in the sierra. New chieftainships were established in these areas. The colonies were called, according to Cuneo Vidal, 'mitmas' by the Incas. It is interesting to note that the practice of the highland kingdoms of relocating populations and establishing colonies in the valleys and the lower mountain regions preceded the Inca Empire. Recently (Rothhammer et al., 1982), we pointed out that archaeologic evidence suggests a continuous cultural contact between the valleys and the highlands, at least after 500 BC. Furthermore, Santoro and Chacama (1982) obtained for Pinuta, an archaeologic site located some 10 kilometers northwest of Putre, a radiocarbon date of 1800 ± 140 BC. It is, therefore, conceivable that the sierra was inhabited by descendants of pre-Tiwanaku cultural groups at the time the Tacna valley Indians were relocated in Socoroma.

It has been hypothesized that the inhabitants of the villages at lower altitudes belonged to highland kingdoms which through a system of colonization maximized the exploitation of natural resources (Murra, 1968). This 'vertical control' system, according to its author, Murra (1972), had also the peculiarity of having the structure of an archipelago, that is to say, that different highland kingdoms controlled 'islands' in the lower mountain region or in the coastal valleys. It is important to bear in mind that this apparent ethnic heterogeneity was political and administrative, and not biological, since all post-Tiwanaku kingdoms shared a common ancestry.

The Spaniards who initiated the conquest of Chile rode from Perú southward using the route along the eastern slope of the Andes and entered Chilean territory through the San Francisco Pass, located near the city of Copiapo. The conquerors, under the command of Diego de Almagro, thus avoided the need to cross the extensive Atacama desert, which in the winter months is extremely cold during the nights and in the summer, hot and dry. The Indians, according to the Spanish chronicler, crossed the desert making use of water supplies that they obtained in 'jagueyes' or springs located at distances between 10 and 40 kilometers apart (Hidalgo, 1972). Advised by the Indians, Diego de Almagro used the desert route on his way back to Perú and conquered the area now occupied by the Aymará in 1535. The Spanish conquest was consolidated by Pedro de Valdivia in 1540.

Captain Juan Maldonado de Buendía, who was sent by Viceroy Francisco de Toledo to visit the city of Arequipa and its jurisdiction, wrote on March 25th of 1575 to the Spanish King that he found 226 little Indian settlements in the province of Collesuyo, which comprised the area between the Arequipa and Loa rivers, covering some 75,000 square kilometers (Hidalgo, 1978). The zone inhabited by the Aymará is included in this area. Captain Maldonado concentrated the Indians in 26 hamlets and established 13 'doctrinas' or collative curateships. This is probably the first historical account of the existence of Aymará villages. Once established, it is reasonable to assume that these villages have not changed their geographical locations.

The Aymará maintained their ethnic and cultural identity first under the Inca and later under the Spaniards. Casquez de Espinosa visited villages in the Lluta Valley, and the villages of Lluta, Socoroma, Putre, Saxamar, Chapiquiña and Codpa, among others in 1618. The communities were very isolated and most Indians had not been baptized. Espinosa burned the village of Isquiliza because he found that the Indians of that village were idolatrous (Hidalgo, 1978).

The Count of Superunda, Viceroy and Governor of Perú and Chile, in 1750, ordered Don Joaquin Xavier de Cardenas to carry out a reinspection of the area which is now the Province of Arica. The census performed by Cardenas was published (Hidalgo, 1978) and provides names, ages and kinships of all Indian

TABLE 1
The sizes of some Aymará districts
as recorded in the reinspection of 1750 and the 1970 national census

District	1750 Reinspection	1970 National Census
Putre	233	408
Socoroma	217	160
Belén	414	325
Tignamar	169	288
Parinacota	271	278
Guallatiri	48	90

inhabitants by village. The total number of Indians listed is 2,758 not markedly different from the number of inhabitants in this area at the time of the 1970 National Census. It is interesting to compare the census of 1750 with the 1970 National Census data. Inspection of Table 1 reveals that village sizes have remained surprisingly constant during the last 220 years. Some villages have increased their sizes slightly, as for example, Putre, and others have diminished; however, the changes are not drastic nor have the fluctuations in population over time been large as censuses between 1750 and 1970 reveal. In 1943, the populations of Belén, Putre, Socoroma, and Tignamar were 338, 485, 264, and 202, respectively (Keller, 1946).

The production of the silver mines of Choquelimpie in the Chilean altiplano, and Oruro and Potosi in Bolivia declined markedly in 1776. This fact and the foundation of the Virreinato del Río de la Plata led, as a consequence, to many Spaniards leaving the area of Arica. The Peruvian census of 1879 lists the villages of the sierra as being exclusively Indian. The territory was taken over by the Chileans in 1880 after the Pacific War. Belén was established as the center of the civil administration. At the beginning of this century a railroad was built from Arica to La Paz, Bolivia, generating some immigration to the highlands, but the area remained basically isolated until some 30 years ago when the first roads were built. Construction of the latter has, however, begun to alter slowly but perceptibly both the coastal valleys and the sierra. Immigration has occurred and ways of life are changing. But the communities of the altiplano remain largely unchanged; it is still a land of traditional Aymará values and alpaca, llama, and their herdsmen.

MARVIN J. ALLISON

Chapter 5
PALEOPATHOLOGY

Introduction

For the purpose of this chapter mummies from the Alto Ramirez, Cabuza Maitas and classical Tiwanaku phase (BC 500-AD 1000) of the Azapa and other valleys of northern Chile will be considered ancestors of the historical Aymará. It is well to bear in mind that these valleys were overflow areas for groups from the interior and their populations may not be entirely representative of the more advanced highland cultures. For more details about prehistory see Chapter 4 (Rothhammer, this volume). All of the individuals studied died on the coast and were buried there; it is possible that many of them never lived on the altiplano even though they maintained their cultural linkage with highland groups. It is important to separate them from the coastal people, the Changos or their predecessors, who were dedicated to fishing and hunting of sea mammals at the openings of the valleys on the ocean. These coastal people at times used artifacts from the Tiwanaku and Inca cultures but were sufficiently different to be separated in most cases. However, they filled a need in the highlanders' economic scheme by supplying guano for fertilizer, peppers, corn, and other coastal products.

Adaptive response to the environment

It is difficult to ascertain the environment(s) where the individuals studied spent most of their lives. Andeans differ from their lowland counterparts in the proportionately larger size of their chest, larger vital capacity, larger lung surface, heavier carotid bodies, a muscularization of the terminal portions of the pulmonary arterial tree, a right ventricular preponderance in infancy and childhood that persists electrocardiographically in many modern adolescents and adult highlanders (see Weidman et al., Chapter 12, this volume). Whether these changes reflect ethnic differences or are evidence of adaptation is debatable but relatively unimportant here so long as the observations are real. While we seek to identify individuals who may have been of highland origin many of the above attributes are not easily measured on mummies but some might prove useful. Table 1 gives some data based on cardiomegaly.

It is clear from the above table that 'coastal' people have a low frequency of enlarged heart, but here, as in the highlands, some enlargement might be due to complications from pulmonary disease. In the case of the highlands it is most probable that the majority of enlarged hearts are related with living at high

William J. Schull and Francisco Rothhammer (eds.), The Aymará: Strategies in Human Adaptation to a Rigorous Environment, 49-61.

TABLE 1
Cardiomegaly seen in four different groups of mummies

Culture	Origin	%
Azapa	Coastal fishing people	3
Alto Ramirez	Highland shepherds	36
Cabuza	Highlanders	29
Tiwanaku	Highlanders	14

altitudes. Often this observation is reinforced by the finding of a 'barrel chest'. Currently, attempts are being made to measure the rib cage but this information is not ready for publication. At this time we must conclude that in the majority of cases it is not possible to determine whether a long term residency in the highlands of a mummified individual did or did not occur, and, therefore, the effects of such a residency on health can only be surmised based on cultural items associated with the burial.

Childbirth and maternal care

Childbirth and maternal care are two areas where information may be obtained from the study of mummies. Tschopik (1963) in his chapter on the Aymará in the Handbook of the South American Indians, describes childbirth in the historic Aymará, and his description suggests interpretations of the pre-Columbian data. Pregnancy among the Aymará is recognized by the cessation of menstruation. The sex of the unborn child is presumably influenced by magical procedures such as placing farm implements under the mother's bed to produce a boy, and cooking utensils, a girl. Birth takes place in the home assisted by female relatives or midwives (these may be male) who receive an extra fee for disposing of the afterbirth. The midwife massages the woman, and tumbles her in a blanket to position the child. The woman delivers in a crouching position supported by her husband. A belt is tightened around her waist above the abdomen when labor has begun and twisted tightly after delivery to expel the placenta; if this does not occur spontaneously, the midwife pulls it out. The placenta receives special attention either by covering it with flowers and burying it or by placing it in a pottery bowl and burning it. It is considered to be dangerous to the eyes and the hands, and after handling it the hands must be rubbed with llama fat and red ocher.

In view of the above, some pre-Columbian observations may be explained. Gravid females are frequently seen among the mummified bodies and it is not uncommon to see them with a sash 2 or 3 inches wide around their swollen abdomen, the placenta still in place and their breasts enlarged. Autopsy of such individuals reveals the pubic symphysis and the ilium-sacral articulations open, and if the woman was multiparous, scars of parturition are seen at these points (Ashworth et al., 1976). These scars, by their length and depth are a rough

TABLE 2
Mortality for females estimated to be between the ages of 18 and 50 years at time of childbirth

Culture	No.	%
Alto Ramirez	40	33
Cabuza	40	20
Colonial Inca	56	16

indication of the number of pregnancies, but do not necessarily represent the carrying to completion of the pregnancy (see, however, the caveats of Kelley, 1979). It is difficult to know at what age sexual intercourse first occurs but the earliest known pregnancy among these Tiwanaku people is 18 years old. This girl died during the delivery of twins. After delivering the first child she attempted to pull out the placenta; the cord was in her hand, and a second child was in the uterus. One is left with the impression that she was unattended during her delivery. The placenta itself also received special attention in pre-Columbian times. 'Placenta pots' have been found in a number of different Tiwanaku excavations. These are usually large pottery vessels either decorated or plain containing one or more placentas; at times with an offering of corn.

Children who died at birth along with the mother are often buried with her; if they were born dead, the cord is still attached. A number of fetuses have been found in utero, and term babies, who were in difficult positions for delivery with primitive obstetrical methods and died, have also been seen. Table 2 gives some figures on female mortality in which death may have been due primarily to childbirth (see also Arriaza, Allison, and Gerszten, 1988).

The figures in Table 2 might seem exceptionally high but they represent values taken from direct observation on mummified bodies with a full complement of organs from women in the Alto Ramirez and Cabuza phases. The lower figure of 16% seen in the colonial Inca is based on the total adult female population even if no organs were present. Several of these skeletons had the remains of children buried at their feet or skeletons of fetuses found in place in the adult. Deaths due to childbirth in the female childbearing years will fall between 16 and 33%.

The baby, if born alive, had only one chance in two of reaching 15 years of age. Tschopik (1963) reports a 34% mortality for children to the pediatric age of 13 in the modern Aymará with an average number of living children of 2.5 per family. It is difficult to estimate the number of children per family in pre-Columbian times but data from an early colonial census gives a figure of two (Ortíz de Zuñiga, 1972).

General evaluation of health status

Evaluations of the health of a given population on the basis of pathology found at autopsy may lead to erroneous impressions since, in general, one is looking at a static picture. If, as is often the case when studying early peoples, we are limited to the skeleton alone, the error is greater since only about 10 to 20% of human diseases will leave stigmata on the bones. Furthermore the reaction of bone is limited and similar, even though the etiological agent may be varied, and as a result, precise diagnoses are difficult if not impossible in many cases. Bones and teeth do serve in a broad way for an evaluation of general health. We are what we eat, or so it is stated, and if so, the skeleton should reflect the effects of nutrition and the analysis of stature will give even more information. The oral cavity also serves as a dietary indicator. In recent times there has been a change in the dimensions of the maxilla and mandibles in Andean people with no reduction in tooth size (Sawyer et al., 1978a; Rothhammer and Rosales, 1990). Since bone size is affected by mechanical stress or lack of it, it is reasoned that the smaller size is due to a softer diet requiring less mechanical force to masticate. There will be a reduction in ramus size as well. The attrition and calculus size on the teeth reflect the consistency of the diet as do subsequent caries and tooth loss. The incidence of antemortem tooth loss rises spectacularly with the transition from a hunting and gathering economy to agriculture. Among Andean agricultural societies those individuals living on the coast had the highest incidence of caries while the highlanders had much less (Sawyer et al. 1978b; Palomino, Chapter 13). Differences were also seen when comparing caries frequency of coastal Peruvians with permanent dentition, where one or more carious lesions were present in 85% of cases, to highland Chileans from the same period who had a caries rate of under 10%. These differences, presumably dietary in origin, may be related to the more extensive use of corn among the Peruvians.

Harris lines

A general indicator of health during childhood are the so-called Harris or growth arrest lines. During bone growth each time the child has a febrile illness, a period of starvation, or certain diseases that interfere with bone metabolism, cartilage formation ceases. However, with recovery, calcium accumulates in the area of renewed or even increased bone growth forming an extra heavy deposit which, in the case of the long bones, is seen on x-ray as a line crossing the marrow cavity (Steinbock, 1976). This line is also readily seen if the bone is sawed in half. Through a simple system of measurements and mathematical calculations it is possible to know when these lines appeared during the person's childhood; thus we have a rough record of childhood health reflected in these lines (Allison and Gerszten, 1982). While it is true there may be some loss of these lines due to bone remodeling, they are still a useful tool to look at childhood health problems in prehistoric populations.

Table 3 gives the frequency of Harris lines from inhabitants of coastal and inland cultures from Perú and Chile. The average number of lines per positive individual (last column) in theory represents the number of bouts of stress (illness or starvation) during the first 16 years of life (the approximate growth

TABLE 3
The frequency of Harris' lines in Andean mummies from coastal and inland cultures[1]

Culture	No.	Positive No.	Positive %	Lines/positive individual
Preceramic	21	5	24	2.2
San Miguel	19	5	26	1.6
Tiwanaku (coastal)	8	0	0	0
Wari	19	9	47	2.2
Ica	12	5	42	2.2
Azapa	23	20	87	6.3
Alto Ramirez	8	6	75	4.6
Atacameños	16	7	44	8.7
Cabuza	14	8	57	2.9
Tiwanaku (highland)	14	5	36	6.8
Maitas	60	47	78	9.0

1 These estimates are based on an opportunistic sample of individuals of both sexes and all ages. Since the growth of the tibia is completed by 16 or so years of age, the data reflect only stresses occurring in the pre-adult years.

period of the tibia). The frequency of positives from individuals living on the coast was 24-47% with an average of 30.3%; the inland people were 36-87% positive with an average of 68.8%. Not only did the inland people have twice as many positives but the number of lines per positive was also higher, at times reaching over 20 lines per individual. As mentioned above these lines can occur during periods of starvation, but it is questionable whether this is a valid etiology for the people studied here since there was an abundance of foodstuff among the burial goods. It would appear more likely that the lines are due to diseases of an infectious nature, possibly in some cases seasonal, suggesting an insect vector. The Arica area throughout colonial times and up until 40 years ago was malarious; in fact the Inquisition in Lima, Perú banished many of its prisoners to Arica where they soon died of malaria. Although we have evidence for a reticuloendotheliosis, causing enlargement of the liver and the spleen, suggesting malaria, we have not been able to find the malaria parasites in mummies as yet.

Mortality

Table 4 reveals that among early hunters of sea mammals, fishermen and gatherers, who were probably living in temporary camps for relatively short periods, there was a loss of around 25% of all children born, whereas the highland shepherds had a mortality of 50% of their children before the age of fifteen (the current generally accepted pediatric age). At the other end of the scale, among the age group of forty and over, the number of survivors in the two populations was approximately the same, 15-18%. As agriculture developed and people lived in villages with 'full' agriculture, there was an improvement in the survival of adults into old age with an average rate of 25% and in one case 40% of the adult population lived to be over forty. It is to be noted that females

TABLE 4
Mortality for pediatric and geriatric populations in coastal and Tiwanaku cultures

Culture	Age at death (%) Before age 14	40 or older
Coastal hunters and gatherers	28	18
Early Tiwanaku	50	15
Late Tiwanaku	49	25

tended to live longer than males even though during the childbearing years they suffered a greater mortality.

Respiratory diseases and their complications

The most common cause of death among individuals of all cultures studied for any time period was acute respiratory disease, generally a bacterial pneumonia (Allison et al., 1983). This is still the major cause of death in all countries of Latin America, outside of the major urban centers. Table 5 gives the type of acute pulmonary disease seen at autopsy in 51 mummies. Approximately 70% had a bilateral pneumonia, predominantly a bronchopneumonia, although typical lobar pneumonias in the red and gray hepatization stages were not uncommon. The structure of the individual inflammatory cells is generally lost in the mummies but the debris of such cells fills the alveolar spaces, often with recognizable bacteria present. It was possible in some cases to identify the etiological agent; these include Streptococci group A, Salmonella group D, as well as a *Bartonella bacilliformis*. Complications of pneumonia were seen in the form of lung abscesses, pericarditis, pleurisy, bacterial endocarditis, and one case of meningitis. The latter was observed in a two and half to three year old child with bronchopneumonia; the autopsy revealed an intact spinal cord in which the cauda equina area was covered with an abundant inflammatory exudate. This case today would be clinically diagnosed as a hemophilus influenza meningitis. Numerous Gram and fluorescent antibody stains were done but were inconclusive in establishing the etiology of this interesting disease. In general, the complications of pneumonia seen in these mummies were similar to those seen in pre-antibiotic era patients and in about the same frequency.

The first dated case of pre-Columbian tuberculosis seen in the Americas was in a child, about 7 years old, who died in Ica, Perú, around 700 A.D. He died with a terminal miliary tuberculosis (Allison et al., 1973). Since then numerous cases have been seen in many different cultures, many with soft tissue lesions and demonstrable acid fast bacilli. The disease was seen in all of its many protean forms from a simple healed Ghon complex to extensive soft tissue pulmonary and bone disease. Among the Tiwanaku people of northern Chile a calcified primary lesion, an active Ghon complex, several cavity pulmonary lesions and several healed vertebral lesions of Pott's disease were noted. Since

TABLE 5
Fifty-one mummies from all cultures with acute pulmonary disease

Gross	
Gross pneumonia, right lung	13.0 %
Gross pneumonia, left lung	17.4
Gross pneumonia, bilateral	69.6
Microscopic	
Microscopic negative	6.8
Microscopic bacteria	9.1
Microscopic inflammation	22.7
Microscopic inflammation plus bacteria	61.4
Pleural exudate	14.8
Atelectasis	9.3
Hemorrhage	13.0
Emphysema	41.0
Anthracosis	5.6
Pulmonary abscess	3.7
Granuloma	3.7
Pleural adhesions	44.4

the populations seen in the small, rural communities distant from large population centers were limited, it is logical that this disease would not be seen as commonly as in the larger pre-Columbian urban centers. Nevertheless, there is archaeological evidence for a large trade network throughout the Andean area that would permit ample contact with a series of 'exotic' diseases with their possible introduction into small local populations. One example of such an 'exotic' import was noted in the form of the South American blastomycosis in a female inhabitant from the Loa River valley in northern Chile from around 290 AD (Allison et al., 1979). This woman died of cavitary disease of the lungs with kidney metastasis and the parasite was seen in both locations.

Gastrointestinal and liver diseases

Gastrointestinal disease is a common cause of illness in the Andean region today. Improper sanitation causes episodes of diarrheal illness, often fatal in young children, and the systemic Salmonelloses, such as typhoid fever, are common. Adults have adopted the European custom of attributing a wide spectrum of symptoms to liver and gallbladder disease, the latter being in reality not extremely common. Looking back in time one sees that recognizable gastrointestional disease was only present in 7% of the coastal population living in the Arica, Chile, area 5,000 years ago, and the first highlanders who settled on the coast around 2,500 years ago had about 2%. These early people, probably did not live in fixed abodes but periodically moved their camp from time to time thus maintaining a certain degree of sanitation. The Cabuza phase apparently had a full agricultural economy along with shepherding that allowed a more sedentary life resulting in small villages. Here for the first time appeared a significant rise in gastrointestinal parasites (Fouant et al., 1982). Cysts of *Endamoeba coli* were seen in about 30% of the individuals examined along with an occasional oxyuris and whipworm. One example of the hookworm, *Ancylostoma duodenale*, was reported in a Wari culture man from the large Ica Valley in Perú (Allison et al., 1974). In general, it appears that the valleys of northern Chile were too small to maintain for any length of time a cyclic parasite, since to conserve arable land, living sites were built on neighboring desert land and the populations were small.

If intestinal parasites were uncommon then it would appear that the intestinal diseases were probably the result of bacterial agents. Two cases of Salmonellosis were identified, one in a Wari man from Ica, Perú, and the other in a Tiwanaku individual from Arica. The Tiwanaku individual had generalized illness with massive hemorrhages into the intestines and appendix with peritonitis and a bilateral bronchopneumonia. The etiological agent was a Gram negative bacillus with peritrichous flagella seen in liver lesions and was identified serologically as a Salmonella Group D.

Liver disease was noted in 5-8% of the population depending on the culture studied. It was often seen as an abnormally large liver with abscesses in about 25% of the cases, and with no spleen present. This was attributed to an infectious process that produced a septic spleen that went quickly to autolysis. Gallbladder disease was rare and only three cases were seen in Tiwanaku people from the Loa River valley who consumed tremendous quantities of algarroba beans, probably in the form of an alcoholic drink (Munizaga et al., 1978). Two of these individuals died from peritonitis induced by cholelithiasis and a cholecystitis. The stones were cholesterol and in one case there were 63 of them varying in size from 3 to 15 mm. Although gallstones have a high incidence among modern Andean inhabitants, and supposedly in Indians in general (see Weiss, Ferrell and Hanis, 1984), it was apparently not a major problem among the pre-Columbian peoples since only one other case was noted and that in an early sea lion hunter and gatherer. However, one must bear in mind that stones are more common among women than men, and although they can appear precociously, that is, in the second decade of life, they do not generally become frequent until the fourth or fifth decade in contemporary populations, and the mummies that have been studied are necessarily an opportunistic sample with regard to these variables, sex and age.

A different type of gastrointestinal disease was seen in a group of 22 mummified bodies from the area of Tarapacá in northern Chile. Pathology suggestive of Chagas disease was present in nine of twenty-two individuals dating from the third or fourth century AD. These individuals had a tremendously enlarged colon (megacolon) containing enormous quantities of feces that in at least some cases produced death due to impaction. One individual had megaesophagus in addition to megacolon. Chagas is an important vector borne disease that probably had its origins in Minas-Gerais, Brazil, and is still common in Chile and southern Perú. The vector, the 'kissing' bug (triatominae), is common in rural dwellings where it lives in the cracks and thatch or mat roofs.

No parasites were seen in these individuals but immunological studies are currently in progress (Rothhammer et al., 1985).

Renal and venereal diseases

Disease of the genitourinary tract made up 8-10% of the health problems seen, about the same percentage encountered in contemporary societies. One case of cystic kidney, various examples of hydroureter, and pyelonephritis and acute kidney abscesses were seen. Chronic infectious kidney disease was noted in the form of tuberculosis and South American blastomycosis. Kidney atrophy was also recorded. Three cases of bladder calculi were noted in Tiwanaku individuals, in one cultural group, representing a frequency of 3.8%.

An examination of the genitalia must of necessity lead to a discussion of venereal disease. It should first be noted that among the Tiwanaku people there was no evidence of circumcision nor did they remove body hair as did some coastal people who removed all hair except that on their head. No genital lesions were seen in any people from any cultural group, but osseous lesions typical of tertiary syphilis were seen in nearly all cultural groups from the coast and the mountains, at times reaching as high as 7%. Since we have no evidence for venereal transmission as yet it is more proper to refer to these lesions as a treponematosis rather than syphilis. The characteristic lesion was an osteitis and periostitis of the calvaria and the tibia (saber shin) as well as lesions resembling gumma located in soft tissue (Allison et al., 1982). To date no specific etiological agent has been found, but such lesions must be considered to be a treponematosis until proven otherwise and it is really immaterial whether it is syphilis, yaws, etc., since they all have a common origin and represent merely a slight modification of the parasite (Hudson, 1965). Certainly the oldest example of these pinta is a typical American disease. Forbes too speculated on the occurrence of 'syphilis' in this population; he noted (pg. 226): 'It would appear probable that syphilis has been known amongst these Indians from a very early period, because they have in their language a name for this disease ('Cchaca-usu', literally translated 'bone-disease' Huanti, a bubo), because they are apparently quite familiar with its treatment, and, lastly, from the occasional occurrence of skulls taken out of graves dating from a period antecedent to the Spanish conquest, on which may be seen depressions or scars pronounced by several medical men to have resulted from syphilitic caries of the bone, and which in two instances which came under my observation afforded proof that the disease had been arrested in its progress and new bone formed during the lifetime of the individual.'

It is also of interest that one of the remedies used in 'modern' medicine had its basis in Andean folk medicine. Sarsparilla was used in a very effective treatment for syphilis on the northern coast of Perú. The treatment consisted of burying the patient up to his neck in the hot desert sands and giving him quantities of sarsparilla tea to drink. He was left for a day in the blazing sun and often his syphilis was cured. The cure when seen by European doctors was attributed to the use of the sarsparilla but in reality this was only a drink to prevent dehydration. The real cure was the production of a high fever (a form of sun stroke) that killed the Treponema. Such therapy was introduced later into modern medicine by the General Electric Company when patients were inoculated with malaria to cure their syphilis by producing a high fever.

The other major venereal disease, gonorrhea, on the basis of circumstantial evidence, was probably a European import. A review of an early Spanish colonial census (Ortíz de Zuñiga, 1972) failed to reveal any blind young adults. Blind adults mentioned in the census were few in number and all were elderly women whose blindness might have been due to cataracts, glaucoma, trauma or possibly trachoma.

Neoplasia

Today, in both North and South America a major problem in health is neoplasia. The increased importance of malignant tumors as a cause of death is alarming, and yet very little is known about their frequency among prehistoric people in general, and in the Americas, less than a dozen cases have been reported. The reason for this, as often glibly stated, is that early Americans did not live long enough to develop tumors. This statement is not valid since in nearly all of the Andean cultures 25% of the population survived over the age of 40. While it is true that for carcinoma of the breast in a modern United States population 48.5 cases per 100,000 would be at risk under the age of 49, seven times that number would be at risk over the age of fifty. Longevity cannot be the only factor; social customs and environment must be considered as well. In modern populations, an environmental factor able to produce a variety of health problems including neoplasia is the presence of arsenic in the drinking water. Long term usage of such water produces cancers of the skin and internal organs after 20 or more years exposure. A recent study of pre-Columbian and modern inhabitants of the same valleys of northern Chile, utilizing the same water supplies contaminated with arsenic, (see Chapter 3: Trace Metals) had a very similar frequency of skin cancer in long term residents; and, in general, the manifestations of other pathologies due to chronic arsenic poisoning were also similar. Considering exposure times the pre-Columbian inhabitants who were probably born and died there had an incidence of disease of over 80%, whereas the modern inhabitants, some of whom left and returned to the contaminated valleys had a frequency of health problems due to arsenic ingestion of over 50%. In both the ancient and modern populations there were some individuals who, even though they were long term residents, showed no signs of disease.

Among the Tiwanaku people a single case of carcinoma was seen in a woman about 45 years old. She died of this disease about 750 AD (Allison et al., 1980). She had a metastatic tumor in nine different bones, namely, the skull, right and left innominate bones, sacrum, right femur, and the eighth thoracic vertebra, the fourth and fifth lumbar vertebrae and the sternum. Although the primary location of the tumor will never be known for certain, due to the lack of soft tissue, the distribution and radiographic appearance of the lesions are suggestive of a mammary carcinoma. A second metastatic tumor in an adult female skull was also seen but since the skeleton was incomplete no further information can be offered.

Benign tumors of the bone were not uncommon and osteomas, osteochondromas and hemangiomas have been seen. Bone lesions produced by soft tissue tumors were also noted, including mucoceles and fibrous dysplasias, that were often dramatic in their untreated, long term appearance.

Skeletal lesions

As previously stated, approximately 10 to 20% of diseases leave a mark on the skeleton; trauma will add another 13 to 35% of recognizable lesions. The frequency of these will vary with the age and activities of the person. It is obvious that the skeleton is a poor medium for the evaluation of disease. Even considering such a chronic disease as untreated carcinomas the frequency of bone lesions may vary from 5 to 70% depending upon the cell type. Among the acute infectious diseases, complications of bone are relatively low and in a chronic infectious disease, such as tuberculosis, the person must have a high resistance to survive the initial pulmonary disease in order to develop the later osseous lesions. Trauma today is high among the western populations due to the automobile and competitive sports; a figure of 35% in our population who have had some accident, damaging one or more bones, is not excessive. Among pre-Columbian people a figure of 5% for accidental fractures is high and 2 to 3% is more reasonable. In general, among the Tiwanaku people an additional 12 to 15% must be added for physical violence, much of this was directed towards women and even children, and involved blows to the face that fracture the nasal bones and the zygomatic arch as well as parry fractures of the forearm. In some cases fractures from blows produced death in small children.

Trauma that might have resulted from warfare was seen among all of the Tiwanaku cultures; these included bodies with the heads missing and cut marks on the cervical vertebrae, skull fractures indicating the taking of trophy heads, skull fractures due to clubbing, projectile points lodged in bone and soft tissue and cutting wounds on the abdomen from knives and axes. One such abdominal wound in a woman's lower abdomen was plugged with a corn cob that was apparently inserted during life, in what was apparently an attempt to close it. A Tiwanaku man had been hit in the throat with a lance that probably felled but did not kill him; he then received an axe wound in the lower abdomen and his intestines spilled out. He died in a vain attempt to push them in with his hand which was in the wound when we found him. Another Tiwanaku warrior was hit in the chest with a lance but survived, and the shaft had been pulled out, the spear head remaining in the thoracic cavity in an essentially normal lung from which it was removed at autopsy some 1,200 years later. There have been a number of arrow wounds with some survivors and some deaths. Perhaps the most fatal shot was into the thoracic cavity where extensive bleeding produced death. Shots that lodged in the vertebrae or other bones were generally not lethal since the bows were not adequate to drive the arrow with enough force to break or penetrate the bone. A throwing spear at a relatively close range had more penetration since a spear point of this type had severed the vertebra and cut the spinal cord resulting in a lingering death in one early warrior.

Perhaps the most common bone lesion was that due to osteoarthritis. This degenerative disease is most commonly associated with the lumbar vertebrae and is part of the aging process as a result, at least in part, of repeated minor trauma. In some pre-Columbian groups this lesion made its appearance at ages in the early twenties and in nearly all cultures it was well established by the forties. One Tiwanaku group had extensive osteoarthritis of the cervical vertebrae due to the use of a special basket that was held in place with a tumpline to the forehead. This basket, which could hold 40 to 50 kilos, also produced a premature closure of the sutures of the skull where it put pressure on the forehead.

Osteoporosis, the most common metabolic disease of women today, was also extremely common in pre-Columbian times in the Andean region. It was also present in some males, although today they are usually exempt from this disease until they are 75 or 80 years old as a result of their greater skeletal mass. In many pre-Columbian women osteoporosis was present before forty years of age, and over 40, collapse of vertebral bodies was seen in relatively young women of 50-60 in 15% of the individuals examined. One point of interest is that in over 3,000 skeletons examined not a single example of osteoporotic fracture of the femoral neck was seen, the most common osteoporotic fracture today.

Pre-Columbian therapy

Since the Andean region has a rich folk medicine and over 2,000 medicinal herbs available, (see, e.g., Penso, 1978; Bastien, 1987) many of which are medicinally useful it is logical to expect to find some material in the excavations related with therapy. Over the years many bags of herbs have been recovered but were more in the form of magical offerings such as coca or sorona, rather than specifics for the person's disease. One interesting case of a specific therapy was seen in a Tiwanaku individual who had an enormous bladder stone that probably caused him to have problems urinating. He was buried with a basket of 'Cola de Caballo' a well known diuretic.

Several items that could be considered aids to make more comfortable chronically ill people were found. One was a type of collar that was found on a child with hydrocephalus that possibly helped him hold up his head during life; another was an adobe seat with a thick cushion molded to fit the paralyzed lower limbs of an eight year old boy. It is interesting to note, however, that the lack of alignment of bones in fractures indicates a failure to attempt to reduce them, despite their commonness. Severe fractures were haphazardly healed often with shortening of the limb. In only one case that we have seen was an attempt made to immobilize the limb. This occurred in an infant who probably suffered the fracture on delivery. His leg was immobilized with a piece of rawhide that was put on wet, sewn in place and allowed to dry. It was as hard as plaster and effectively immobilized the limb.

Conclusions

To date, these studies have not revealed any new or exotic diseases different from those afflicting the present, modern local indigenous population. The Aymará are currently plagued with respiratory diseases, especially tuberculosis, and may have an increased susceptibility to these due to their larger lung volume – a result of highland living, but undoubtedly chronic malnutrition and poor medical care contribute importantly too. Perhaps the most interesting aspect of paleopathology is the collection of epidemiological data over thousands of years, by direct observation, and the ability to relate these with changing ways of life. In many cases, these early Americans provide the only record on the development of human disease, and coping behaviors. And this record may help solve some of the problems seen in their modern counterparts, a good example of this is environmental studies such as that of chronic arsenic poisoning. Moreover, the recent development of techniques to study genetic changes, specifically the use of the polymerase chain reaction to amplify and ultimately characterize sequences of DNA, holds promise of the reconstruction of the relationship of particular genes to the diseases of the pre-Columbian inhabitants of the north of Chile (Roberts, 1989).

SARA A. BARTON, NELIDA CASTRO WILLIAMS,
ITA BARJA, AND FEDERICO MURILLO

Chapter 6

NUTRITIONAL CHARACTERISTICS OF THE AYMARA OF NORTHERN CHILE

Traditional Aymará foodstuffs

Archaeological and anthropological research have provided some insight into pre-Columbian central Andean foods. Prior to the Spanish conquest a variety of plants were cultivated; there was, however, a greater dependency on potatoes, and quinoa than followed the introduction of wheat and cereals such as barley (Sauer, 1963 and Murra, 1960). Crop cultivation depended, of course, on the local environment and above 4500 meters little farming was attempted. Potatoes were the staple crop generally, although quinoa was the most important grain. Quinoa represents a near perfect food in that it contains nearly all life sustaining nutrients and will grow at extremely high altitudes. It thrives in cold as well as hot sunny locations (high solar radiation), under sparse rainfall, and poor soil conditions. Its leaves are boiled like spinach or used for animal fodder. Its stalks are made into ash for chewing with coca leaves or burned for fuel, and its seeds, prepared much like rice, are used for a gruel. Oca, ulluco and anu were also common crops and cañihua, a grain related to quinoa, could be grown in the lower valleys. Corn was widely cultivated in the lower altitudes, and in the warmer valleys, chili peppers, cotton, gourds, peanuts, beans, lima beans, sweet manioc, tomatoes, avocados, and sweet potatoes were commonly planted (Rowe, 1963). The need for guano as a fertilizer is said to be the reason the Aymará expanded to the coast of northern Chile and southern Perú (LaBarre, 1948). Guano is produced by seagulls and pelicans, and along the coast their rookeries are common. Bennett (1963, see also Núñez, 1974) reports that the plants cultivated by the Inca at the time of the conquest had long been known and included maize, squash, cotton, sweet potatoes, peppers, peanuts, manioc, oca, quinoa, cañihua, potatoes, coca, achira, mashua, ulluco, jiquima, yacon, and lupines as well as such fruits as pepino (cucumber), pacae, lucuma, tuna (cactus), algarrobo, chirimoya, guanabana, tumbo, papaya, pineapple, palta (avocado), and melons (see Table 1). In addition to these plants the meat of llama, alpaca, guinea pig, and dog were available. Europeans introduced wheat, barley, oats, rice, onions, garlic, broad beans, oranges, grapes and bananas, and such animals as cattle, horses, goats, sheep, burros, and pigs.

Keller (1946) and Marquez (1967) provide further information on the important cultivated plants in northern Chile in the 20th century. The Lluta valley produced alfalfa and corn, squash, artichokes, cauliflower, potatoes, garden vegetables, legumes, cotton, curaguilla and, until the Pacific War, wheat

William J. Schull and Francisco Rothhammer (eds.), The Aymará: Strategies in Human Adaptation to a Rigorous Environment, 63-74.

TABLE 1
Selected prehistoric or contemporary agricultural plants in the Andes

Common name	Botanical name	Originally cultivated
TUBERS AND ROOTS		
achacana	*Neowedermannia vorwecki*	Highlands
archira	*Canna edulis*	Coast
arrachacha	*Arracacia xanthorryza*	Lowlands
camote	*Hipomea batatas*	Lowlands to 2400 m
cuchuchu	*Xantocsy laceae*	Highlands
isaño (mashua)	*Tropaelum tuberosum*	Lake Titicaca region & valleys below 3000 m
maca	*Lepidium meyen*	Highlands
ñoque	*Ruellia suberránea-balano-phoracea*	Highlands
oca	*Oxalis tuberosum*	Highlands
papa	*Solanum tuberosum*	Coast
	Solanum andigenum	Highlands
totora	*Scirpus riparius*	Highlands
ullucu (papalisa)	*Ullucus tuberosus*	Highlands
yacon	*Polymnia sonchifolia*	Temperate foothills to 2000 m
CONDIMENTS AND MISCELLANEOUS		
ajíes	*Capsicum*	Temperate valleys
red & yellow	*C. pendelum*	Temperate valleys
green	*C. chinense*	High valleys of Cochabamba to 2567 m
ulupica	*C. eximium*	Dry regions 1800-2200 m
lokoto	*C. pubescens*	Sierra
quillquina	*Porophyllum puderale*	Sierra
CEREALS AND GRAINS		
maíz	*Zea mays*	Generally in lowlands with rain
kañahua (cañihua)	*Chenopodium pallidicaule*	Highlands
lupine	*Lupinus tauris*	Highlands
millmi, coimi	*Amaranthus caudatus*	Highlands
quinua	*Chenopodium quinoa*	Highlands

(continued)

crops were sufficiently abundant to send flour to the altiplano. Production was limited, however, by the poor water quality of the river as previously described (Chapter 3). The Azapa valley produced potatoes, alfalfa, corn, oregano, chiles, squash, bananas, guayabos, grapefruit, papaya, mangoes, garden vegetables, olives, oranges, watermelons, and, on a smaller scale, sugar cane. In the sierra, while farming was more limited, quinoa and garden vegetables, principally legumes, artichokes, onions, celery, green beans, cabbage, garlic, carrots, and oregano, were produced, but alfalfa was of most importance. In antiquity, quinoa was grown throughout northern Chile and as late as the 1940s on a reduced scale in the sierra at Putre. Corn, the most important cereal prior to the arrival of the Spanish, has diminished in production and in the sierra, is only cultivated in Putre now. The coastal valleys, and the areas around Putre and Belén have sufficient milk to produce some cheese. Meat is eaten infrequently and usually

TABLE 1 (continued)
Selected prehistoric or contemporary agricultural plants in the Andes

Common name	Botanical name	Originally cultivated
FRUITS		
aceitunilla	*Vitex pseudolea*	Highlands
achuma de La Paz	*Trichocereus bridgesii*	Arid areas
capuli	*Physalis peruviana*	Adapted to the coast of northern Chile
chañar	*Gourliaea decorticans*	Low valleys of Pacific
granadilla	*Passiflora ligularis*	800 to 3000 m
hulunchu	*Cereus huilunchud*	Arid areas
kalapari	*Neocardenasia herzogianad*	Arid areas
kari-kari	*Robus roseusd*	Preferably grown 2800-3300 m
kcusa-kcusa	*Corryocactus melanotrichusd*	Arid areas
pepino dulce	*Solanum muricatum*	Highlands, varieties adapted to the coast
puca, ulala, velo	*Cereus hankeanus*	Arid areas
sitikiras	*Cereus sp.*	Arid areas
tumbo	*Passiflora mollissima*	Sierra
tuna	*Opuntia ficus*	Sierra
tunilla	*Opuntia cordobensis*	Well developed in high altitude valleys
ulala, pasakana	*Eriocereus tephrancathus*	Arid areas
EDIBLE LEGUMES		
achokkcha, caygua	*Cyclanthera pedata*	Coast
canavalia	*Canavalia ensiformis*	Coast
escario	*Cucurbita pepo*	Widely distributed
lacayote	*C. ficifolia*	Widely distributed
pacay	*Inga feuillei*	To 2500 m; in northern Chile archaeological evidence in oasis & valleys 1000-1500 m
purutu, frejol	*Phaseolus sp.*	Lowlands, sierra
tauri, tarhui	*Lupinos mutabilis*	Between 2500-3600 m
tiako, algarrobo	*Prosopis sp.*	Interandean valleys between 1500-2600 m
zapallo	*Cucurbita máxima*	Interandean valleys of the Cordillera; adapted to the coast

Adapted from Núñez (1974), pp. 96-116; Bennett (1963), Table 1, Vol 2, p. 5.

broiled over wood or dung chips, llareta or whatever scarce fuel source is available.

A common source of protein is dried, salted strips of freshly slaughtered sheep, llama or alpaca meat, called charqui. Potatoes are preserved in the form of chuño, moraya (or moray), or tunta. Although descriptions of the making of chuño vary somewhat from author to author, possibly reflecting local differences in its preparation, basically it involves the placing of uncooked bitter potatoes well spaced on a layer of grass and exposing them to heavy frosts to freeze them. The frozen potatoes are thawed in the sun on the following day, and then stamped with the feet with a twisting motion to squeeze out any water and to encourage the splitting and sloughing of the skins. The potatoes are left to dry in the sun, and become shriveled and shrunken. When the process is finished, they are black in color and will keep almost indefinitely. Tunta is made in much the same way as chuño, but the potatoes, preferably the frost-hardy species *Solanum ajanhuiri*, are kept in the shade (not the sun) for about 30 days and the shading accounts for their white color. Consumption is possible after soaking in water or grinding into a white flour (Tschopik, 1963; La Barre, 1948; Murillo, personal communication). Although in some areas of the altiplano the word moraya is used as if synonymous with tunta, in regions of Bolivia, at least, it can also refer to a preservation technique using poor quality potatoes and placing these in a pit with water for fermentation or by placing them in a sack and submerging the latter in a pond. After which time the resulting starchy matter is dried in the sun and stored. Customarily, chuño, moraya, and tunta are prepared in the winter, June and July, when the coldest weather and strongest frosts occur. The nutritive value of these various products depends not only on the preservation technique itself but upon the variety of potato used (Christiansen, 1977).

THE NUTRITIONAL SURVEY AND ITS METHODS

Data collection

An enumeration of all persons normally living in a sample of houses, including nonbiological relatives, but excluding temporary visitors, was made, and then two dietary questionnaires were completed, one for the household, the Dietary History Questionnaire, and the second, the Dietary Recall Questionnaire, an in-depth account of the previous day's food consumption for the specific family member providing the household dietary information. Professional nutritionists from the Universidad de Chile, Departamento de Nutricion, Facultad de Medicina, developed the dietary questionnaires on the basis of their previous work in 1968 (Arteaga et al. 1968 and Castro et al. 1972) when 70 Aymará families (459 individuals) were interviewed in three of the same sierran villages in which the current study is based. The nutritionists (NCW and IB) were experienced in the use of the dietary history and recall forms, in inquiring about dishes eaten at each meal and the ingredients within a dish, in measuring the units of food consumed, and in converting these into grams per day.

The Dietary History Questionnaire was administered to the wife, or the person who usually prepared the meals for the household. This history recorded by age group (males 15 years of age or older, females of these same ages, pregnant women, children 4 to 14 years of age and under three), the frequency with which family members consumed milk and milk products, cheese, eggs, cereal and cereal products, dry beans, potatoes, bread, meat and poultry, fish, fruit, and vegetables, as well as specifics about breast feeding and the solid food habits of the last three infants. Information was also sought on the use of oils, butter and salt in food preparation.

The Dietary Recall Questionnaire was designed to elicit the exact foods and beverages and amounts of each consumed during the course of the previous day at breakfast, lunch, afternoon tea, supper, between meals and after supper. For each meal, the person interviewed was asked to specify the contents of the meal and the ingredients within each dish. There were 124 different foods reported to have been eaten. These foods or the ingredients in a dish, if it contained several foods, were then weighed. If it was not possible to make the weight determinations, weight was estimated from the University of Chile's Department of Nutrition Measurement Tables. Measuring cups and rulers were provided to approximate standard measurements of quantity of consumption. These data were coded and the average number of milligrams of nutrients per 100 grams of food consumed calculated using the Table of Chemical Composition of Chilean Foods developed by the University of Chile's Department of Nutrition.

Limits are imposed on the interpretation of our data, of course, by the methodology we were obliged to use and the problems inherent in the ascertainment of nutrition generally. While these prevent exact evaluation of intakes common to a modern society, the data are useful in comparing the diets of indigenous peoples.

Participation and sample characterization

Limited resources made it impracticable to visit the homes of everyone examined in the study (n=2,096 in Chile). Accordingly, using the census for each village prepared prior to the initiation of the study and the fertility histories completed during the examination process, the homes of the larger families were consciously selected so as to obtain dietary information on more individuals.

Two hundred and forty-three homes were visited during the spring season. Collectively these homes represented 1,297 individuals, or an average of 6.2, 4.6, and 5.1 persons per household in the two coastal areas, the four sierran, and the four altiplano villages, respectively. The households interviewed include 91 on the coast, 79 in the sierra, and 73 in the altiplano. However, 93 individual dietary recalls were completed on the coast, two houses had two persons interviewed. In the valleys the principal occupation was farming, with a transition to farming and herding in the sierra and to predominantly herding in the altiplano. Females commonly provided the dietary information for the family (79.3%) because of our desire to interview, if possible the person most knowledgeable about the family dietary habits, i.e., the person cooking for the family, and the more frequent availability of the housewife rather than her husband.

The composition of the 243 sampled households varied across the altitudinal niches (see Table 2). On the coast, 98% of the households contained one or more adult males in comparison to 92% and 90% in the sierra and altiplano, respectively. Adult females were similarly distributed per household, namely, 89%, 96%, and 86%, respectively. Few households had a pregnant woman present. The highest number was on the coast (14) with only four in the sierra and eight in the altiplano. Households having children 3 years of age or younger present were more common on the coast (56%) and altiplano (59%) than in the sierra (35%).

As shown in Table 3, the 243 households interviewed represented 1,297 persons. Across altitudes, the sierra (52.5%) has the highest percentage of adults, followed by the altiplano (50.1%) and coast (48.9%). The coast (37.1%)

TABLE 2
Household composition: Number of households by altitude of residence

	Coast	Sierra	Altiplano
Adult females	81	76	63
Adult males	89	73	66
Pregnant women	14	4	8
Children: 4-14 years	75	45	50
0- 3 years	51	28	43
Households interviewed	91	79	73

TABLE 3
Number of persons represented in the 243 households

	Coast	Sierra	Altiplano
Adults	278	189	185
Children: 4-14 years	211	134	124
0- 3 years	79	37	60
No. persons living in house	568	360	369

and sierra (37.2%) are virtually equal in their representation of children age 4 to 14 years; whereas the frequency of individuals in this age group in the altiplano is 33.6%. The percentage of children 3 years of age and younger represented in the altiplano is higher (16.3%) than either the coast (13.9%) or the sierra (10.3%).

RESULTS, DISCUSSION AND COMPARISON WITH OTHER DATA

On a daily basis, food habits of the general population are unvarying, particularly in the sierra and altiplano, where only a limited variety of foods, especially fresh fruits and vegetables, are normally available. At the time of our survey, none of these villages had a foodstore. Customarily an order for those staples, such as coffee, tea, salt or fresh fruits, not produced in the mountains, is placed with an itinerant merchant when his truck makes its circuit tour through the villages, and one's requests are delivered when next the truck returns. One needs bear in mind that during the spring rains the sierran and altiplano roads, which are not all-weather surfaced, become impassable and foodstuffs from the coast cannot be imported.

Although substantial variability exists between the different meals of the day, and the same meal in the various villages, breakfast commonly consists of tea or coffee with sugar and bread. Only on the coast is this limited fare supplemented with butter, jelly, meat slivers, or, at times, eggs and milk. On the coast, the noon meal consists of two dishes normally, soup and salad or a casserole made of rice

TABLE 4
Average number of grams of each food group consumed per person per day by altitude of residence

Food Group		Coast (n=93)	Sierra (n=79)	Altiplano (n=73)
		Altitude of residence		
Milk and milk products		113.3	129.4	41.2
Animal products, fresh		44.7	54.4	73.9
Animal products, dry		2.6	21.4	38.3
Fish		21.4	2.6	1.4
Eggs		8.6	3.2	3.0
Legumes		13.8	10.7	2.3
Potatoes		110.3	143.9	116.4
Vegetables, fresh		94.9	25.3	30.4
Fruits, fresh, canned		27.4	10.7	11.1
Cereal and cereal products:	Bread	229.7	252.6	332.2
	Cereals	59.6	56.0	72.0
Sugar and sweet products		30.3	33.7	39.1
Fats and oils		11.1	7.9	8.2
Beverages: carbonated		14.3	3.2	3.4
alcoholic		2.2	1.4	1.4
miscellaneous		0.7	0.8	0.3

or spaghetti with vegetables and some meat. Occasionally eggs or fruit are eaten at lunch. Only one dish is usually served in the sierra – a soup with dried meat and a mixture of rice and cereal to which vegetables are sometimes added. In the altiplano, only a soup of rice and other cereals, with the occasional addition of freeze dried potatoes (chuño) or dried llama or alpaca, is eaten. For afternoon tea, tea or coffee and bread are consumed. Sometimes afternoon tea is omitted or taken later, in which case supper is not eaten. For the last meal of the day – supper – leftovers from lunch are commonly used. It is usually a light meal of small quantity and without meat; complemented again with tea or coffee and bread. It is not customary to eat between meals. Most of the schools served powdered milk and cookies to the school children.

Daily meals in Turco and Toledo were somewhat different, largely reflecting differences in food availability and the regional rural cultivars. They are usually eaten cold, and consist of cooked potatoes, chuño, beans, boiled dry corn, and a hot sauce (ají). In both communities, as much as ten percent of the daily caloric intake consisted of quinoa. Little grease or lard is used in cooking, for neither cattle nor pigs are commonly husbanded; however, the mutton that is consumed is exceptionally greasy.

Dietary recall

In comparing amounts of different food groups consumed in school at the various altitudes, one needs to consider that local availability and means to preserve food affect school lunches substantially (Table 4). In the sierra and

TABLE 5
Interpretation of Aymará nutrient intake data using ICNND standards

Nutrient (per day)	Altitude of residence: Coast	Sierra	Altiplano	ICNND Survey[1]: Total Chile	Arica/Calama Iquique	ICNND Suggested intake/day[2]: Deficient or low	Acceptable or high
Calories	1458	1723	2123	2280	2285	2348 required[3]	
Protein (gm)	46.6	55.5	72.4	72.0	65.0	63.6 required[3]	
Calcium (gm)	0.35	0.31	0.26	0.70	0.58	0.30-0.39	0.4-0.8
Iron (mg)	12.8	12.5	15.4	17.6	14.3	6-8	9-12
Thiamine (mg/1000 cal)	0.89	0.87	0.85	0.61	0.48	0.20-0.29	0.3-0.5
Riboflavin (mg)	0.9	0.9	1.0	1.7	1.2	0.7-1.1	1.2-1.5
Niacin (mg)	10.7	10.0	11.6	16.4	15.2	5-9	10-15
Ascorbic acid (mg)	50.8	43.3	35.8	50.0	41.0	10-29	30-50
Vitamin A (mg)	2.2	0.1	1.2	4.2	3.3	1.2-2.1	2.1-3.0
Sample size (n)	93	79	73	1647	199		

[1] Table 70. Interdepartmental Committee on Nutrition for National Defense (ICNND). Chile Nutrition Survey: March-June, 1960, Washington, DC: U.S. Government Printing Office, 1961.
[2] Appendix C. op. cit.
[3] Table 67. op. cit.

altiplano, for example, in the 1970s there were no refrigerators in the homes to preserve foods over longer periods of time. Fuel for cooking and heating was also limited. Save for small quantities of queñua and llareta and manure chips, wood is nonexistent and only a few families have propane bottled gas stoves. Moreover, if a product is not locally produced, it must be trucked into the region or, as in the case of one altiplano village (Visviri), arrive by train from the coast. The majority of the sources of milk and milk products consumed on the coast and in the sierra were from fresh cow and goat milk. There are virtually no cows and few goats in the Chilean altiplano, and the dairy products consumed are powdered milk, condensed canned milk, and cheese. In contrast, domesticated llama and alpaca are more abundant in the altiplano, and as a consequence, more meat is eaten (73.9 gm and 38.3 gm, fresh and dried, respectively), than in the sierra (54.4 gm and 21.4 gm) and especially the coast (44.7 gm and 20.0 gm) where the price of beef is prohibitive for many families. As would be expected, fresh fish are eaten more frequently on the coast (21.4 gm) than in the mountains – 2.6 gm in the sierra and 1.4 gm in the altiplano.

Table 5 gives the daily intake per person of calories, protein and other nutrients by level of altitude of residence. It should be noted that the values here described for the sierra are consistently lower than those earlier reported by Arteaga et al. (1968) for the villages of Belén, Chapiquiña, and Socoroma. While this may reflect differences in sampling, it also warrants note that these differences may be real, for our data were obtained at a time when inflation was rampant in Chile, and the economic situation had been worsened by the instability of the Allende government. To return to Table 5, one observes that

TABLE 6
Body mass index by age and altitude of residence: Females

Age Group (yrs.)	Coast No.	Coast kg/m^2	Sierra No.	Sierra kg/m^2	Altiplano No.	Altiplano kg/m^2
10-19	3	2.51	1	2.16	4	2.34
20-29	12	2.40	11	2.54	10	2.30
30-39	19	2.65	9	2.39	11	2.46
40-49	6	2.44	13	2.70	9	2.42
50-59	2	3.15	5	2.33	5	2.70
60-69	4	3.05	7	2.54	1	2.54
70+	1	3.19	3	2.71	0	0
Total	47	2.62	49	2.54	40	2.43

the daily intake is related to crop and animal production; fruits and vegetables in the coastal valleys and meat, potatoes, and bread in the mountains. Caloric intake is higher in the altiplano (2123) than in the sierras (1723) or along the coast (1458). This was anticipated, given the fact that this niche reported eating the most dried and fresh meat, bread, cereal and sugar, and is in accord with Castro and collaborators (1972) previous finding of 2,400 calories. However, the caloric level for each altitude is below the Chilean national average (2,280 calories, n = 1,647), and the Calama, Iquique, Arica combined area findings (2,285 calories, n = 199) in a dietary survey of civilian families (ICNND, 1961, Nutrition Survey, Chile). It is also below the ICNND 2,348 required. All nutrient values, with the exception of calcium, phosphorus and vitamins A and C, are higher in the altiplano than in the sierra, and higher in the sierra than on the coast; for these exceptions the values are highest on the coast and may reflect the greater consumption of fruit. The higher values seen in the altiplano in other respects most likely reflect the higher meat consumption, except in regard to vitamin C, and the sierra's higher consumption of fresh potatoes. All altitudes are below the ICNND acceptable levels of calcium and riboflavin, and the coast and sierra are below the ICNND 63.6 gms of required protein. The sierra and altiplano diets are severely deficient in Vitamin A.

Of interest is a comparison of the persons for whom we have both a dietary recall interview and anthropometric measurements (from the physical examination). Table 6 compares the body mass index (defined as kg/m^2) by age, and altitude among women. Unfortunately, too few males had all of the necessary observations to make a meaningful comparison. It will be noted that among females, for most age groups, the body mass index of the coast residents is larger than that of the highland residents, and in general, body mass in the sierra is larger than in the altiplano.

TABLE 7
Salt consumption by altitude: grams per person per day

Consumption gms/person/day	Coast No.	Coast %	Sierra No.	Sierra %	Altiplano No.	Altiplano %
0.0- 4.9	13	16.9	3	5.6	5	9.6
5.0- 9.9	38	49.4	16	29.7	14	26.9
10.0-14.9	17	22.1	16	29.7	15	28.8
15.0-19.9	5	6.5	7	13.0	6	11.5
20.0-24.9	2	2.6	4	7.4	5	9.6
25.0-29.9	1	1.3	2	3.7	1	1.9
30.0-34.9	1	1.3	0	0.0	1	1.9
35.0-39.9	0	0	5	9.3	1	1.9
41.7	0	0	1	1.9	2	3.8
50.0	0	0	0	0	1	1.9
66.7	0	0	0	0	1	1.9
Mean gms/person	8.94		12.37		15.86	
No. reporting households	77		54		52	

Dietary history

As the household dietary history reveals, the three altitudinal niches share one similarity – the majority of families eat four meals a day, respectively, on the coast (61.5%), sierra (60.8%), and the altiplano (75.3%). However, they report very different amounts of salt consumed daily per person per household. The average daily per capita consumption of salt in the altiplano is 15.9 grams; whereas in the sierra and coast per capita consumption is 12.4 and 8.9 grams, respectively (Table 7). There is more uniformity between altitudes in reporting the number of days needed to use a kilo of salt (data not shown); the majority being 10 to 14 days, with the altiplano (17.3%) exhibiting the fewest days (5 to 9) in comparison to five percent of the households in the coast and sierra needing up to two months. The higher apparent consumption of salt in the altiplano undoubtedly reflects to some degree its use in the preparation of charqui. To the extent that the salt used in this preservative process is not subsequently ingested, our figures obviously overestimate daily salt intake but by how much is moot.

From the household dietary history, at all altitudes and age groups, the majority of the households did not have anyone consuming cheese. This was especially true in the altiplano where more than 75% of all age groups did not eat cheese. However, if cheese was consumed, it was rarely eaten more often than twice a week and often less than once a month by all age groups except children three years old or younger who tended to eat cheese more frequently if they lived on the coast or in the sierra although less than 20% of the altiplano three year olds ate cheese. These differences in consumption patterns must

TABLE 8
Comparison of nutrient intake

Study	Place	No. House-holds	Month study	Alti-tude (m)	Total intake (kcal)	Pro-tein (g)	Fat (g)	Carbohy-drates (g)	Cal-cium (mg)	Phos-phorus (mg)	Iron (mg)	Vit. C (mg)
PERU*												
Collazos (1954)	Vicos	40	Jul	2747	1509	44.4	11.2	308.8	125	---	17.3	70.6
Collazos (1954)	Vicos	37	Feb		1481	35.2	---	---	138	---	12.1	76.9
Collazos (1954)	Chacán	43	Dec	3416	1194	31.3	11.3	292.5	426	---	16.6	43.0
Collazos (1954)	Chacán	39	Jul		1404	34.8	---	---	76	---	12.8	68.0
Mazess (1964)	Nuñoa	39	Jul	4000	3204	69.0	16.0	696.0	441	2119	22.0	113.6
Gursky (1969)	Nuñoa		Jul	4000	1479	46.4	17.7	283.6	465	761	12.4	10.9
Gursky (1969)	Sincata		Jul	4000	2447	65.5	24.3	491.5	870	1706	31.8	54.7
Gursky (1969)	Chillihua		Dec	4300	1494	59.9	21.5	265.1	289	1106	19.8	24.9
CHILE												
Arteaga (1968)	Sierra	70	Jan	3000-4000	2400	60.0	64.0	400.0	390	---	18.9	40.0
current (1974)	Coast	93	Nov	0-2500	1458	46.6	28.5	260.8	345	757	12.8	50.8
	Sierra	78	Nov	2500-4000	1723	55.5	49.5	273.3	314	789	12.5	43.3
	Altiplano	74	Nov	>4000	2123	72.4	62.9	326.8	264	768	15.4	35.8

*Data reported in Picón-Reátegui (1978).

reflect the availability of cheese, but they may also be ascribable to some extent to a higher frequency of lactose intolerance among the Aymará as contrasted with non-Aymará. Two studies of the Aymará in Bolivia report 62.3% lactose intolerance (see Roychoudhury and Nei, 1988) and 77% with lactose restriction (Flatz, 1989); for a general discussion of lactose malabsorption, its biology and history, see Johnson, Kretchner, and Simmons, 1974.

At all altitudes and age groups, eggs are most commonly eaten only 2-3 times per week. However, in the altiplano (28-35%) significantly more households do not eat eggs than on the coast (4-12%) or in the sierra (11-21%). Again, the virtual absence of chickens in the altiplano and their limited number in the sierra affect egg consumption.

When comparing the nutritional characteristics of the Aymará of northern Chile with other high altitude populations one must keep in mind that environmental factors – temperature, altitude, soil conditions, rainfall, as well as latitude and slope orientation which influences the sun's rays – alter the variety and quantity of food crops produced. Moreover, the month in which a dietary survey is conducted, in relation to yearly harvest, greatly affects the food consumption that is reported (see Mazess and Baker, 1964 for seasonal consumption of major foods in Nuñoa, Perú). In addition, the isolation of the village, bartering capabilities, socioeconomic status, and concentration on herding cattle, sheep, llama, and alpaca influence food status.

Reported number of meals consumed per day varies from four in northern Bolivia to three in the south (Esquef, 1972) and usually two in the District of Nuñoa in southern Perú (Pícon-Reátegui, 1978). Whereas in northern Chile the majority of the households report eating four meals a day. The Aymará of northern Chile appear to eat a greater variety of foods than is true in two areas studied in Bolivia and Perú, with the exception of the lack of eating barley, quinoa, cañihua, and highland tubers, ano and ulluco. These latter foods are no longer grown in northern Chile.

Comparison of nutrient intake among high altitude populations is difficult for a variety of reasons. There has been no standardization of the measures of diet, the season of the year at which surveys have been conducted, the sex and age of the individuals interviewed – all of which influence the differences that have been reported. However, in reviewing Table 8 one outstanding comparison is the higher fat intake and lower iron ingestion reported by the two Chilean surveys than was seen in sierran and altiplano villages in Perú. There is also a larger protein intake with higher altitude of residence of the settlement. Fresh potatoes can contribute importantly to the intake of ascorbic acid (Vitamin C). However in the preparation of chuño a substantial amount of the Vitamin C normally present is lost (1.7 mg/100 g versus 20.5 mg/100 g; Pícon-Reátegui, 1978). Thus, the variability in the various reported amounts of vitamin C ingested could merely reflect the different seasons of the year in which the studies occurred since fresh potatoes are most available from June to August (harvesting usually occurs in April and May). Similarly, as Leonard and Thomas (1989) and Leonard (1989) have stressed, total caloric intake varies in relationship to the time of harvest. In the town of Nuñoa, Perú, for example, they report ingestion of 1150 calories per day prior to harvest and 1519 after the harvest which is similar to previous studies in the same town (see Table 8). These authors also document the variation in energy intake with age. They observed little seasonal variation in the consumption of food by children, presumably because of their year round use in many of the productive activities of the household, and a conscious effort to 'protect' the children from the seasonal scarcities of food.

WILLIAM J. SCHULL, ROBERT E. FERRELL, AND SARA A. BARTON

Chapter 7
THE CHILEAN AYMARA AND THEIR REPRODUCTIVE PATTERNS

Introduction

When Francisco and Hernando Pizzaro, and their erstwhile ally and fellow countryman, Diego de Almagro, led their intrepid bands of opportunists into Perú, and subsequently Chile most, if not all of the indigenous populations they encountered were undoubtedly increasing in number, albeit slowly. Soon thereafter, as contemporary censuses reveal, most of these populations underwent a decline, precipitously in some instances, more slowly in others. Presumably these changes reflected exposure to new diseases, and deaths occasioned by warfare and rebellion as well as the physical exploitation by the Spanish. Little is accurately known of the changes in reproductivity that may have occurred, but apocryphal anecdotes abound. Monge and Monge (1966; see also Monge, 1948) cite statements of Father Cobo (1891-2) to the effect that 'The Indians are healthiest and where they multiply the most prolifically is in these same cold air-tempers, which is quite the reverse of what happens to children of the Spaniards, most of whom when born in such regions do not survive. But where it is most noticeable is in those who have half, a quarter, or any admixture of Indian blood; better they survive and grow; so that it is now a common saying based on everyday experience that babes having some Indian in them run less risk in the cold regions than those not having this admixture.' and that 'the birth of the first Spaniard did not take place until fifty-three years after the founding of Potosi (4500 m or 14,900 feet).' The latter remark, if true is difficult to explain on the basis of present knowledge of the effects of the hypoxia of altitude on fertility.

Reproductive capacity is nevertheless a particularly sensitive indicator of the success or failure of adaptation in an individual, or in a population, as Clegg and Harrison (1971) have noted. Its assessment, however, is complex for one must consider the whole life cycle, beginning with gametogenesis and terminating with sexual maturity. Each of the many components which comprise this process is undoubtedly influenced by biological, cultural and socioeconomic factors. Thus, their evaluation is difficult under the best of circumstances, and virtually impossible in most field studies. Accordingly, we find ourselves obliged to be opportunistic, to assess those components which appear feasible and to infer the probable values of those that cannot be directly estimated from experimental data or other epidemiological studies. But this pathway is studded with pitfalls for the comparability of such data may be tenuous at best. Even assertions about altitudinal and ethnic differences in fertility based on national censuses have prompted strikingly disparate interpretations (see, e.g., Stycos, 1963; Heer, 1964;

William J. Schull and Francisco Rothhammer (eds.), The Aymará: Strategies in Human Adaptation to a Rigorous Environment, 75-86.

Whitehead, 1968 and Bradshaw, 1969). Often such differences are inferred from observations which are indirect; for example, it has been argued that hypoxia of altitude reduces fertility because the total number of children born increases with migration from high to low altitudes (Abelson, Baker and Baker, 1974; Abelson, 1976). But obviously there are other explanations in most such situations that are difficult to exclude.

The purpose of this chapter is to describe the reproductive performances of the Aymará women we encountered. Our review of the literature will make no attempt to be comprehensive; we doubt whether the experiences in Colorado, Ethiopia or Nepal have much relevance to the reproductive performance of the women of northern Chile in the absence of suitable control of the cultural and socioeconomic factors which separate these regions. We shall, however, examine those anatomic, biochemical, hormonal and physiologic factors that may provide insight into the observations we shall report. We present our data in the spirit of Baker's remark (1978) 'the fertility data on high-altitude peoples present a complex picture from which obvious conclusions do not emerge.'

Anatomic, biochemical and hormonal changes at altitude which may impinge on reproductive patterns

Menarche is delayed at altitude (Donayre, 1966). In a Peruvian study, the greatest change was seen at 13 years of age where a significantly larger proportion of schoolgirls were menstruating at sea level, 73%, than at high altitude, 38%. The mean ages at menarche in the two groups were 12.58 and 13.58 years, respectively. It has been conjectured that this may reflect a difference in maturation of the hypothalmic-pituitary-gonadal axis. In both sexes, it appears, however, that the development of secondary sexual characteristics is markedly delayed at high-altitude (Donayre, 1966; Peñaloza, 1971). Such contrasts between highlanders and lowlanders frequently confound socioeconomic differences (the highlanders are the poorest), and poor nutrition in early life, commonly part of such differences, leads to later ages at menarche (Leistol, 1982). There is evidence too that children from smaller families mature earlier than those from large ones (Douglas and Simpson, 1964; Valsik, 1965; Douglas, 1966), and family size differences do obtain between lowland and highland residents. As further evidence of the probable role of extraneous sources of variation in these comparisons, Kashiwazaki and his colleagues (1988) have reported that menarche among Japanese residents in La Paz actually occurs later than in their ethnic counterparts in the eastern Bolivian lowlands (Santa Cruz), and this comparison involves individuals who are relatively better placed socioeconomically.

Evidence of altitudinally mediated changes of an hormonal nature in men or women is not more persuasive. Donayre (1966; see Sobrevilla et al., 1967) has reported the levels of urinary gonadotropins to be the same (1.25 versus 1.14 mg/24hr NIH-HPG-UPM-1) in highland and lowland males, and Guerra-Garcia, Velasquez and Whittembury (1965) found no significant differences in urinary excretion of testosterone in men residents at sea level and at 14,300 feet (4300 m). But these two groups do appear different in the effects of human chorionic gonadotropin (HCG) on testicular function as measured in urinary excretion of testosterone. The latter appears significantly diminished at altitude (work of Guerra-Garcia, cited by Donayre, 1966), a finding which resembles the corticoid response to ACTH stimulation (Moncloa, 1966). Pituitary gonadal hormones are not decreased in natives from high compared to low altitudes (Bangham and Hackett, 1978). In the female, measurements of luteinizing hormones indicate that adult values in girls are attained one year later at high altitude than at sea level (Llerena, 1973). However, levels of pregnanediol excretion during the menstrual cycle are similar (Moncloa, quoted by Sobrevilla et al., 1967). Thus, as Clegg and Harrison (1971) have noted, altitude apparently does not significantly affect steroid production in humans. The sample sizes on which these various findings rest are small and other potential sources of variation may not always have been adequately removed. However, there appears to be no impairment of spermatogenesis among native high altitude males (Sobrevilla et al., 1967).

It is generally conceded now that infants born at high altitude are, on average, smaller than those born in the lowlands (see, e.g., Lichty et al., 1957; McClung, 1969; Beall, 1976; Haas, 1976; Haas et al., 1980), presumably because of fetal growth retardation, and more frequently succumb during the neonatal and infantile periods than is to be expected (Mazess, 1965). This difference in birth weight does not appear to be related to ethnicity, however, as Kashiwazaki, Suzuki, and Takemoto (1988) have recently shown. In a study of children born to Japanese residing in Santa Cruz (lowland Bolivia) and La Paz (highland Bolivia), the La Paz born infants were consistently smaller, 422 grams on average, than their lowland counterparts in Santa Cruz (or in Japan, for that matter). This difference is consistent with that reported for traditional Andean populations.

Highland born infants also present signs of neurological and behavioral immaturity more often than newborns at low altitude (Sacro-Pollitt, 1981) although it has been questioned whether these findings connote immaturity or growth retardation (see Haas et al., 1980). Some of these effects seem more pronounced in male than in female infants. Irrespective of sex, however, the reasons for the diminished growth, apparent immaturity and higher mortality are not fully known but it seems reasonable to presume that they may be related to fetal oxygenation. The latter is, of course, critically dependent on maternal oxygen supply.

It is commonly assumed that the fetus of a gravid woman, even one in an hypoxic environment has its oxygen needs met preferentially as it were. A variety of mechanisms are thought to make this possible. Thus, for example, women who have sickle cell anemia and whose hemoglobin values are often only 6-8 grams have children who show little, if any evidence of oxygen deprivation. It is argued that a cardiac compensation occurs which makes this possible, but as Moore and her colleagues have shown in another connection (Moore et al., 1982b) hyperventilation may also be involved. The latter investigators have demonstrated that at high altitude (Leadville, Colorado) ventilation and hemoglobin concentrations are both important variables contributing to oxygen transport during pregnancy (see also, e.g., Hellegers et al., 1961). Subsequently, in studies of pregnant women in Cerro de Pasco, Perú, Moore and her associates (1982c, 1986) have shown that increased hypoxic ventilatory responsiveness raised maternal ventilation and arterial oxygen saturation, and that the increase in responsiveness, although varying among women, correlated ($r=0.44$) with infant birth weight. The factors responsible for this increasing hypoxic responsiveness during pregnancy are not known. However, based on these findings, they argue that 'maternal characteristics that affect oxygen transport during pregnancy may be important adaptations for maintaining fetal growth and, by extension, well-being at high altitude.'

Moore (see Moore et al., 1982a) has also suggested that pre-eclampsia may compromise fetal well-being at altitude. She notes that a failure in maternal oxygen transport is involved in the etiology of pre-eclampsia for an altitude-associated rise in blood pressure occurs even in normal pregnancies and there is an inverse relationship between maternal arterial oxygen saturation and the degree of hypertension present. These inferences rest on findings with regard to residents in Leadville, Colorado, and it may be argued that these are an unadapted people, in the evolutionary sense. Similar studies on the Aymará and Quechua would be interesting.

Other factors which could influence fetal oxygenation are (a) an increased tissue unloading of oxygen in the mother, (b) an increase, at least relatively if not absolutely, in placental size and vascularity, (c) greater oxygen avidity on the part of the fetus, and (d) increased fetal tissue utilization of oxygen. Evidence of an increased tissue unloading is sparse although a priori it is reasonable to presume that an increase in 2,3-diphosphoglycerate would enhance the unloading of oxygen in the placenta. It is known that this organic phosphate along with temperature and pH affect the oxygen-hemoglobin dissociation curve. 2,3-DPG binds to deoxygenated hemoglobin but not to oxyhemoglobin, and thus an increase in 2,3-DPG shifts the reaction to the right with the consequent liberation of more oxygen. Efforts to test this supposition directly are limited.

Clegg (1978) has reviewed placental morphological and functional variation at high altitude and suggests several mechanisms by which the placenta responds to hypoxia. Most studies of placental weight have failed to find significant differences between high and low altitude pregnancies. However, Kruger and Arias-Stella (1970), in a comparison of placental weights among lowland and highland pregnancies, have shown that the average weight of the placenta at 4600 m was 12 per cent higher than that seen in Lima (561 versus 501 grams) although the newborns on the coast were 15% heavier than those at Río Pallange (3490 versus 2946 grams). These authors went to substantial lengths to minimize potentially significant extraneous sources of variation. Thus, their attention was restricted to mestizos at both altitudes; only term pregnancies were studied; and pregnancies that terminated in an abnormal child were excluded. Most other early studies failed to pay attention to these possible sources of confusion.

Kruger and Arias-Stella believe too that the histological structures of the placenta are more densely distributed per unit volume of placenta at high altitudes. McClung (1969) had earlier reported that in proportion to birth weights, placental weights were high in Peruvian high altitude residents. This increase in placental ratio (placental weight/birth weight) has been confirmed by other investigators, including Kruger and Arias-Stella. More recent studies of the histological composition of highland placentae reveal them to be substantially different from lowland ones in that, on average, they had a more voluminous intervillous space but reduced volumes of villi, juxtavillous fibrin and non-parenchyma (Jackson, Mayhew, and Haas, 1987). These structural differences extended to ethnic groups where these authors have also found that Amerindian placentae tend to possess more trophoblast and villous stroma than is seen in non-Indian placentae (op. cit.).

Fetal hemoglobin has a greater affinity for oxygen than does adult hemoglobin and this facilitates the flow of oxygen from a mother to her fetus. Interestingly, the cause of this greater affinity is the poor binding of 2,3-DPG by the gamma chains which replace the beta chains in fetal hemoglobin. Adult hemoglobin appears in the fetus at about the 20th week of gestation when the bone marrow first begins to function. At birth, about 20% of the circulating hemoglobin is of the adult type, and this amount increases steadily with the cessation of production of fetal hemoglobin. Some retardation of this process in the final weeks of gestation could increase the transfer of oxygen to the fetus, and presumably be beneficial at higher altitudes. Ballew and Haas (1986) have provided some evidence, based on cord blood obtained at parturition, that the newborn infant at high altitude exhibits an enhanced erythropoiesis, and that the proportion of fetal hemoglobin is higher than that seen among newborns at low altitudes. They interpret their findings as supporting the notion that the high altitude fetus experiences a greater degree of hypoxia in utero than does the low altitude fetus. However, direct, comparative studies of fetal oxygenation in the course of pregnancy have apparently not been made, and would be interesting in the light of Moore's findings on hypoxic ventilatory responsiveness previously described.

Patterns of reproduction

Fertility histories were obtained on 417 women, fifteen years of age or older. Very detailed questioning was employed in an effort to identify all pregnancies recognized by these women and to record their fates, that is, whether a given pregnancy terminated in a fetal death, stillbirth or live-born child. Special attention was paid to intergenesic intervals of three or more years. Despite these efforts, some under reporting undoubtedly occurred; its extent is uncertain. We can only estimate it crudely, and then largely from the work of others. For example, Plank and Milanesi (1973) have commented on the amount of recognizable pregnancy wastage which goes unreported in Chile, especially in the rural communities; they contend it can be large, but depends in part upon the

TABLE 1
The distribution of numbers of pregnancies and live births
by the ages of the mothers at the time of interview and the altitudinal niches of their residence

	Coast			Sierra			Altiplano		
Age	No. Women	No. live births	No. preg-nancies	No. Women	No. live births	No. preg-nancies	No. Women	No. live births	No. preg-nancies
15-19	4	8	8	4	5	5	10	17	17
20-24	22	44	50	7	16	18	16	36	37
25-29	20	51	60	19	66	67	11	33	36
30-34	17	74	87	8	46	46	10	59	60
35-39	16	77	87	14	78	82	14	102	107
40-44	6	33	36	18	109	119	17	122	127
45-49	9	43	43	16	129	149	14	95	102
50-54	5	19	21	19	149	163	12	91	95
55-59	1	10	10	8	47	53	8	56	60
60-64	3	16	19	12	90	102	3	20	20
65-69	2	19	20	12	81	89	5	31	31
70+	3	19	22	17	92	101	8	54	54
Total	108	413	463	154	908	994	128	716	746

method of ascertainment. In this latter connection, Marckwardt (1973) has evaluated several different methods of gathering fertility data in Perú, a situation presumably analogous to ours in northern Chile and finds that a short interview tends to under record live births as contrasted with a traditional, in-depth approach by about ten per cent. Interestingly, there was no deterioration with advancing age in reports on number of live births nor was there a consistent difference in the two interview techniques in the proportions of children born alive who had died before age one.

Twenty-five of the 417 women interviewed reported no pregnancies; whereas 392 stated that they had had one or more (the maximum number was 16). Collectively, they recalled 2,203 pregnancies (ave., 5.6), resulting in 2,039 live births (ave., 5.2). Histories were either not obtained on 114 women, age 15 or older, or were deemed inadequate or inappropriate for analysis. This number includes those women who had not resided in the study area throughout the bulk of their reproductive years; most of the latter individuals were teachers, or the wives of teachers or members of the carabineros, the national police force.

Analysis and interpretation of these reproductive histories are complicated somewhat because of migration and the fact that not all of the reproductive performances were complete. To mitigate these effects we shall, first, emphasize our findings on those women whose reproductive performances can be presumed to be complete. We shall arbitrarily assume women who were 45 years of age or older had effectively completed their reproductive lives. One hundred and ninety women fell into this category. The bulk of these (148 of the 179 with complete reproductive data) were between the ages of 45 and 69. Second, in the tables to follow, unless otherwise stated, each woman has been assigned to that environmental niche where the bulk of her children were born, and presumably conceived. Of the 392, 131 had not lived in the niche of their examination throughout their reproductive years.

Table 1 sets forth the number of pregnancies and of live births for all of the women based upon their age at examination and the niche within which they resided for most of their reproductive years. Patently the number of women interviewed at the various altitudes differs somewhat by age, and since numbers of children are related to the age of the mother, simple comparison between the altitudinal niches is unwarranted. Moreover, it should be noted that a negative correlation exists between total number of pregnancies and age when mothers of all ages from 45 onwards are considered. This is not an uncommon phenomenon; it has often been observed from census data that women, particularly those over the ages of 35 or so, apparently under report the number of children they have borne. The relative error rises with increasing age. We presume that the older women have poorer recall but it must be borne in mind too that the same effect would occur if survivorship was related to previous reproductive performance. Child-bearing is not a riskless undertaking, particularly in remoter areas where medical care is limited, if it exists at all. Be this as it may, this correlation with age is essentially zero over the range 45 through 69. We were tempted to restrict the data to these ages, but since the decline in numbers of pregnancies among women 70 or more at the time of examination was independent of the ethnic origin of the woman interviewed, we have elected to present the larger body of data. It should be borne in mind, however, that the means and variances to be presented in subsequent tables may be underestimates of the 'true' values.

Table 2 summarizes the reproductive performances of these women with completed fertilities in terms of the average number of pregnancies, of live births, and of live-born children surviving the first twelve months of life by ethnic group, by altitude for one ethnic group, the mestizos, and by ethnic groups for one altitude, the sierra. The latter two comparisons were chosen because the mestizos are better represented at all three altitudes (there are relatively few Aymará in the coastal sample, and even fewer non-Aymará in the altiplano one), and the sierra, though relatively few non-Aymará are represented, has a broader representation of the three ethnic groups than either the coast or the altiplano.

Observe, first, that among the three ethnic groups the Aymará have had the most pregnancies, on average, and that the mestizos have had more than the non-Aymará. The average number of live births follows this same gradient, as does the average number of live-born children who have survived the first year of life. Mestizo newborns have somewhat poorer prospects of survival than the Aymará who, in turn, do more poorly than the non-Aymará. The differences are, however, small and not statistically significant; indeed, expressed as product-moment correlations, the association of number of live births with the number surviving through the first year of life varies from 0.94 to 0.96. Couched in terms of relative risk of death, using the non-Aymará as the standard, the relative risk

TABLE 2
The reproductive performances of those women who were 45 years of age or older at the time of their examinations in 1973-1974

Group	No.	Average number of pregnancies	Average number of live births	Average number of liveborn children surviving one year	Percentage surviving
ALL WOMEN					
Aymará	77	7.55 (0.41)	6.99 (0.36)	6.18 (0.35)	88
Mestizos	69	7.01 (0.40)	6.36 (0.38)	5.46 (0.33)	86
Non-Aymará	33	6.27 (0.58)	5.70 (0.60)	5.21 (0.53)	91
Total	179	7.10 (0.26)	6.51 (0.24)	5.73 (0.22)	88
ONLY MESTIZOS					
Coast	13	5.08 (0.83)	4.62 (0.84)	4.23 (0.84)	92
Sierra	40	7.58 (0.55)	6.73 (0.52)	5.80 (0.45)	86
Altiplano	16	7.19 (0.72)	6.88 (0.64)	5.63 (0.50)	82
ONLY SIERRA					
Aymará	38	8.11 (0.64)	7.11 (0.54)	6.42 (0.49)	90
Mestizos	40	7.58 (0.55)	6.73 (0.52)	5.80 (0.45)	86
Non-Aymará	7	6.71 (1.60)	6.43 (1.59)	5.71 (1.34)	89

( ) The standard errors of the various means are given in parentheses.

for the Aymará is 1.29 and for the mestizos, 1.47. Second, although the average number of children born to mestizos is greater in the sierra than in either the altiplano or the coast, relatively more survive the infantile period on the coast than in the other two altitudinal niches. The poorest survival is seen in the altiplano. Finally, within the one niche, the sierra, where the three ethnic groups can be compared, the Aymará have more pregnancies and more surviving children than either the mestizos or the non-Aymará. Analyses of variance reveal these differences between the ethnic means when altitude is ignored, between altitudes when the comparison is restricted to the mestizos and between ethnic groups when the altitudinal niche is fixed to be marginally significant at most ($P < 0.10$). Parenthetically, it warrents noting that the average number of pregnancies of Aymará women in Chile is slightly, but not significantly higher than the number seen in our studies in Bolivia or reported by Tichauer (1963). Survivorship through the first year of life is, in our experience, approximately the same in Turco and Toledo as in the Chilean altiplano.

Cruz-Coke and his colleagues (1966) studied 128 families drawn from the villages of Belén, Chapiquiña and Guallatiri and the Azapa and Lluta valleys in the spring of 1965 and autumn of 1966. Some of their findings, for the four villages or locales where comparisons can be made are summarized in Table 3. The average number of pregnancies ranges from 5.8 in Belén to 8.5 in Chapiquiña; these are values very similar to our own in the same areas (see Table 3). Given that less than a decade intervened between their study and our own, some overlap in our samples seems certain to have occurred. It warrants

TABLE 3
Comparison of the fertility findings of Cruz-Coke et al. (1966) in 1965-66 with ours in 1973-74

	Coast		Sierra				Altiplano	
	Azapa		Belén		Chapiquiña		Guallatiri	
	'65-66	'73-74	'65-66	'73-74	'65-66	'73-74	'65-66	'73-74
Mean pregnancy no.	6.4	6.2	5.8	6.7	8.5	7.8	7.3	8.5
Surviving (%)	96	92	87	91	87	91	96	92
Live births (%)	83	87	90	82	99	92	99	96

note, however, that in Chile between 1969 and 1974 the birth rate declined by 10 per cent and the infant mortality rate by no less than 18 per cent (Cabrera, 1980). Indeed, between 1950 and 1980, infant mortality in Chile fell from 123 deaths per thousand live births to about 33 (Behm, 1983; Castillo et al., 1983), and the northern area of Chile participated in these changes. Thus, there is a basis for a difference to exist in our findings. Cruz-Coke et al. also report a decreasing gradient in natality and mortality from the altiplano to the coast, and using Crow's Indices of Selection conclude that 'total selective opportunities decrease in correlation to cultural evolution, but the fertility component increases.' Haas (1981), however, has observed that in Bolivia indigenous women appear better adapted to childbearing than non-indigenous women although newborn infants at this altitude exhibit a significant growth retardation suggesting that the maternal adaptation to the stress of pregnancy is not complete.

Most current models of the 'natural' reproductive pattern of a woman, that is, one unmodified by contraception, assume that at the beginning of cohabitation she is in a non-pregnant, but fecundable state, and after a random length of time passes into a pregnant state which ultimately terminates in an abortion, a still-birth, or a live birth with a given probability (see, e.g., Perrin and Sheps, 1964; Potter, 1963). Each pregnancy is followed by an infecundable period attributable to an episode of amenorrhoea directly following the previous birth and one or more menstrual cycles which are anovulatory. Eventually, of course, the woman returns to the fecundable, non-pregnant state. Both the number of anovulatory cycles and the period of amenorrhoea can vary as a function of the nature of the pregnancy outcome, that is, whether it terminates in an abortion, stillbirth, or live-born infant. More generally, the duration of stay in each of these various states is assumed to be a random variable whose distribution depends upon the state into which the woman will pass next as well as the one currently occupied. These probabilities undoubtedly reflect many other factors too – genetic, hormonal, socio-cultural, environmental, previous disease experience and the like. In the main, they are not directly knowable, but some are estimable in a non-contracepting population through the study of birth intervals.

TABLE 4
Average age (years) at first pregnancy by altitude

Age (in yrs)	Coast No.	Coast Age	Sierra No.	Sierra Age	Altiplano No.	Altiplano Age
15-19	4	15.5	4	15.5	10	16.0
20-24	22	18.9	7	18.4	16	18.4
25-29	20	20.8	19	19.8	10	20.8
30-34	15	21.6	8	19.7	10	19.1
35-39	15	22.9	14	20.7	14	19.9
40-44	6	21.3	18	20.8	14	22.2
45+	20	23.8	59	23.4	44	23.3

As Potter (1963) has pointed out, partition of the birth interval in this manner has a number of uses, not the least of which is the more subtle characterization of differences in fertility among different groups within a society or among societies in the absence or near absence of family limitation. This general approach to the study of reproduction has been limited by the scarcity of sufficiently detailed data on birth intervals, and the difficulty in identifying non-contracepting populations. Several lines of evidence suggest that in the absence of lactation the average birth interval (unmodified by known pregnancy wastage) should be approximately 18 months, and with prolonged lactation 27 months (Potter, 1963). Average birth intervals in societies where it is reasonable to assume on cultural and historical grounds that little or no birth control is or was practiced vary from approximately 24 to somewhat less than 36 months. The Hutterites of the western United States and Canada have an average birth interval of 25.5 months (Tietze, 1957), and the Amish of western Indiana an interval of 25.7 months (Juberg, 1966), for example.

Efforts to obtain comparable data on the Aymará are complicated by a less well-developed sense of time – mothers tend to place little value upon the exact date of birth of a child, particularly one now dead – and the understandable problems posed in the remembrance of events which have seemingly little social relevance to the person interviewed. Accordingly, our data are restricted to the average age at the first pregnancy within the various altitude niches based on the present ages of the women on whom reproductive histories exist. Table 4 clearly shows these ages to differ trivially across the various altitudes for women of the same age.

Reproductive performance and glycolytic intermediates

Of the women with fertility histories to whom we have alluded in the previous section, there exist adenosine triphosphate (ATP) and 2,3-diphosphoglycerate (2,3-DPG) determinations on 263 (see Clench, Ferrell and Schull, 1982 for a description of the methods used). These determinations were, of course, not made at the time of specific pregnancies, and can, therefore, serve only as guides

TABLE 5
The correlation between the glycolytic intermediates, adenosine triphosphate and 2,3-diphosphoglycerate, and total number of pregnancies

	No.	ATP	DPG
Coast	30	-0.17	0.26
Sierra	14	-0.11	-0.28
Altiplano	44	0.06	0.26+
All women	88	-0.07	0.23*

* Significant at $P < 0.05$
+ Significant at $P < 0.10$

TABLE 6
The relationship of age, altitude, ethnicity and 2,3-diphosphoglycerate to the number of pregnancies for women with completed fertility.
The entries are partial regression coefficients; their standard errors are given in parentheses.

			P
Age	-0.071	(0.039)	0.07
Altitude	0.708	(0.467)	0.25
Ethnicity	0.549	(0.543)	0.62
2,3-DPG	0.329	(0.190)	0.17

The increments (or decrements) of change are per year of life (after 45 years), per 1500 m, per unit of ethnicity (scale = 1, 2, 3) and per micromole of DPG per gram of hemoglobin.

to the values which probably obtained on these latter occasions. Both of these intermediates have been shown to be under genetic control (Brewer, 1967; Chakraborty et al., 1983; Gilroy, Brewer and Sing, 1978) and, therefore, an individual's level at one point in time should be correlated with that at another. We shall exhibit two analyses, however, one which assumes the single determination on any particular woman is indicative of her value throughout her reproductive career, and the other which merely assumes that the value available to us is reasonably close to the value which obtained at her last pregnancy – assuming that the latter did not occur more than five years prior to our measurement. Our analyses will be based upon rank order statistics, and thus this assumption merely implies that a woman's rank with respect to her reproductive peers is more or less invariant with time. This seems more likely to be true than the assumption that the value itself will not change with time. Again we will emphasize the findings based upon the 88 women with completed fertilities among the 178 on whom measurements of the glycolytic intermediates are available. Attention will be called to the observations on the women who had not as yet completed their reproductive spans only when these seem at variance with the data on completed reproductive performances.

Table 5 gives the correlations between ATP and 2,3-DPG and the total number of pregnancies for all women, and for those residing in the specified altitudinal niche. Note that ATP is not significantly correlated with number of pregnancies for all women or for those in a specific niche. 2,3-DPG is, however, significantly and positively associated with number of pregnancies among all women, and is marginally so among altiplano women as well. Simple correlations are difficult to interpret, however, for levels of 2,3-DPG increase with altitude and as we have seen Aymará women have more pregnancies. Thus, a significant correlation may merely reflect the association of Aymará women with that altitude at which DPG levels are highest. To address this possibility, the number of pregnancies was regressed on age, altitude, ethnicity and 2,3-DPG level. The partial regression coefficients to emerge from this analysis are shown in Table 6. Note that level of 2,3-DPG continues to be positively associated with the number of pregnancies after the effects of altitude and ethnicity have been removed. This regression coefficient is not significantly different from zero, however ($P = 0.17$).

To examine this issue further, we include now the women whose reproductive performances were not complete at the time of interview. This increases the sample from 88 to 229, or almost two and a half-fold. The partial regression coefficients are now:

	Constants	Standard errors
2,3-DPG	0.242	0.129
Ethnicity	0.443	0.389
Altitude	0.767	0.318
Age	0.091	0.016

As was to be anticipated, both age and altitude are significantly and positively related to the number of pregnancies; 2,3-DPG is marginally so ($P=0.14$) and ethnicity is not. Patently, the increase in sample size does not resolve the association, if real, of 2,3-DPG with number of pregnancies; however, it seems clear that the experience of those women who have not completed their fertility is similar to that of women who have. But what does this mean? Are women with higher DPGs more fecund? Or do they merely manage to carry all (most) of their pregnancies longer, and thus are more aware of them. If, as has been reported 25 to 50%, perhaps, of pregnancies are spontaneously aborted very early in pregnancy (Hertig, Rock, and Adams, 1956; Abramson, 1971; Wilcox et al., 1988), a relatively modest change in this pregnancy wastage could be important in the present context.

To summarize briefly our findings, differences in the number of children born to the three ethnic groups are seen when altitude is ignored (or fixed), and between altitudes when the comparison is restricted to the mestizos, on whom the largest amount of data are available. These differences are small, marginally significant statistically, and it is moot whether they are attributable to the hypoxia of altitude or to extraneous sources of variation.

Chapter 8
ECOLOGIC DETERMINANTS OF THE HEALTH OF AYMARA CHILDREN

Introduction

Although the study we describe was concerned with the health of all individuals in the Departamento de Arica, as reflected in an altitudinal cross-section of the region's residents, the health of the young was a matter of special concern. We justify this focus and this chapter as follows: Forty-two percent of the population of Latin America is less than 14 years of age (Galofre, 1979). There are 3.6 million children in Chile under fifteen years of age (37.7% of the total population); 1.4 million of these are less than five years old. If the present fertility rate of 4.1 live births per woman continues, in the year 2000 there will be 6.5 million children in Chile, almost 50 percent of the total population (International Demographic Tapes, 1980). Many of these children will live in households of extreme poverty with potentially adverse effects on physical and mental growth and development. In South American countries, a strong positive correlation exists between the number of young children (less than five years of age) and the percentage of households below the absolute poverty line. The Economic Commission for Latin America (CEPAL) defines absolute poverty as per capita income below the amount required to purchase the foods necessary to meet basic nutritional requirements (Piñera, 1979; Molina and Piñera, 1979). The coefficient of correlation between the gross national product (GNP) of South American countries and their infant and preschool population (0-6 age group) is -0.61 (Pollitt, 1980). Countries with higher standards of living and low levels of internal, economic disparity have fewer youngsters to care for; whereas those with high internal inequity and a lower GNP have large numbers of young children to shepherd.

Not only is poverty a health impediment, but when the risk of death between birth and two years is examined in terms of the mother's education, little between-country differences exist, if the mother has at least 10 years of education (all mortality rates are less than 50 deaths per 1,000 live births); however for the illiterate mother, mortality soars to over 200 in Perú and Bolivia, and 130 in Chile (UNICEF/CEPAL, 1979).

The health status of children in rural communities is worse, particularly those of indigenous origin. Infant mortality rates in rural Chilean localities (areas with less than 20,000 people) are more than twice those of urban communities; several rural communities have infant mortality rates that exceed 120 (Solimano and Hakim, 1978). When the risk of death between birth and two years of age is matched to ethnicity, indigenous children have a far higher risk of death. This is

William J. Schull and Francisco Rothhammer (eds.), The Aymará: Strategies in Human Adaptation to a Rigorous Environment, 87-100.

TABLE 1
Frequency of ICDA codes compatible with overt infection

ICDA code	Infection Category	Frequency
020 - 136.9	General and parasitic	30
000 - 009.9	Intestinal	9
360 - 369.9	Eye	19
380 - 384.9	Ear	27
460 - 466	Acute respiratory	170
480 - 486	Pneumonia	6
490 - 491	Bronchitis	7
500	Hypertrophy of tonsils and adenoids	79
502 - 502.1	Pharyngitis and nasopharyngitis	5
010 - 019.9, Y030	Tuberculosis	6
680 - 689.9	Skin and subcutaneous tissue	9
782.7	Lymph node enlargement	166

reduced somewhat if they live in urban areas, but even then, their mortality risk remains substantially higher than that of non-indigenous children living in rural areas. The chance an indigenous child will have the same mortality risk as that of a non-indigenous child is directly correlated to the years of maternal schooling (UNICEF/CEPAL, 1979).

Fifty-five percent of all children in Latin America are undernourished; whereas only 27.4 percent of the adult population is (Selowsky, 1978). The origin of this difference, and indeed of malnutrition more generally is ecologic and complex (see May and McLellan, 1974); however, malnutrition has startling effects on health. The Pan American Health Organization (PAHO) analysis of 35,094 death certificates and autopsy reports of children under five in the Americas found a pre-existing nutritional deficiency or immaturity (defined as a severe growth deficit) to be the underlying or associated cause of death in 19,994 (57%) of the deceased preschool age population (Puffer and Serrano, 1975). Even though infection was the leading cause of death (58% of the 35,094 deaths were attributed directly to infection), 61 percent of the children who died of infection also had a nutritional deficiency (Puffer and Serrano, 1975). In Chile infection causes 43 percent of the deaths in the one to four age group (UNICEF/CEPAL, 1979). Undoubtedly nutritional deficits preceded a large percentage of these deaths.

Malnutrition and infection are synergistic, and notably so among children, where infection is a radically different process than that seen in an adult. Children become ill and recover faster, have higher fevers, lose proportionally more fluid, and develop greater electrolyte imbalances than do adults. Their smaller anatomical structures lie closer together, allowing infections to spread rapidly; only children experience febrile seizures (Barnett and Einhorn, 1980; Chow et al., 1979; Kempe et al., 1982).

Malnutrition and infection affect the vast majority of children in developing countries. Because infection is usually a short term problem, and malnutrition a

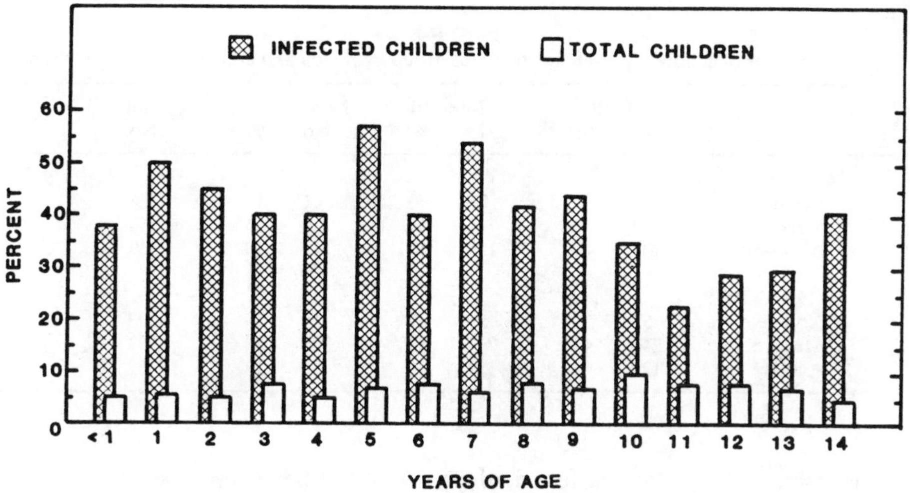

FIGURE 1. Percentage distribution of infected children within each age (hatched bars) compared with percentage distribution of number of children in each age group (open bars)

chronic state of ill health, age-specific prevalence rates of infection are considered crucial indicators of health status and are used to measure the health condition of Aymará children.

Infection rates

Medical examinations were completed on 2096 individuals of whom 988 were children, age 15 days to 14 years. Their examination schedule included (1) anthropometric measures, (2) audiometric examination, (3) medical history, (4) ophthalmoscopic examination, (5) physical examination, (6) pulmonary function tests, and (7) residential history. All of the children were classified as Aymará, mestizo or non-Aymará (Spanish) and by permanence of residence as previously described (see Chapter 1: Ancestry and residence).

After the physical examination all medical findings were converted to ICDA codes; codes compatible with overt infection are listed in Table 1 along with their frequency. The majority of overt infections (34%) involve the respiratory system followed by a smattering among sensory (9%), skin (2%), and digestive systems (2%). Some 6% of the infections were classified as general and 31% of the codes implicated lymph node enlargement. Because stool samples were not evaluated for the presence of parasites nor were other laboratory tests performed to assess the burden of covert disease, the reported prevalence of childhood infection is conservative and an underestimation of true morbidity.

When the physical examinations of the 988 children in the survey were evaluated for the presence of ICDA codes compatible with infection (see Table 1), 393 children (40%) presented one or more infections, 175 (18%) exhibited one or more non-infectious disorders (e.g., chronic alterations in neurologic,

TABLE 2
Number of children in each health status group by region and ethnicity category

	Well		Infected		Non-Infected		Total
	No.	%	No.	%	No.	%	No.
REGION							
Coast	159	56	85	30	41	14	286
Sierra	127	35	148	41	89	24	364
Altiplano	134	40	159	47	45	13	338
ETHNICITY							
Non-Aymará	52	56	27	29	14	15	93
Mestizo	240	40	247	42	106	18	593
Aymará	128	42	119	39	55	18	302

cardiovascular, or metabolic functioning), and 420 (42%) were well and free of disease. The distribution of infection within each age class appears in Figure 1. The percentage of children infected remains high for all age groups, never dropping below 20% and only receding below 30% for the 11 and 12 year groups. Interestingly, youngsters aged 14 have an infection rate comparable to children aged three, four and six. For children in this survey, infection does not decrease appreciably with age.

Children were further sorted by region of residence and ethnicity. Table 2 sets forth the number of children in each health status class, i.e., well and free of disease, infected, or non-infectious disorder, by region and ethnicity.

It is non-Aymará (Spanish) children residing on the coast who are most likely to be well and free of disease. Highland children have the highest rates of infection. The prevalence of non-infectious disorders shows little ethnic variability and no appreciable difference between coast and altiplano regions. Figure 2 presents age-specific prevalence rates of infection by region and ethnicity. Aymará children, from birth to two years of age, living in the altiplano, have the highest infection rate (60%). Coastal and sierran children, age 0-2, have similar infection rates; however 40% of young mestizos are infected as compared to only 27% of Spanish youngsters. Children, age 3-5 and 6-8 have similar infection rates, regardless of ethnicity or region of residence. Infection rate varies appreciably as a function of region and ethnicity for the very young (age 0-2) as well as the older child (age 9-14).

To summarize the relationship between well and infected youngsters and their region and ethnicity, the 175 youngsters with a non-infectious disorder were eliminated from analysis and Kendall's tau correlations were computed on the remaining 813 children. This correlation is a measure of the strength of the relationship between two variables, such as the health status (well or infected) and a child's region of residence. Once computed, the tau values can be used to compare the strength of the association between variables for one group with variables from a second group, e.g., the health status and region of residence of children age 9-11. Kendall's tau correlations were computed using the program

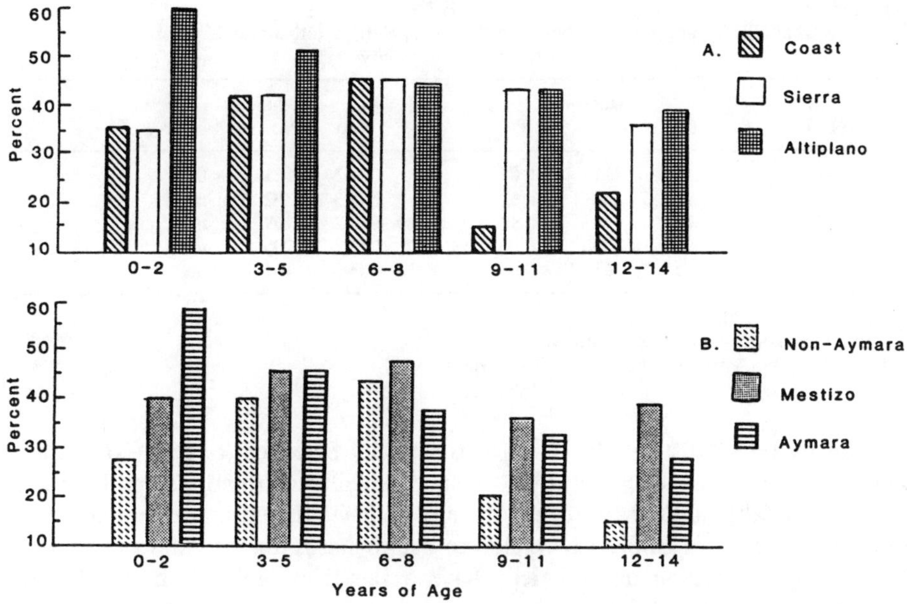

FIGURE 2. Age-specific prevalence rates of infection (per 100 children) by region and ethnicity

TABLE 3
Kendall's Tau correlations between the age-specific health status of children and region and ethnicity

Age (yrs.)	Region Tau	Region No.	Region P	Ethnicity Tau	Ethnicity No.	Ethnicity P
0-2	0.177	121	<0.05	0.163	121	<0.05
3-5	0.129	162	n.s.	0.073	162	n.s.
6-8	-0.035	169	n.s.	-0.112	169	n.s.
9-11	0.316	200	<0.001	0.082	200	n.s.
12-14	0.155	161	<0.05	-0.006	161	n.s.

Health status: 1 = well, 2 = infected
Region: 1 = coast, 2 = sierra, 3 = altiplano
Ethnicity: 1 = non-Aymará, 2 = mestizo, 3 = Aymará

provided by the Statistical Package for the Social Sciences (SPSS) (Nie et al., 1975) and are set forth in Table 3. We note significant relationships between region and health status as well as ethnicity and health status for the child 0-2 years; only region is significantly related to health status for the child age 9-11 or 12-14. Neither region nor ethnicity have a significant relationship to health status for the child age 3-5 or 6-8.

To recapitulate, age-specific infection rates are significantly related to region. Children living in the altiplano and sierra have a far higher prevalence of infection than coastal youngsters, regardless of ethnicity. Obviously, the different rates of childhood infections between the three regions cannot be explained by a single factor or agent, or even a multifactorial analysis of the child's region. Child health is ecological, in the sense that it relates to the total environment that surrounds the child, the physical ecosystem that determines agro-economic practices, occupations, and life styles, as well as the social and political systems that determine distribution and availability of resources and services.

Associations between infection rates and family socio-economic variables:

Family health variables abstracted from the Multinational Andean Health Program are enumerated in Table 4 along with the breakdown scheme of each variable. Maternal age and education as well as the father's occupation were abstracted directly from the residential record and demographic history. Maternal age ranged from 17 to 62 years; the median was 35 years. To derive a measure of economic status, or wealth, each household was scored according to the number of animals and acreage owned. The scoring system is set forth in Table 5 and was derived following frequency and distribution analysis. The wealth scoring matrix appears biased towards agrarian families; however, regional statistics document that an equal percentage of households in each of the three regions derive their livelihood from farming and/or animal husbandry. Actual family income was not sought. Understandably, complete information on income is difficult to obtain and because of the extensive use of barter exchange,

TABLE 4
Family health variables

Variable	Variable classes			
Socio-economic				
Maternal education	1 = None	2 = Elementary	3 = Secondary	
Maternal age	1 = <35 years	2 = ≥35 years		
Paternal occupation	1 = non-agrarian	2 = agrarian		
Family wealth	1 = score of <15	2 = score of ≥15		
Parental health				
Father's health	1 = well	2 = infected		
Mother's health	1 = well	2 = infected		
Maternal demographics				
Gravida	Number of pregnancies			
Parity	Number of children borne			
Early child health				
Birth order	Ordinal placement			
Birth condition	1 = normal	2 = abnormal		
Birth color	1 = normal	2 = abnormal		
Birth problems	1 = present	2 = absent		
Was child nursed	1 = yes	2 = no		
Length of nursing	1 = <1 wk	2 = 1-2 wk	3 = 2-3 wk	4 = 3-4 wk
	5 = 1-6 mo	6 = 6-12 mo	7 = >1 yr	
Did child nurse eagerly	1 = yes 2 = no			
Birth attendant	1 = physician	2 = paramedical	3 = trained midwife	
	4 = lay midwife	5 = family	6 = unattended	
Did child gain weight properly	1 = no	2 = yes		
Family composition				
Number of children living in the household				
Number of under 6 years living in the household				
Child presently living with the mother	1 = yes	2 = no		

TABLE 5
Family wealth scoring system

Llamas	1 = none	2 = 1-10	3 = 11-30	4 = 31-50	5 = 51-100	6 = 101+
Sheep	1 = none	2 = 1-5	3 = 6-10	4 = 11-30	5 = 31-50	6 = 51+
Goats	1 = none	2 = 1-5	3 = 6-10	4 = 11-30	5 = 31-50	6 = 51+
Donkeys	1 = none	2 = 1	3 = 2-3	4 = 4-5	5 = 6-10	6 = 11+
Mules	1 = none	2 = 1	3 = 2-3	4 = 4-5	5 = 6-10	6 = 11+
Cattle	1 = none	2 = 1	3 = 2-3	4 = 4-5	5 = 6-10	6 = 11+
Land*	1 = none	2 = 1	3 = 2-3	4 = 4-5	5 = 6-10	6 = 11+

* Land holdings in hectares.

TABLE 6
Kendall's Tau correlation between region specific health status of children aged 0-14 years and socio-economic-health variables

	Health status							
	Total		Coast		Sierra		Altiplano	
Variable	Tau	No.	Tau	No.	Tau	No.	Tau	No.
Socio-economic:								
Maternal education	-.105**	532	-.066	143	-.077	204	-.019	185
Maternal age	-.068*	532	-.166*	143	+.074	204	-.067	185
Paternal occupation	-.002	344	-.018	73	+.027	123	-.017	148
Family wealth	-.022	562	-.017	145	+.0	197	-.112*	220
Parental Health:								
Father's health	+.120*	255	-.090	63	+.207*	91	+.108	101
Mother's health	+.208**	291	+.239*	64	+.196*	130	+.188*	97

*P < 0.05; **P < 0.01
Health status (at time of physical examination):

	1 = well and free of disease,	2 = presence of one or more infections	
Maternal education:	1 = none,	2 = elementary,	3 = secondary
Maternal age:	1 = < 35 years,	2 = ≥ 35 years	
Parental occupation:	1 = non-Agrarian,	2 = Agrarian	
Family wealth:	1 = < median,	2 = ≥ median	
Father's health:	1 = well and free of disease,	2 = infected	
Mother's health:	1 = well and free of disease,	2 = infected	

monetary income might merely reflect social and professional status, rather than the economic resources available to the household. Wealth scores ranged from 8 to 32; the median was 15.

Parental health was scored using the algorithm set forth earlier to classify child health. For purposes of the present study, only those parents and children classified as well or infected are considered for analysis.

All family variables were abstracted from parental records and then matched and attached to the appropriate child's file. Numerous children were siblings and hence shared identical values for family socioeconomic, parental health, and maternal demographic variables. Because of existing covariation between siblings (and to a lesser degree other relatives), the measured variances underestimate the true variances. This bias is expected to exert no systematic impact on the statistical computations, the resulting direction, or sign of the test, or non-significant associations. However, when results are statistically significant, the existence of correlated observations can act to inflate the attained level of significance and thus deserve consideration. To correct for covariation effects, only family variables that achieved a high significance level were considered for further analysis. All remaining variables are child-specific and therefore free of covariation bias.

Table 6 sets forth Kendall's tau correlations between the health status of children and the socio-economic-health variables of their families. Values are calculated first for the total pediatric population, and then for children living

TABLE 7
Kendall's Tau correlations between region of residence and ethnicity of children aged 0-14 years and socio-economic health variables

Variable[1]	Region Tau	Region No.	Region P	Ethnicity Tau	Ethnicity No.	Ethnicity P
Socio-economic:						
Maternal education	-.203	649	0.001	-.104	649	0.001
Maternal age	+.069	655	0.05	+.106	655	0.005
Paternal occupation	-.019	414	n.s.	+.158	414	0.001
Family wealth	+.152	668	0.001	+.161	668	0.001
Parental Health:						
Father's health	+.102	299	0.05	+.011	299	n.s.
Mother's health	+.054	350	n.s.	+.080	350	n.s.

Region: 1 = coast, 2 = sierra, 3 = altiplano
Ethnicity: 1 = non-Aymará, 2 = mestizo, 3 = Aymará
[1] Refer to Table 6 for the coding of the remaining variables.

within each region. To interpret the correlation values in Table 6, refer to the key and accompanying ordinal values assigned to each variable. For example, maternal education is statistically and significantly negatively related to child health. Maternal education is ranked as: 1 = no education, 2 = elementary, and 3 = secondary. Child health is ranked as: 1 = well and 2 = infected. Therefore, a negative relationship between health and maternal education implies that well children (ranked as 1) are likely to have a mother with a secondary education (rank 3) and children infected (rank 2) are most likely to have a mother with no education (rank 1).

Any correlation may be a mere reflection of other variables which are more powerfully related to child health. In addition, variables with no apparent relationship to child health (e.g., paternal occupation) may be correlated to other variables, such as ethnicity or region, which are related to child health. To see whether such relationships were operant, additional correlations were computed between family ethnicity. Table 7 lists the tau value, sample size and significance level.

To summarize the results of the tau analyses from Tables 6 and 7: Maternal education and age are significantly related to health status, region, and ethnicity; their effect on child health appears direct. Paternal occupation and family wealth are not significantly related to child health. Maternal health is highly correlated with child health and maintains a significant relationship with each region. The father's health does not follow a similar pattern; rather paternal health is significantly correlated to child health for the total population, but not for each region. Maternal health emerges as the most vital socio-economic-health variable that directly affects child health, regardless of region. Paternal health, maternal education, and maternal age, while significantly affecting the total pediatric population, do not consistently correlate significantly with child health within each region.

TABLE 8
Results of maternal and child health analysis

Variable[1]	Factor 1	Factor 2	Factor 3	Factor 4	Factor 5
Parity	+.962	+.103	+.007	-.116	-.087
Gravida	+.958	+.095	+.006	-.160	-.085
Birth order	+.861	+.048	+.119	-.307	-.083
Birth condition	-.243	+.783	+.338	-.064	-.230
Birth color	+.270	+.771	-.351	+.128	+.215
Birth problem	+.087	-.305	+.307	+.389	-.121
Was child nursed	.000	.000	.000	.000	.000
Length of nursing	+.314	-.009	+.463	+.400	+.331
Did child nurse eagerly	+.023	+.490	-.074	+.158	+.494
Did child gain weight properly	+.085	+.309	-.300	-.255	+.662
Birth attendant	+.375	-.004	+.486	+.356	+.217
Is child living with mother	+.011	-.169	+.353	+.020	+.079
No. children in household	+.566	+.280	-.464	+.341	-.211
No. children in household < 6 yrs	+.014	+.311	-.399	+.717	-.129
% of variance	25	14	11	10	8
Eigen value	3.29	1.86	1.39	1.31	1.04

Sample Size = 350
[1] Refer to Table 4 for the coding of the variables.

Many of the fourteen maternal, early child health, and family size variables (refer to Table 4) are highly correlated with each other (e.g., parity and gravida, birth condition and birth color) and are difficult to interpret or to relate to the child's present health status. To derive a few meaningful, and independent measures of fertility and early child health, routine factor analysis with quartimax rotation was used. Five factors were derived and are presented in Table 8 with their correlation values. To summarize each of these briefly: Factor 1 is a general fertility index that includes parity, gravida, and birth order. Factor 2 reflects the child's birth condition and birth color. Factor 3 indicates length of nursing and birth attendant. Factor 4 deals with the number of children in the household less than 6 years of age and Factor 5 deals primarily with weight gain. In principle, the factors extracted by such an analysis are orthogonal (statistically independent), so that their effects are additive.

Each factor analysis program derives a factor-scoring matrix that can be used to compute, for each child, a score on each factor. In this study, factor analysis reduced the original 14 variables to five factors (described above) that were then 'scored' for each child. These factor scores are standardized deviates with a zero mean and a standard deviation of one.

To determine whether the mean factor values varied significantly as a function of health status, region, or ethnicity, analyses of variance of factors one through five were performed; the F-ratios are displayed in Table 9. None of the five factors varied significantly as a function of health status; factor 5, the child's weight gain, approached significance ($F = 2.82$, $df = 286$, $P < 0.10$) but did not reach the level set for this study ($P < 0.05$). To better understand the data, Figure 3 shows the standardized mean factor score (horizontal bars) and the 95

TABLE 9
Analysis of variance of maternal and early child health factors testing for the effects of health status (well vs infected), region of residence (coast, sierra, altiplano), and ethnicity (Aymará, Mestizo, Spanish)

	Main effects					
	Health	Residual	Region	Residual	Ethnicity	Residual
df	1	286	2	347	2	347
Dependent variable:						
Factor 1 (fertility)						
Sum of squares	.03	294.60	8.45	340.53	2.04	346.93
F-ratio	.03		4.31**		1.02	
Factor 2 (birth condition)						
Sum of squares	.96	268.83	10.54	338.50	2.57	346.45
F-ratio	1.00		5.40**		1.29	
Factor 3 (nursing length)						
Sum of squares	.04	296.44	74.04	275.23	37.98	311.29
F-ratio	.04		46.67**		21.17**	
Factor 4 (no. children < 6 yrs)						
Sum of squares	.15	281.56	5.35	343.86	.32	348.88
F-ratio	.15		2.70		.16	
Factor 5 (weight gain)						
Sum of squares	2.90	293.89	7.07	341.89	.85	348.10
F-ratio	2.82		3.59*		.43	

*P <0.05; **P <0.01

percent confidence interval for the sample mean score (vertical bars), first for the total pediatric population of a region, second for well children and lastly for infected youngsters.

Regional differences are significant for fertility, birth condition, length of nursing, and the child's weight gain. Fertility increases with altitude and birth condition worsens. Factor 3 demonstrates that coastal children are nursed for the shortest period of time, altiplano youngsters for the longest. Highly significant is the weight gain differential between well and infected coastal children. When compared to the weight gain of well youngsters, mothers of infected children report poor, unsatisfactory weight increments.

CONCLUSIONS AND IMPLICATIONS

To establish the health status of Aymará children of northern Chile living at the three studied altitudes, medical examinations were classified according to the presence of overt infection. Some 393 (40%) of the youngsters harbored one or more overt infections and when sorted by region and ethnicity, indigenous children of the highlands had infection rates 50% higher than those of Spanish descent living near the coast. Age-specific infection rates were significantly related to region; however, ethnicity was not a significant determinant of infection except for the very young child 0-2 years of age. Children living in the altiplano and sierra have far higher rates of infection than coastal youngsters

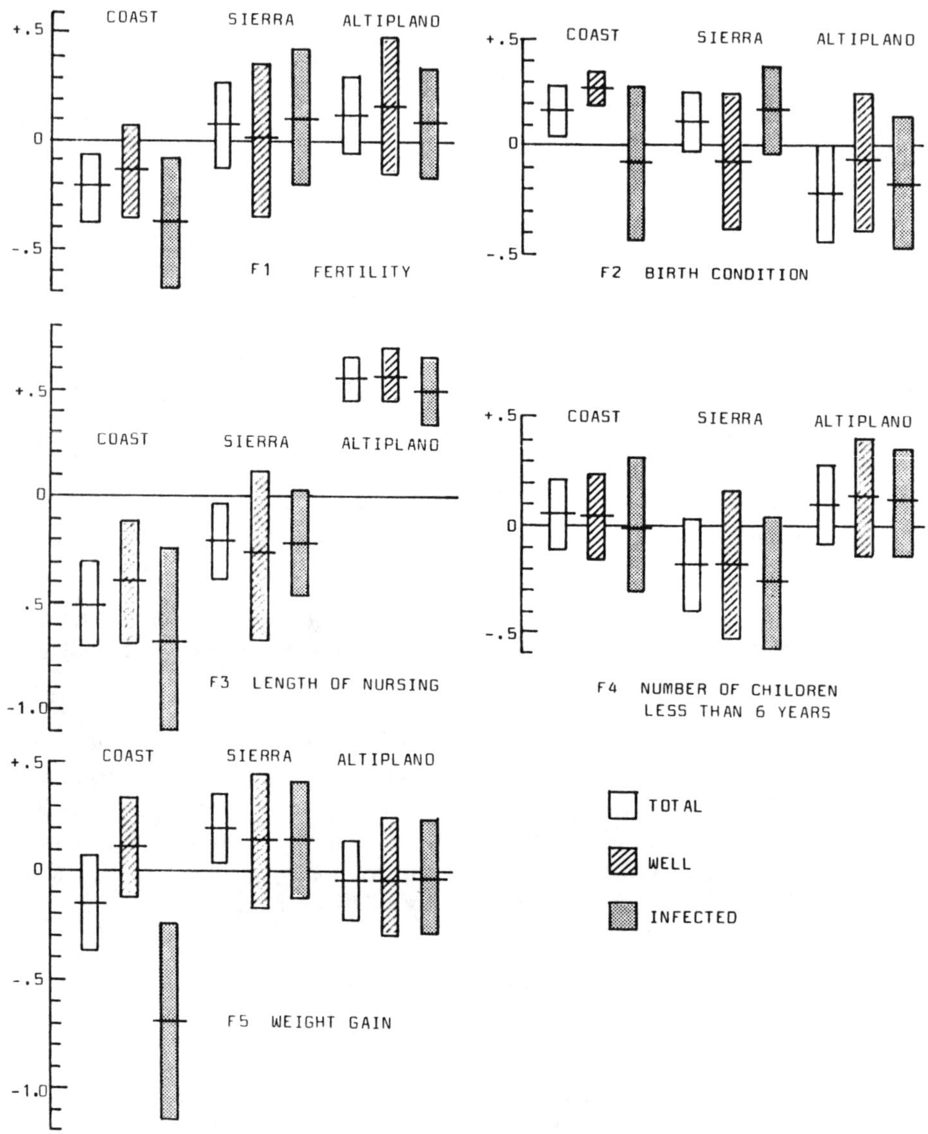

FIGURE 3. Maternal and early child standardized mean factor scores (horizontal bars), and 95 percent confidence interval (vertical bars), for the total pediatric population of each region (open bar), and for well (diagonal stripe) and infected youngsters (stipple)

regardless of ethnicity. Because region embraces politico-economic factors as well as a set climatic and demographic state, a region-specific analysis of the relationship between select familial socio-economic variables and child health was completed.

The results of the region specific analysis are summarized as follows

In comparison to children free of infection and well at the time of a standard physical examination, children with the presence of one or more infections were more likely to be cared for by a mother who was presently infected, below the age of 35, and with minimal or no education. A significant number of infected youngsters in the altiplano reside in homes below the median wealth index; however, wealth does not differentiate between the health status of sierra or coastal children; neither does the father's occupation. Only among sierra children does the father's health correlate significantly with child health. None of the five factors deduced from the 14 maternal demographic and early child health indices varied significantly as a function of health status, although each changed as region changed.

Many of these results agree with previous reports; some differ markedly. The young, uneducated mother is consistently linked to child morbidity (Galofre, 1979; Molina and Piñera, 1979; Pollitt, 1980). The results herein concur. Several studies (Freij and Wall, 1977; 1979; UNICEF/CEPAL, 1979) link family income to child morbidity. In this study family wealth, measured as land and animal holdings, varied significantly as a function of health status in one region only, the altiplano. Health of children in sierra and coastal communities did not fluctuate as a function of wealth. Studies report a positive correlation between the number of children less than five years of age in a household and infection rate; the connection is logical and straightforward. However, in this analysis family size, maternal demographics, and early child health variables did not change significantly as a function of health status. Inability to measure a direct association between certain variables and child health is not surprising considering the within region homogeneity of many variables, such as parity. If indeed traditional variables of child health, for example, family wealth and size, act synergistically to forestall or intensify illness, then the separate impact of each variable may be impossible to measure.

Two types of variables emerge from the analysis: one group defines and sets the environment within which the child must adapt if he or she is to survive (these variables will be referred to as conditioning factors of child health). Examples of such conditioners are family wealth, parental age and education level; each of these determines the family's access to basic needs. A second group of variables are catalytic in function (to be referred to as risk factors of morbidity) and, when present, can lead to infection, if a certain set of conditioning forces is present. For example, the mother with infection places all other family members at risk to infection (indeed maternal infection is the single most decisive determinant of child infection); however, if the family has access to health care, determined by such family variables as paternal occupation and family wealth, then the mother's risk potential may be quickly mitigated.

The health status of children is set by both conditioners and risk variables. Conditioning variables are generally interrelated and stem from the economic structure, political organization, and social values of a nation which, in turn, dictate distribution and access to basic needs of communities and families. Birth weight, weaning age and foods, and intra-family health, are some of the specific variables that determine a child's risk of illness. Risk factors are mitigated by optimum conditioning variables (e.g., access to sanitation, and health care) and aggravated by unfavorable conditioners (e.g., inadequate sanitation and health care).

Aggregate morbidity rates, at least in the short run do not measure the survival or adaptive state of children or a population. An ecological approach that relates both conditioning and risk factors is necessary to unravel the mechanisms by which a community, a family, or a given child cope with or succumb to the negative, nonadaptive effects of infection. To sift out contributing versus confounding variables, a process is needed that establishes both conditioning and risk forces and seeks to quantify their synergistic effects. For example, how does a physical variable (e.g., altitude) interface with a biological one (birth weight) and a family conditioner (access to weaning foods; plus an associated risk variable, maternal health) to determine child health at varying ages and stages of development? It is essential to go beyond easy-to-measure traditional variables if we are to develop a model of child health which accounts for a major proportion of the variance exhibited by any sample of children (see, e.g., Solimano and Vine, 1980).

BIFFRET DIAZ, DANIEL GALLEGOS, FEDERICO MURILLO, VIVIAN LUNNY LENART, WILLIAM H. WEIDMAN, AND ROBERT I. GOLDSMITH

Chapter 9

DISEASE AND DISABILITY AMONG THE AYMARA

Introduction

Few systematic, community-wide studies have been published that provide a clear perspective on acute and chronic disease and disability among people indigenous to altitudes of 4000 meters or more. Morococha (4500 meters) in Perú has been studied by the staff of San Marcos University's Institute of Andean Biology and by members of Cayetano Heredia University. Buck and colleagues (1968) have examined health status in four Peruvian villages, of which one (Pusi, population 500) was at an elevation of 3500 meters. And, finally, Omran, McEwen, and Zaki (1967) have reported findings derived from the study of eight Bolivian communities, three of which (Compi, San Miguel, and Penas) are in the altiplano. However, most of what is known about high-altitude disease and disability involves risks associated with special occupations or age groups, and there is a paucity of information on disease and disability in the typical highland Aymará or Quechua village or town. Some data are available, of course, from cities such as La Paz, Cuzco, and Arequipa, but these are generally based upon hospital admissions, an uncertain guide where the vast majority of people have little access to medical attention. Nonetheless, these observations appear to confirm higher morbidity and mortality from respiratory, gallbladder, and liver disease.

Andean men and women are generally presumed to have adapted effectively to the lessened oxygen, rigorous temperatures, and low humidity that go with life in the highlands where they reside (Hurtado, 1964; Monge and Monge, 1966; and Frisancho, 1975). However, some of their apparent adaptations may have deleterious health effects in the long run. For example, increased hematopoiesis can lead to a higher frequency of gallbladder and liver disease, and to an elevated serum uric acid level stemming from increased red blood cell destruction (Lewis and Gardner, 1960; Page et al., 1974). Higher serum uric acid levels, in turn, appear to be a coronary risk factor in some populations, although admittedly not a certain one (Hall, 1965; Jacobs, 1972; McEwin et al., 1974; and Klein et al., 1973; but see also, for example, Ciswicka-Sznajderman et al., 1972 or Allard and Goulet, 1973). Elevated hemoglobin and hematocrit, both characteristic of high-altitude dwellers, have been associated with an increased risk of coronary heart disease in Framingham (Dawber, 1963), an association confirmed by Heyden and colleagues (1971) among white residents of Evans County, Georgia. Similarly, polycythemia predisposes to thrombus formation

William J. Schull and Francisco Rothhammer (eds.), The Aymará: Strategies in Human Adaptation to a Rigorous Environment, 101-131. ©1990 *by Kluwer Academic Publishers.*

(Erf, 1956) and physiologic evidence suggests that increased blood viscosity, as measured by hematocrit levels, could increase the risk of coronary heart disease.

Pulmonary edema is a recognized hazard for the high-altitude dweller upon his or her return to altitude after a stay at sea level (Hurtado, 1937), and the seemingly acute loss of adaptation known as Monge's disease, which appears to threaten all indigenous inhabitants, must add to the perils of highland life (Monge and Monge, 1966). Similarly, the miner's scourge, pneumoconiosis, causes respiratory insufficiency at sea level, and its occurrence among miners at the higher altitudes would seem especially threatening. However, the functional effects of this disorder appear to be different at high altitudes than at sea level. Hurtado (1944, see also Cosio, 1973) reports no reduction in residual air among high-altitude miners with this disease (there is a reduction in vital capacity); this contrasts with the diminution seen at sea level. But, simple comparisons based solely upon altitude differences are hazardous, for it is now recognized that the impact of pneumoconiosis upon the miner depends on the nature of the dust that he inhales (Morgan et al., 1972a; Marek and Kujawska, 1973). Indeed, the risk itself appears to be related to smoking as well as to other extraneous factors which may condition the symptomatology of the disease as well as its incidence and prevalence (Morgan et al., 1972a; Morgan et al., 1972b).

But these observations, often necessarily opportunistic, are a weak platform on which to assess public health needs or base public health policy in an area so unique. Accordingly, one of the aims of this study was to provide data on a more representative cross-section of the health needs of sierran and altiplano residents.

The present study

The standardized clinical examination described in Chapter 1 called for comments on 1) general appearance, 2) the skin, 3) the head (including the face, mouth, and throat, nose, and ears – the latter including the eardrums, cerumen type, and general observations), 4) the neck (including venous engorgement and the thyroid), 5) the lymphatics, 6) the abdomen, 7) the bones and joints, 8) the spine and other parts of the musculoskeletal system, 9) the extremities, and 10) the nervous system (a neurological appraisal).

Special attention was given to the chest and lungs, since one of the program's other objectives was evaluation of pulmonary and cardiovascular changes and relationships between altitude and cardiopulmonary status. This portion of the examination required comments on the subject's respiratory rate, tachypnea, posterior-anterior diameters, decrease in diaphragm motion, percussion, breath sounds, adventitious sounds, pulse and apical rate, apical impulses (including character and location), thrills, heart tones, rhythm, systolic murmurs (both significant and insignificant), diastolic murmurs, and quality of arterial pulsations. Two blood pressure measurements, made with a mercury sphygmomanometer having an appropriate size cuff, were recorded from the right arm with the subject sitting. (Korotkoff sounds I, IV, and V were recorded.

Korotkoff IV was used for diastolic blood pressure.) Finally, a resting 12 lead electrocardiogram was recorded with the subject supine using a portable Hewlett-Packard Sanborn machine.

All of the evaluations of the chest, lungs, and heart in Chile were made by one cardiologist (Weidman); six physicians (four in 1973 and two in 1974) conducted the remainder of the examinations. In Bolivia, the examinations of the chest and lungs were performed by a cardiologist (Lenart), and the general clinical appraisals by several physicians from Bolivia.

Diagnostic standards

Given the traditional metrics of clinical medicine, the capacity to recognize and describe properly the presence of disease can vary widely from one physician to another. So it is important in a study such as ours, which attempts to examine differences in the 'burden' of disease and disability as a function of hypoxia, to be able to demonstrate that no systematic diagnostic biases exist. As previously stated, seven different physicians participated in our clinical evaluations in Chile and an additional four in Bolivia; so there was clearly ample opportunity for systematic biases which might fortuitously affect the data so as to suggest altitude differences. We have, therefore, examined the general frequencies of disease and disability encountered at different altitudes (the coast and sierra) in the years 1973 and 1974 when different physicians were involved in the general examinations. While individual diagnoses differed (but in a manner wholly explicable by chance), the overall rates in the two years were comparable. In 1973, 1.40 diagnoses were made for each individual examined; in 1974, this figure was 1.34. Within ecological niches in Chile, these values were 1.20 versus 1.19 for the coast, and 1.44 versus 1.92 for the sierra. It bears noting that the proportion of males seen in the years 1973 and 1974 did not differ significantly, nor did the proportion of children. Tables 1 through 6 give the number of occurrences of various diagnoses and diagnostic rubrics for children (<15 years of age) and adults (≥15 years of age) at the different altitudes and for the different ethnic groups. Tables 1 through 3 are for permanent residents and Tables 4 through 6 for non-permanent residents.

Some of the diagnoses in these tables are matters of clinical judgment, while others, such as the diagnosis of hypertension, are matters of convention. In the latter connection we recorded two events, namely, 'frank' and 'borderline' hypertension. We defined 'borderline' hypertension among individuals 15 years of age or older as a systolic pressure of 140-159 mm of mercury and/or a diastolic pressure of 90-94, while 'frank' hypertension represented a systolic pressure of 160 or greater and/or a diastolic pressure of 95 or more. Hypertension, frank or borderline, is less clearly defined in children (subjects under 15 years of age) and the definition is likely age-dependent; but experience suggests that systolic pressures over 140 mm or diastolic pressures over 90 are abnormal. Though these standards do not adequately recognize cardiovascular disease at high altitude in our view, we accepted them for purposes of

Table 1a
Distribution of diseases and disorders among the Aymará children[1]
examined in the population of the Departments of Arica, Chile and Oruro, Bolivia
by sex and ecological niche (permanent residents of each niche only)

		Coast		Sierra		Altiplano Chile		Altiplano Bolivia		Total	
Disease category	ICDA code	M	F	M	F	M	F	M	F	M	F
Infective and parasitic	*000-136*	-	-	1	-	5	6	5	3	11	9
Neoplasms	*140-239*	-	-	-	-	1	-	-	-	1	-
Malignant	140-209	-	-	-	-	-	-	-	-	-	-
Benign or unspecified	210-239	-	-	-	-	1	-	-	-	1	-
Endocrine, nutritional, metabolic	*240-279*	1	1	1	1	3	2	-	1	5	5
Diabetes	250	-	-	-	-	-	-	-	-	-	-
Blood, blood forming organs	*280-289*	1	-	-	-	-	-	1	-	2	-
Mental disorders	*290-315*	-	-	-	2	-	-	-	-	-	2
Nervous system, sense organs	*320-389*	-	-	1	4	7	-	1	-	9	4
Nervous system	320-358	-	-	-	-	2	-	1	-	3	-
Eye	360-379	-	-	1	1	3	-	-	-	4	1
Ear, mastoid process	380-389	-	-	-	3	2	-	-	-	2	3
Circulatory system	*390-458*	1	-	6	-	-	2	-	2	7	4
Acute hypertension (≥160/95)	401	-	-	-	-	-	-	-	-	-	-
Borderline hypertension (≥140/90)	401.0	-	-	-	-	-	1	-	-	-	1
Acute MI	410	-	-	-	-	-	-	-	-	-	-
Other ischemic heart disease	411-414	-	-	-	-	-	-	-	-	-	-
All other heart disease	390-429	1	-	6	-	-	1	0	2	7	3
CVA	430-438	-	-	-	-	-	-	-	-	-	-
Respiratory system	*460-519*	-	2	8	9	29	29	11	3	48	43
Acute resp. infect.; except influenza tonsillitis, sinusitis	460-466	-	1	5	5	19	22	11	3	35	31
Pneumonia	480-486	-	-	-	-	-	2	-	-	-	2
Acute tonsillitis, hypertrophy of tonsils and adenoids	463,500	-	-	3	2	8	5	-	-	11	7
Digestive system	*520-577*	-	-	3	-	2	4	-	-	5	4
Inguinal hernia	550,552	-	-	-	-	-	-	-	-	-	-
Cholelithiasis, cholecystitis	574,575	-	-	-	-	-	-	-	-	-	-
Genitourinary system	*580-629*	-	-	-	-	1	-	-	-	1	-
Urinary system	580-599	-	-	-	-	-	-	-	-	-	-
Hyperplasia of prostate	600	-	-	-	-	-	-	-	-	-	-
Disorders of menstruation	626	-	-	-	-	-	-	-	-	-	-
Complications of pregnancy	*630-678*	-	-	-	-	-	-	-	-	-	-
Skin, subcutaneous tissue	*680-709*	1	-	11	14	12	12	1	-	25	26
Musculoskeletal, connect. tissue	*710-738*	-	-	2	1	1	2	1	1	4	4
Arthritis, all forms	710-718	-	-	-	-	-	-	-	-	-	-
Congenital anomalies	*740-759*	-	1	5	-	5	5	3	-	13	6
Symptoms, ill-defined conditions	*780-796*	1	1	10	4	20	13	-	-	31	18
Accidents	*800-999*	-	-	3	1	1	-	-	-	4	1
Conditions, exams w/o sickness	*793, Y00-Y13*	-	-	-	-	-	2	-	-	-	2
Total all diagnoses (italics)		5	5	51	36	87	77	23	10	166	128
People examined		5	6	37	33	87	82	39	33	168	154

Adapted from Díaz et al. (1978) and Murillo et al. (1980).
\- = 0
[1] Subjects less than 15 years of age.

Table 1b
Distribution of diseases and disorders among the Aymará adults[1]
examined in the population of the Departments of Arica, Chile and Oruro, Bolivia
by sex and ecological niche (permanent residents of each niche only)

Disease category	ICDA code	Coast M	Coast F	Sierra M	Sierra F	Altiplano Chile M	Altiplano Chile F	Altiplano Bolivia M	Altiplano Bolivia F	Total M	Total F
Infective and parasitic	*000-136*	-	-	*1*	*1*	*4*	*1*	*5*	*9*	*10*	*11*
Neoplasms	*140-239*	-	-	-	-	*3*	*2*	*2*	*1*	*5*	*3*
Malignant	140-209	-	-	-	-	-	-	1	1	1	1
Benign or unspecified	210-239	-	-	-	-	3	2	1	-	4	2
Endocrine, nutritional, metabolic	*240-279*	*1*	*1*	*2*	-	*3*	*9*	-	*2*	*6*	*12*
Diabetes	250	-	-	-	-	-	-	-	-	-	-
Blood, blood forming organs	*280-289*	-	-	-	-	-	*1*	-	-	-	*1*
Mental disorders	*290-315*	-	-	*1*	*1*	-	-	-	-	*1*	*1*
Nervous system, sense organs	*320-389*	*1*	-	*7*	*10*	*14*	*5*	*15*	*10*	*37*	*25*
Nervous system	320-358	1	-	1	-	-	-	2	1	4	1
Eye	360-379	-	-	1	3	5	2	5	1	11	6
Ear, mastoid process	380-389	-	-	5	7	9	3	8	8	22	18
Circulatory system	*390-458*	*2*	-	*8*	*16*	*18*	*16*	*12*	*9*	*40*	*41*
Acute hypertension (≥160/95)	401	-	-	2	2	3	1	1	2	6	5
Borderline hypertension (≥140/90)	401.0	1	-	2	5	8	4	-	4	11	13
Acute MI	410	-	-	-	-	-	-	-	-	-	-
Other ischemic heart disease	411-414	-	-	-	-	-	-	1	1	1	1
All other heart disease	390-429	1	-	1	1	3	7	7	1	12	9
CVA	430-438	-	-	-	-	-	-	-	-	-	-
Respiratory system	*460-519*	-	-	*3*	*8*	*9*	*9*	*4*	*7*	*16*	*24*
Acute resp. infect.; except influenza tonsillitis, sinusitis	460-466	-	-	1	2	3	-	1	5	5	7
Pneumonia	480-486	-	-	1	3	-	2	-	-	1	5
Acute tonsillitis, hypertrophy of tonsils and adenoids	463,500	-	-	-	1	2	4	-	-	2	5
Digestive system	*520-577*	-	-	*1*	*6*	*8*	*11*	*9*	*8*	*18*	*25*
Inguinal hernia	550,552	-	-	1	-	-	-	2	-	3	-
Cholelithiasis, cholecystitis	574,575	-	-	-	-	-	3	-	2	-	5
Genitourinary system	*580-629*	-	-	-	*2*	*2*	*1*	-	*4*	*2*	*7*
Urinary system	580-599	-	-	-	1	-	-	-	-	-	1
Hyperplasia of prostate	600	-	-	-	-	1	-	-	-	1	-
Disorders of menstruation	626	-	-	-	-	-	-	-	3	-	3
Complications of pregnancy	*630-678*	-	-	-	-	-	-	-	*2*	-	*2*
Skin, subcutaneous tissue	*680-709*	-	-	*7*	*9*	*16*	*18*	*8*	*16*	*31*	*43*
Musculoskeletal, connect. tissue	*710-738*	*2*	-	*3*	*5*	*8*	*8*	*3*	*4*	*16*	*17*
Arthritis, all forms	710-718	-	-	1	2	1	2	1	2	3	6
Congenital anomalies	*740-759*	*1*	-	*1*	*1*	*3*	*3*	*2*	-	*7*	*4*
Symptoms, ill-defined conditions	*780-796*	*2*	*1*	*11*	*19*	*28*	*27*	*9*	*6*	*50*	*53*
Accidents	*800-999*	-	-	*3*	*2*	*4*	*3*	-	-	*7*	*5*
Conditions, exams w/o sickness	*793, Y00-Y13*	-	-	-	-	*1*	*5*	-	*4*	*1*	*9*
Total all diagnoses (italics)		*9*	*2*	*48*	*80*	*121*	*119*	*69*	*82*	*247*	*283*
People examined		5	1	21	38	59	69	41	53	126	161

Adapted from Díaz et al. (1978) and Murillo et al. (1980).
- = 0

[1] Subjects 15 years of age and older

Table 2a
Distribution of diseases and disorders among the mestizo children[1]
examined in the population of the Departments of Arica, Chile and Oruro, Bolivia
by sex and ecological niche (permanent residents of each niche only)

		Coast		Sierra		Altiplano Chile		Altiplano Bolivia		Total	
Disease category	ICDA code	M	F	M	F	M	F	M	F	M	F
Infective and parasitic	*000-136*	*6*	*5*	*1*	*5*	*5*	*2*	*8*	*5*	*20*	*17*
Neoplasms	*140-239*	-	-	*1*	-	*2*	-	-	-	*3*	-
Malignant	140-209	-	-	-	-	-	-	-	-	-	-
Benign or unspecified	210-239	-	-	1	-	2	-	-	-	3	-
Endocrine, nutritional, metabolic	*240-279*	*4*	*3*	*5*	*2*	-	*1*	-	-	*9*	*6*
Diabetes	250	-	-	-	-	-	-	-	-	-	-
Blood, blood forming organs	*280-289*	*4*	-	-	-	-	-	-	*1*	*4*	*1*
Mental disorders	*290-315*	-	-	*1*	*2*	-	-	-	-	*1*	*2*
Nervous system, sense organs	*320-389*	*5*	*1*	*8*	*7*	*4*	*5*	*10*	*3*	*27*	*16*
Nervous system	320-358	-	-	-	1	-	-	-	-	-	1
Eye	360-379	2	-	3	1	4	4	5	1	14	6
Ear, mastoid process	380-389	3	1	5	5	-	1	5	2	13	9
Circulatory system	*390-458*	*5*	*5*	*8*	*5*	*3*	-	-	*4*	*16*	*14*
Acute hypertension (≥160/95)	401	-	-	-	-	-	-	-	-	-	-
Borderline hypertension (≥140/90)	401.0	1	-	-	-	1	-	-	1	2	1
Acute MI	410	-	-	-	-	-	-	-	-	-	-
Other ischemic heart disease	411-414	-	-	-	-	-	-	-	-	-	-
All other heart disease	390-429	4	5	8	5	2	-	-	3	14	13
CVA	430-438	-	-	-	-	-	-	-	-	-	-
Respiratory system	*460-519*	*8*	*20*	*28*	*30*	*23*	*22*	*9*	*5*	*68*	*77*
Acute resp. infect.; except influenza tonsillitis, sinusitis	460-466	6	12	16	16	14	13	9	4	45	45
Pneumonia	480-486	-	1	-	1	2	-	-	-	2	2
Acute tonsillitis, hypertrophy of tonsils and adenoids	463,500	1	5	10	11	6	9	-	1	17	26
Digestive system	*520-577*	*1*	*3*	*2*	-	*2*	*1*	*1*	*4*	*6*	*8*
Inguinal hernia	550,552	-	-	-	-	-	-	-	-	-	-
Cholelithiasis, cholecystitis	574,575	-	-	-	-	-	-	-	-	-	-
Genitourinary system	*580-629*	*1*	*1*	-	-	*1*	-	-	-	*2*	*1*
Urinary system	580-599	-	-	-	-	-	-	-	-	-	-
Hyperplasia of prostate	600	-	-	-	-	-	-	-	-	-	-
Disorders of menstruation	626	-	1	-	-	-	-	-	-	-	1
Complications of pregnancy	*630-678*	-	-	-	-	-	-	-	-	-	-
Skin, subcutaneous tissue	*680-709*	*6*	*4*	*33*	*32*	*3*	*5*	*1*	*1*	*43*	*42*
Musculoskeletal, connect. tissue	*710-738*	*1*	*2*	-	*2*	*2*	*4*	*3*	*1*	*6*	*9*
Arthritis, all forms	710-718	-	-	-	-	-	-	-	-	-	-
Congenital anomalies	*740-759*	*3*	*2*	*2*	*7*	*5*	*4*	*7*	*1*	*17*	*14*
Symptoms, ill-defined conditions	*780-796*	*17*	*6*	*25*	*28*	*19*	*14*	*6*	*2*	*67*	*50*
Accidents	*800-999*	*1*	-	*2*	-	*1*	*1*	*2*	-	*6*	*1*
Conditions, exams w/o sickness	*793, Y00-Y13*	-	-	-	-	-	-	-	-	-	-
Total all diagnoses (italics)		*62*	*52*	*116*	*120*	*70*	*59*	*47*	*27*	*295*	*258*
People examined		78	73	96	104	59	69	73	63	306	309

Adapted from Díaz et al. (1978) and Murillo et al. (1980).
- = 0
[1] Subjects less than 15 years of age

Table 2b
Distribution of diseases and disorders among the mestizo adults[1] examined in the population of the Departments of Arica, Chile and Oruro, Bolivia by sex and ecological niche (permanent residents of each niche only)

		Coast		Sierra		Altiplano Chile		Altiplano Bolivia		Total	
Disease category	ICDA code	M	F	M	F	M	F	M	F	M	F
Infective and parasitic	*000-136*	-	1	1	7	1	1	5	7	7	16
Neoplasms	*140-239*	1	2	-	2	-	1	1	-	2	5
Malignant	140-209	-	-	-	-	-	-	-	-	-	-
Benign or unspecified	210-239	1	2	-	2	-	1	1	-	2	5
Endocrine, nutritional, metabolic	*240-279*	-	5	2	2	1	4	-	1	3	12
Diabetes	250	-	-	-	-	-	-	-	1	-	1
Blood, blood forming organs	*280-289*	1	1	-	-	-	1	1	4	2	6
Mental disorders	*290-315*	-	1	2	1	-	-	-	-	2	2
Nervous system, sense organs	*320-389*	1	-	5	4	2	4	17	14	25	22
Nervous system	320-358	-	-		-	-	-	1	-	1	-
Eye	360-379	-	-	2	-	1	2	12	5	15	7
Ear, mastoid process	380-389	1	-	3	4	1	2	4	9	9	15
Circulatory system	*390-458*	12	6	9	9	10	12	9	7	40	34
Acute hypertension (≥160/95)	401	1	2	-	3	2	1	-	-	3	6
Borderline hypertension (≥140/90)	401.0	5	3	3	1	1	2	2	3	11	9
Acute MI	410	-	-	-	-	-	-	-	-	-	-
Other ischemic heart disease	411-414	-	-	-	1	-	-	2	-	2	1
All other heart disease	390-429	5	1	2	3	5	7	3	4	15	15
CVA	430-438	-	-	1	-	-	-	-	-	1	-
Respiratory system	*460-519*	-	1	3	9	5	6	3	1	11	17
Acute resp. infect.; except influenza tonsillitis, sinusitis	460-466	-	-	-	3	-	1	2	1	2	5
Pneumonia	480-486	-	-	1	3	-	-	-	-	1	3
Acute tonsillitis, hypertrophy of tonsils and adenoids	463,500	-	-	2	3	-	-	1	-	3	3
Digestive system	*520-577*	4	1	-	-	2	4	6	5	12	10
Inguinal hernia	550,552	-	-	-	-	1	-	3	-	4	-
Cholelithiasis, cholecystitis	574,575	-	-	-	-	-	-	2	3	2	3
Genitourinary system	*580-629*	-	1	-	2	1	2	1	8	2	13
Urinary system	580-599	-	-	-	-	-	-	-	-	-	-
Hyperplasia of prostate	600	-	-	-	-	1	-	-	-	1	-
Disorders of menstruation	626	-	1	-	1	-	-	-	-	-	2
Complications of pregnancy	*630-678*	-	-	-	-	-	-	-	-	-	-
Skin, subcutaneous tissue	*680-709*	4	7	7	10	5	14	10	8	26	39
Musculoskeletal, connect. tissue	*710-738*	2	2	8	2	7	2	9	4	26	10
Arthritis, all forms	710-718	-	-	1	1	-	-	3	2	4	3
Congenital anomalies	*740-759*	1	-	3	3	1	3	2	2	7	8
Symptoms, ill-defined conditions	*780-796*	4	1	7	16	8	10	9	4	28	31
Accidents	*800-999*	-	-	2	1	3	-	2	-	7	1
Conditions, exams w/o sickness	*793, Y00-Y13*	-	-	-	1	-	2	-	8	-	11
Total all diagnoses (italics)		30	29	49	69	46	66	75	73	200	237
People examined		30	23	30	33	22	30	41	42	123	128

Adapted from Díaz et al. (1978) and Murillo et al. (1980).
- = 0
[1] Subjects 15 years of age and older

Table 3a
Distribution of diseases and disorders among the non-Aymará children[1] examined in the population of the Departments of Arica, Chile and Oruro, Bolivia by sex and ecological niche (permanent residents of each niche only)

		Coast		Sierra		Altiplano Chile		Altiplano Bolivia		Total	
Disease category	ICDA code	M	F	M	F	M	F	M	F	M	F
Infective and parasitic	*000-136*	*1*	*1*	-	-	-	-	-	-	*1*	*1*
Neoplasms	*140-239*	-	-	-	-	-	-	-	-	-	-
Malignant	140-209	-	-	-	-	-	-	-	-	-	-
Benign or unspecified	210-239	-	-	-	-	-	-	-	-	-	-
Endocrine, nutritional, metabolic	*240-279*	*2*	-	-	-	-	-	-	-	*2*	-
Diabetes	250	-	-	-	-	-	-	-	-	-	-
Blood, blood forming organs	*280-289*	-	-	-	-	-	-	-	-	-	-
Mental disorders	*290-315*	-	-	*1*	-	-	-	-	-	*1*	-
Nervous system, sense organs	*320-389*	-	*1*	-	*1*	-	-	-	-	-	*2*
Nervous system	320-358	-	-	-	1	-	-	-	-	-	1
Eye	360-379	-	-	-	-	-	-	-	-	-	-
Ear, mastoid process	380-389	-	1	-	-	-	-	-	-	-	1
Circulatory system	*390-458*	*4*	*2*	-	-	-	-	-	-	*4*	*2*
Acute hypertension (≥160/95)	401	-	-	-	-	-	-	-	-	-	-
Borderline hypertension (≥140/90)	401.0	-	1	-	-	-	-	-	-	-	1
Acute MI	410	-	-	-	-	-	-	-	-	-	-
Other ischemic heart disease	411-414	-	-	-	-	-	-	-	-	-	-
All other heart disease	390-429	4	1	-	-	-	-	-	-	4	1
CVA	430-438	-	-	-	-	-	-	-	-	-	-
Respiratory system	*460-519*	*6*	*4*	*2*	*1*	-	-	-	-	*8*	*5*
Acute resp. infect.; except influenza tonsillitis, sinusitis	460-466	2	2	2	-	-	-	-	-	4	2
Pneumonia	480-486	-	-	-	-	-	-	-	-	-	-
Acute tonsillitis, hypertrophy of tonsils and adenoids	463,500	3	2	-	1	-	-	-	-	3	3
Digestive system	*520-577*	-	-	-	-	-	-	-	-	-	-
Inguinal hernia	550,552	-	-	-	-	-	-	-	-	-	-
Cholelithiasis, cholecystitis	574,575	-	1	-	-	-	-	-	-	-	-
Genitourinary system	*580-629*	*1*	-	-	-	-	-	-	-	*1*	-
Urinary system	580-599	-	-	-	-	-	-	-	-	-	-
Hyperplasia of prostate	600	-	-	-	-	-	-	-	-	-	-
Disorders of menstruation	626	-	-	-	-	-	-	-	-	-	-
Complications of pregnancy	*630-678*	-	-	-	-	-	-	-	-	-	-
Skin, subcutaneous tissue	*680-709*	*3*	*6*	-	-	-	-	-	-	*3*	*6*
Musculoskeletal, connect. tissue	*710-738*	-	-	-	-	-	-	-	-	-	-
Arthritis, all forms	710-718	-	-	-	-	-	-	-	-	-	-
Congenital anomalies	*740-759*	-	*2*	-	-	-	-	-	-	-	*2*
Symptoms, ill-defined conditions	*780-796*	*5*	*5*	*1*	-	-	-	-	-	*6*	*5*
Accidents	*800-999*	-	-	-	-	-	-	-	-	-	-
Conditions, exams w/o sickness	*793, Y00-Y13*	-	-	-	-	-	-	-	-	-	-
Total all diagnoses (italics)		*22*	*21*	*4*	*2*	-	-	-	-	*26*	*23*
People examined		29	40	1	4	1	-	3	1	34	45

Adapted from Díaz et al. (1978) and Murillo et al. (1980).
- = 0
[1] Subjects less than 15 years of age

Table 3b
Distribution of diseases and disorders among the non-Aymará adults[1] examined in the population of the Departments of Arica, Chile and Oruro, Bolivia by sex and ecological niche (permanent residents of each niche only)

Disease category	ICDA code	Coast		Sierra		Altiplano Chile		Altiplano Bolivia		Total	
		M	F	M	F	M	F	M	F	M	F
Infective and parasitic	*000-136*	-	-	-	-	-	-	-	*1*	-	*2*
Neoplasms	*140-239*	*2*	*1*	-	-	-	-	-	-	*2*	*1*
Malignant	140-209	-	1	-	-	-	-	-	-	-	1
Benign or unspecified	210-239	2	-	-	-	-	-	-	-	2	-
Endocrine, nutritional, metabolic	*240-279*	*3*	*13*	-	*1*	-	-	-	-	*3*	*14*
Diabetes	250	-	-	-	-	-	-	-	-	-	-
Blood, blood forming organs	*280-289*	*4*	*1*	-	-	-	*1*	-	-	*4*	*2*
Mental disorders	*290-315*	*2*	*3*	-	-	-	-	-	-	*2*	*3*
Nervous system, sense organs	*320-389*	*10*	*1*	*4*	*3*	-	-	*1*	*1*	*15*	*5*
Nervous system	320-358	3	-	-	-	-	-	-	-	3	-
Eye	360-379	2	-	2	1	-	-	1	-	5	1
Ear, mastoid process	380-389	5	1	2	2	-	-	-	1	7	4
Circulatory system	*390-458*	*20*	*28*	*3*	*1*	*3*	-	-	-	*26*	*29*
Acute hypertension (≥160/95)	401	3	9	-	-	1	-	-	-	4	9
Borderline hypertension (≥140/90)	401.0	9	6	1	1	-	-	-	-	10	7
Acute MI	410	-	-	-	-	-	-	-	-	-	-
Other ischemic heart disease	411-414	-	1	-	-	-	-	-	-	-	1
All other heart disease	390-429	5	5	-	-	-	-	-	-	5	5
CVA	430-438	-	-	-	-	-	-	-	-	-	-
Respiratory system	*460-519*	*9*	*5*	*1*	*5*	-	-	-	-	*10*	*10*
Acute resp. infect.; except influenza tonsillitis, sinusitis	460-466	4	3	1	2	-	-	-	-	5	5
Pneumonia	480-486	1	-	-	1	-	-	-	-	1	1
Acute tonsillitis, hypertrophy of tonsils and adenoids	463,500	-	1	-	-	-	-	-	-	-	1
Digestive system	*520-577*	*5*	*5*	-	-	*2*	*1*	*1*	-	*8*	*6*
Inguinal hernia	550,552	1	-	-	-	-	-	-	-	1	-
Cholelithiasis, cholecystitis	574,575	-	-	-	-	-	-	-	-	-	1
Genitourinary system	*580-629*	*2*	*1*	-	-	-	-	-	-	*2*	*1*
Urinary system	580-599	-	1	-	-	-	-	-	-	-	1
Hyperplasia of prostate	600	1	-	-	-	-	-	-	-	1	-
Disorders of menstruation	626	-	-	-	-	-	-	-	-	-	-
Complications of pregnancy	*630-678*	-	-	-	-	-	-	-	-	-	-
Skin, subcutaneous tissue	*680-709*	*7*	*13*	*2*	*2*	-	-	*1*	*1*	*10*	*16*
Musculoskeletal, connect. tissue	*710-738*	*9*	*10*	*2*	*1*	*2*	-	-	*1*	*13*	*12*
Arthritis, all forms	710-718	2	2	-	-	1	-	-	1	3	3
Congenital anomalies	*740-759*	*1*	-	-	-	*1*	-	-	-	*2*	-
Symptoms, ill-defined conditions	*780-796*	*15*	*6*	*5*	*1*	*4*	-	*1*	-	*25*	*7*
Accidents	*800-999*	-	-	-	-	-	*1*	-	-	-	*1*
Conditions, exams w/o sickness	*793, Y00-Y13*	*1*	-	-	-	-	-	-	-	*1*	-
Total all diagnoses (italics)		*90*	*87*	*17*	*14*	*12*	*3*	*4*	*4*	*123*	*108*
People examined		49	52	7	6	3	1	2	2	61	61

Adapted from Díaz et al. (1978) and Murillo et al. (1980).
- = 0
1 Subjects 15 years of age and older

Table 4a
Distribution of diseases and disorders among the Aymará children[1]
examined in the population of the Departments of Arica, Chile and Oruro, Bolivia
by sex and ecological niche (non-permanent residents of each niche only)

		Coast		Sierra		Altiplano Chile		Altiplano Bolivia		Total	
Disease category	ICDA code	M	F	M	F	M	F	M	F	M	F
Infective and parasitic	*000-136*	-	-	-	*1*	-	*1*	-	-	-	*2*
Neoplasms	*140-239*	-	-	-	-	-	-	-	-	-	-
Malignant	140-209	-	-	-	-	-	-	-	-	-	-
Benign or unspecified	210-239	-	-	-	-	-	-	-	-	-	-
Endocrine, nutritional, metabolic	*240-279*	-	-	*1*	-	-	-	-	-	*1*	-
Diabetes	250	-	-	-	-	-	-	-	-	-	-
Blood, blood forming organs	*280-289*	-	-	-	-	-	-	-	-	-	-
Mental disorders	*290-315*	-	-	-	-	-	-	-	-	-	-
Nervous system, sense organs	*320-389*	-	-	*1*	*1*	-	-	-	-	*1*	*1*
Nervous system	320-358	-	-	-	-	-	-	-	-	-	-
Eye	360-379	-	-	-	1	-	-	-	-	-	1
Ear, mastoid process	380-389	-	-	1	-	-	-	-	-	1	-
Circulatory system	*390-458*	-	-	*2*	-	-	-	-	-	*2*	-
Acute hypertension (≥160/95)	401	-	-	-	-	-	-	-	-	-	-
Borderline hypertension (≥140/90)	401.0	-	-	-	-	-	-	-	-	-	-
Acute MI	410	-	-	-	-	-	-	-	-	-	-
Other ischemic heart disease	411-414	-	-	-	-	-	-	-	-	-	-
All other heart disease	390-429	-	-	2	-	-	-	-	-	2	-
CVA	430-438	-	-	-	-	-	-	-	-	-	-
Respiratory system	*460-519*	-	-	*1*	*1*	*4*	*1*	-	-	*5*	*2*
Acute resp. infect.; except influenza tonsillitis, sinusitis	460-466	-	-	1	1	1	1	-	-	2	2
Pneumonia	480-486	-	-	-	-	-	-	-	-	-	-
Acute tonsillitis, hypertrophy of tonsils and adenoids	463,500	-	-	-	-	3	-	-	-	3	-
Digestive system	*520-577*	-	-	-	-	-	-	-	-	-	-
Inguinal hernia	550,552	-	-	-	-	-	-	-	-	-	-
Cholelithiasis, cholecystitis	574,575	-	-	-	-	-	-	-	-	-	-
Genitourinary system	*580-629*	-	-	-	-	-	-	-	-	-	-
Urinary system	580-599	-	-	-	-	-	-	-	-	-	-
Hyperplasia of prostate	600	-	-	-	-	-	-	-	-	-	-
Disorders of menstruation	626	-	-	-	-	-	-	-	-	-	-
Complications of pregnancy	*630-678*	-	-	-	-	-	-	-	-	-	-
Skin, subcutaneous tissue	*680-709*	-	*1*	*1*	*3*	*1*	*1*	-	-	*2*	*5*
Musculoskeletal, connect. tissue	*710-738*	-	-	-	-	-	-	-	-	-	-
Arthritis, all forms	710-718	-	-	-	-	-	-	-	-	-	-
Congenital anomalies	*740-759*	-	-	-	-	*1*	-	-	-	*1*	-
Symptoms, ill-defined conditions	*780-796*	-	-	*3*	-	*1*	*1*	-	-	*4*	*1*
Accidents	*800-999*	-	-	-	-	-	-	-	-	-	-
Conditions, exams w/o sickness	*793, Y00-Y13*	-	-	-	-	-	-	-	-	-	-
Total all diagnoses (italics)		-	*1*	*9*	*6*	*7*	*4*	-	-	*16*	*11*
People examined		2	4	13	6	9	5	-	1	24	16

Adapted from Díaz et al. (1978) and Murillo et al. (1980).
- = 0
[1] Subjects less than 15 years of age

Table 4b
Distribution of diseases and disorders among the Aymará adults[1]
examined in the population of the Departments of Arica, Chile and Oruro, Bolivia
by sex and ecological niche (non-permanent residents of each niche only)

		Coast		Sierra		Altiplano Chile		Altiplano Bolivia		Total	
Disease category	ICDA code	M	F	M	F	M	F	M	F	M	F
Infective and parasitic	*000-136*	*2*	*1*	*1*	-	*2*	*2*	*1*	*3*	*6*	*6*
Neoplasms	*140-239*	-	*1*	-	*2*	-	*1*	-	-	-	*4*
Malignant	140-209	-	-	-	-	-	-	-	-	-	-
Benign or unspecified	210-239	-	1	-	2	-	1	-	-	-	4
Endocrine, nutritional, metabolic	*240-279*	*4*	*2*	*1*	*1*	-	-	-	-	*5*	*3*
Diabetes	250	-	-	-	-	-	-	-	-	-	-
Blood, blood forming organs	*280-289*	-	*2*	*1*	*1*	-	-	-	-	*1*	*3*
Mental disorders	*290-315*	-	-	*2*	*1*	-	*1*	-	-	*2*	*2*
Nervous system, sense organs	*320-389*	-	*3*	*12*	*5*	*3*	*1*	*2*	*4*	*17*	*13*
Nervous system	320-358	-	-	-	2	-	-	-	-	-	2
Eye	360-379	-	2	3	1	1	1	1	1	5	5
Ear, mastoid process	380-389	-	1	9	2	2	-	1	3	12	6
Circulatory system	*390-458*	*9*	*4*	*20*	*18*	*5*	*2*	*1*	*2*	*35*	*26*
Acute hypertension (≥160/95)	401	3	-	2	4	-	-	-	-	5	4
Borderline hypertension (≥140/90)	401.0	2	3	8	5	3	-	1	-	14	8
Acute MI	410	-	-	-	-	-	-	-	-	-	-
Other ischemic heart disease	411-414	-	-	-	-	-	-	-	-	-	-
All other heart disease	390-429	2	-	4	5	2	1	-	1	8	7
CVA	430-438	-	-	-	-	-	-	-	-	-	-
Respiratory system	*460-519*	-	*1*	*15*	*10*	*2*	*3*	*1*	-	*18*	*14*
Acute resp. infect.; except influenza tonsillitis, sinusitis	460-466	-	1	7	5	2	1	1	-	10	7
Pneumonia	480-486	-	-	1	3	-	-	-	-	1	3
Acute tonsillitis, hypertrophy of tonsils and adenoids	463,500	-	-	2	-	-	2	-	-	2	2
Digestive system	*520-577*	*3*	*4*	-	*3*	*2*	*1*	*3*	*3*	*8*	*11*
Inguinal hernia	550,552	-	1	-	-	-	-	-	-	-	1
Cholelithiasis, cholecystitis	574,575	-	1	-	-	-	-	1	2	1	3
Genitourinary system	*580-629*	-	-	*2*	*2*	-	*1*	-	*2*	*2*	*5*
Urinary system	580-599	-	-	1	-	-	-	-	-	1	-
Hyperplasia of prostate	600	-	-	1	-	-	-	-	-	1	-
Disorders of menstruation	626	-	-	-	1	-	1	-	-	-	2
Complications of pregnancy	*630-678*	-	-	-	-	-	-	-	-	-	-
Skin, subcutaneous tissue	*680-709*	*6*	*5*	*9*	*16*	*9*	*3*	*3*	*4*	*27*	*28*
Musculoskeletal, connect. tissue	*710-738*	*5*	*4*	*5*	*7*	*2*	*2*	-	*1*	*12*	*14*
Arthritis, all forms	710-718	2	1	1	2	1	-	-	1	4	4
Congenital anomalies	*740-759*	-	*1*	-	*1*	*2*	*3*	-	-	*2*	*5*
Symptoms, ill-defined conditions	*780-796*	*2*	*5*	*32*	*15*	*15*	*9*	-	*1*	*49*	*30*
Accidents	*800-999*	-	*1*	-	-	*1*	-	-	*1*	*1*	*2*
Conditions, exams w/o sickness	*793, Y00-Y13*	-	*3*	-	*1*	*2*	*2*	-	*1*	*2*	*7*
Total all diagnoses (italics)		*31*	*37*	*100*	*83*	*45*	*31*	*11*	*22*	*187*	*173*
People examined		26	22	55	47	31	22	5	7	117	98

Adapted from Díaz et al. (1978) and Murillo et al. (1980).
\- = 0

[1] Subjects 15 years of age and older

Table 5a
Distribution of diseases and disorders among the mestizo children[1]
examined in the population of the Departments of Arica, Chile and Oruro, Bolivia
by sex and ecological niche (non-permanent residents of each niche only)

		Coast		Sierra		Altiplano Chile		Altiplano Bolivia		Total	
Disease category	ICDA code	M	F	M	F	M	F	M	F	M	F
Infective and parasitic	*000-136*	*1*	*1*	-	-	-	*1*	-	-	*1*	*2*
Neoplasms	*140-239*	-	-	-	-	-	-	-	-	-	-
Malignant	140-209	-	-	-	-	-	-	-	-	-	-
Benign or unspecified	210-239	-	-	-	-	-	-	-	-	-	-
Endocrine, nutritional, metabolic	*240-279*	*1*	-	-	-	*1*	-	-	-	*2*	-
Diabetes	250	-	-	-	-	-	-	-	-	-	-
Blood, blood forming organs	*280-289*	*1*	-	-	-	-	-	-	-	*1*	-
Mental disorders	*290-315*	-	-	-	-	-	-	-	-	-	-
Nervous system, sense organs	*320-389*	*1*	*1*	*2*	*2*	*1*	*2*	-	-	*4*	*5*
Nervous system	320-358	-	-	-	-	-	-	-	-	-	-
Eye	360-379	-	-	2	-	-	-	-	-	2	-
Ear, mastoid process	380-389	1	1	-	2	1	2	-	-	2	5
Circulatory system	*390-458*	*4*	*2*	*4*	*5*	-	-	-	-	*8*	*7*
Acute hypertension ($\geq$160/95)	401	-	-	-	-	-	-	-	-	-	-
Borderline hypertension ($\geq$140/90)	401.0	-	-	-	-	-	-	-	-	-	-
Acute MI	410	-	-	-	-	-	-	-	-	-	-
Other ischemic heart disease	411-414	-	-	-	-	-	-	-	-	-	-
All other heart disease	390-429	4	2	4	5	-	-	-	-	8	7
CVA	430-438	-	-	-	-	-	-	-	-	-	-
Respiratory system	*460-519*	*3*	*6*	*6*	*9*	*7*	*3*	-	-	*16*	*18*
Acute resp. infect.; except influenza tonsillitis, sinusitis	460-466	1	3	3	6	4	2	-	-	8	11
Pneumonia	480-486	-	-	-	-	-	-	-	-	-	-
Acute tonsillitis, hypertrophy of tonsils and adenoids	463,500	1	3	2	2	3	1	-	-	6	6
Digestive system	*520-577*	-	-	*1*	-	-	-	-	-	*1*	-
Inguinal hernia	550,552	-	-	-	-	-	-	-	-	-	-
Cholelithiasis, cholecystitis	574,575	-	-	-	-	-	-	-	-	-	-
Genitourinary system	*580-629*	-	-	-	-	-	-	-	-	-	-
Urinary system	580-599	-	-	-	-	-	-	-	-	-	-
Hyperplasia of prostate	600	-	-	-	-	-	-	-	-	-	-
Disorders of menstruation	626	-	-	-	-	-	-	-	-	-	-
Complications of pregnancy	*630-678*	-	-	-	-	-	-	-	-	-	-
Skin, subcutaneous tissue	*680-709*	-	-	*9*	*12*	*3*	*1*	-	-	*12*	*13*
Musculoskeletal, connect. tissue	*710-738*	*1*	-	-	-	*1*	-	-	-	*2*	-
Arthritis, all forms	710-718	-	-	-	-	-	-	-	-	-	-
Congenital anomalies	*740-759*	*2*	*1*	*1*	*1*	-	-	-	-	*3*	*2*
Symptoms, ill-defined conditions	*780-796*	*2*	*2*	*6*	*7*	*6*	*2*	-	-	*14*	*11*
Accidents	*800-999*	-	-	-	-	-	-	-	-	-	-
Conditions, exams w/o sickness	*793, Y00-Y13*	-	-	-	-	-	-	-	-	-	-
Total all diagnoses (italics)		*16*	*13*	*29*	*36*	*19*	*9*	*0*	*0*	*64*	*58*
People examined		20	21	26	28	11	8	0	1	57	58

Adapted from Díaz et al. (1978) and Murillo et al. (1980).
- = 0

[1] Subjects less than 15 years of age

Table 5b
Distribution of diseases and disorders among the mestizo adults[1]
examined in the population of the Departments of Arica, Chile and Oruro, Bolivia
by sex and ecological niche (non-permanent residents of each niche only)

		Coast		Sierra		Altiplano Chile		Altiplano Bolivia		Total	
Disease category	ICDA code	M	F	M	F	M	F	M	F	M	F
Infective and parasitic	*000-136*	*4*	*3*	*1*	-	*3*	*1*	-	-	*8*	*4*
Neoplasms	*140-239*	-	*1*	*1*	*2*	-	-	-	-	*1*	*3*
Malignant	140-209	-	-	-	-	-	-	-	-	-	-
Benign or unspecified	210-239	-	1	1	2	-	-	-	-	1	3
Endocrine, nutritional, metabolic	*240-279*	*2*	*8*	*4*	*3*	*2*	*3*	-	-	*8*	*14*
Diabetes	250	-	-	-	-	-	-	-	-	-	-
Blood, blood forming organs	*280-289*	-	*2*	-	*2*	-	-	-	-	-	*4*
Mental disorders	*290-315*	-	-	*1*	-	*1*	-	-	*1*	*2*	*1*
Nervous system, sense organs	*320-389*	*7*	*4*	*8*	*4*	*2*	*1*	*1*	*2*	*18*	*11*
Nervous system	320-358	-	1	1	1	-	-	-	-	1	2
Eye	360-379	3	-	1	1	1	-	1	2	6	3
Ear, mastoid process	380-389	4	3	6	2	1	1	-	-	11	6
Circulatory system	*390-458*	*15*	*7*	*17*	*22*	*7*	*3*	*1*	*3*	*40*	*35*
Acute hypertension (≥160/95)	401	6	-	6	5	2	-	-	-	14	5
Borderline hypertension (≥140/90)	401.0	3	4	5	1	3	1	-	-	11	6
Acute MI	410	-	-	-	-	-	-	-	-	-	-
Other ischemic heart disease	411-414	1	-	-	-	-	-	1	1	2	1
All other heart disease	390-429	2	1	4	5	2	1	-	2	8	9
CVA	430-438	-	-	-	-	-	-	-	-	-	-
Respiratory system	*460-519*	*4*	*6*	*10*	*5*	*4*	*3*	*2*	*2*	*20*	*16*
Acute resp. infect.; except influenza tonsillitis, sinusitis	460-466	2	1	5	3	1	-	2	-	10	4
Pneumonia	480-486	1	-	-	-	-	-	-	-	1	-
Acute tonsillitis, hypertrophy of tonsils and adenoids	463,500	1	1	-	1	1	-	-	-	2	2
Digestive system	*520-577*	*3*	*8*	*5*	*5*	*1*	*1*	-	*2*	*9*	*16*
Inguinal hernia	550,552	-	-	1	-	-	1	-	-	1	1
Cholelithiasis, cholecystitis	574,575	-	3	-	-	-	-	-	1	-	4
Genitourinary system	*580-629*	*2*	*2*	*1*	*3*	-	-	-	*3*	*3*	*8*
Urinary system	580-599	-	-	-	1	-	-	-	-	-	1
Hyperplasia of prostate	600	-	-	1	-	-	-	-	-	1	-
Disorders of menstruation	626	-	-	-	1	-	-	-	1	-	2
Complications of pregnancy	*630-678*	-	-	-	-	-	-	-	-	-	-
Skin, subcutaneous tissue	*680-709*	*12*	*18*	*3*	*9*	*5*	*7*	*1*	*2*	*21*	*36*
Musculoskeletal, connect. tissue	*710-738*	*9*	*3*	*1*	*3*	*2*	*1*	-	-	*12*	*7*
Arthritis, all forms	710-718	3	1	-	2	-	-	-	-	3	3
Congenital anomalies	*740-759*	-	*1*	*3*	-	*2*	-	*1*	-	*6*	*1*
Symptoms, ill-defined conditions	*780-796*	*16*	*14*	*30*	*10*	*9*	*2*	-	*2*	*55*	*28*
Accidents	*800-999*	*1*	-	*1*	-	*1*	-	-	-	*3*	-
Conditions, exams w/o sickness	*793, Y00-Y13*	-	*5*	-	*3*	-	*1*	-	-	-	*9*
Total all diagnoses (italics)		*75*	*82*	*86*	*71*	*39*	*23*	*6*	*17*	*206*	*193*
People examined		55	46	55	52	17	12	4	9	131	119

Adapted from Díaz et al. (1978) and Murillo et al. (1980).
\- = 0

[1] Subjects 15 years of age and older

Table 6a
Distribution of diseases and disorders among the non-Aymará children[1] examined in the population of the Departments of Arica, Chile and Oruro, Bolivia by sex and ecological niche (non-permanent residents of each niche only)

Disease category	ICDA code	Coast		Sierra		Altiplano Chile		Altiplano Bolivia		Total	
		M	F	M	F	M	F	M	F	M	F
Infective and parasitic	*000-136*	-	-	-	-	-	-	-	-	-	-
Neoplasms	*140-239*	-	-	-	-	-	-	-	-	-	-
Malignant	140-209	-	-	-	-	-	-	-	-	-	-
Benign or unspecified	210-239	-	-	-	-	-	-	-	-	-	-
Endocrine, nutritional, metabolic	*240-279*	-	-	-	-	-	-	-	-	-	-
Diabetes	250	-	-	-	-	-	-	-	-	-	-
Blood, blood forming organs	*280-289*	-	-	-	-	-	-	-	-	-	-
Mental disorders	*290-315*	-	-	-	-	-	-	-	-	-	-
Nervous system, sense organs	*320-389*	-	-	-	-	-	-	-	-	-	-
Nervous system	320-358	-	-	-	-	-	-	-	-	-	-
Eye	360-379	-	-	-	-	-	-	-	-	-	-
Ear, mastoid process	380-389	-	-	-	-	-	-	-	-	-	-
Circulatory system	*390-458*	-	-	-	*2*	-	-	-	-	-	*2*
Acute hypertension (≥160/95)	401	-	-	-	-	-	-	-	-	-	-
Borderline hypertension (≥140/90)	401.0	-	-	-	-	-	-	-	-	-	-
Acute MI	410	-	-	-	-	-	-	-	-	-	-
Other ischemic heart disease	411-414	-	-	-	-	-	-	-	-	-	-
All other heart disease	390-429	-	-	-	2	-	-	-	-	-	2
CVA	430-438	-	-	-	-	-	-	-	-	-	-
Respiratory system	*460-519*	-	-	*2*	*5*	-	*1*	-	-	*2*	*6*
Acute resp. infect.; except influenza tonsillitis, sinusitis	460-466	-	-	1	2	-	1	-	-	1	3
Pneumonia	480-486	-	-	-	-	-	-	-	-	-	-
Acute tonsillitis, hypertrophy of tonsils and adenoids	463,500	-	-	1	3	-	-	-	-	1	3
Digestive system	*520-577*	-	-	-	-	-	-	-	-	-	-
Inguinal hernia	550,552	-	-	-	-	-	-	-	-	-	-
Cholelithiasis, cholecystitis	574,575	-	-	-	-	-	-	-	-	-	-
Genitourinary system	*580-629*	-	-	-	-	-	-	-	-	-	-
Urinary system	580-599	-	-	-	-	-	-	-	-	-	-
Hyperplasia of prostate	600	-	-	-	-	-	-	-	-	-	-
Disorders of menstruation	626	-	-	-	-	-	-	-	-	-	-
Complications of pregnancy	*630-678*	-	-	-	-	-	-	-	-	-	-
Skin, subcutaneous tissue	*680-709*	-	-	*2*	*1*	-	-	-	-	*2*	*1*
Musculoskeletal, connect. tissue	*710-738*	-	-	-	-	-	-	-	-	-	-
Arthritis, all forms	710-718	-	-	-	-	-	-	-	-	-	-
Congenital anomalies	*740-759*	-	-	-	-	-	-	-	-	-	-
Symptoms, ill-defined conditions	*780-796*	-	-	*2*	*1*	-	*2*	-	-	*2*	*3*
Accidents	*800-999*	-	-	-	*1*	-	-	-	-	-	*1*
Conditions, exams w/o sickness	*793, Y00-Y13*	-	-	-	-	-	-	-	-	-	-
Total all diagnoses (italics)		-	-	*6*	*10*	-	*3*	-	-	*6*	*13*
People examined		3	1	7	6	-	1	-	-	10	8

Adapted from Díaz et al. (1978) and Murillo et al. (1980).
- = 0
[1] Subjects less than 15 years of age

Table 6b
Distribution of diseases and disorders among the non-Aymará adults[1] examined in the population of the Departments of Arica, Chile and Oruro, Bolivia by sex and ecological niche (non-permanent residents of each niche only)

		Coast		Sierra		Altiplano Chile		Altiplano Bolivia		Total	
Disease category	ICDA code	M	F	M	F	M	F	M	F	M	F
Infective and parasitic	*000-136*	*1*	*1*	-	-	-	-	-	-	*1*	*1*
Neoplasms	*140-239*	-	-	*1*	-	-	-	-	-	*1*	-
Malignant	140-209	-	-	-	-	-	-	-	-	-	-
Benign or unspecified	210-239	-	-	1	-	-	-	-	-	1	-
Endocrine, nutritional, metabolic	*240-279*	*5*	*5*	*2*	*1*	-	-	-	-	*7*	*6*
Diabetes	250	-	-	-	-	-	-	-	-	-	-
Blood, blood forming organs	*280-289*	-	*2*	-	-	-	-	-	-	-	*2*
Mental disorders	*290-315*	-	*1*	*2*	-	*1*	-	-	-	*3*	*1*
Nervous system, sense organs	*320-389*	*3*	*2*	*5*	-	*3*	*1*	-	-	*11*	*3*
Nervous system	320-358	2	-	1	-	-	-	-	-	3	-
Eye	360-379	-	-	-	-	2	-	-	-	2	-
Ear, mastoid process	380-389	1	2	4	-	1	1	-	-	6	3
Circulatory system	*390-458*	*17*	*8*	*27*	*2*	*6*	*1*	-	-	*50*	*11*
Acute hypertension (≥160/95)	401	5	3	7	-	5	-	-	-	17	3
Borderline hypertension (≥140/90)	401.0	5	1	11	-	1	1	-	-	17	2
Acute MI	410	-	-	-	-	-	-	-	-	-	-
Other ischemic heart disease	411-414	4	-	2	-	-	-	-	-	6	-
All other heart disease	390-429	2	2	3	-	-	-	-	-	5	2
CVA	430-438	-	-	-	-	-	-	-	-	-	-
Respiratory system	*460-519*	*2*	*1*	*3*	-	*2*	*1*	-	-	*7*	*2*
Acute resp. infect.; except influenza tonsillitis, sinusitis	460-466	1	1	-	-	-	1	-	-	1	2
Pneumonia	480-486	-	-	-	-	1	-	-	-	1	-
Acute tonsillitis, hypertrophy of tonsils and adenoids	463,500	-	-	3	-	-	-	-	-	3	-
Digestive system	*520-577*	*1*	*3*	*1*	-	-	-	-	*1*	*2*	*4*
Inguinal hernia	550,552	-	-	-	-	-	-	-	-	-	-
Cholelithiasis, cholecystitis	574,575	-	-	-	-	-	-	-	-	-	-
Genitourinary system	*580-629*	*1*	*2*	-	-	-	*1*	-	-	*1*	*3*
Urinary system	580-599	-	1	-	-	-	-	-	-	-	1
Hyperplasia of prostate	600	-	-	-	-	-	-	-	-	-	-
Disorders of menstruation	626	-	-	-	-	-	-	-	-	-	-
Complications of pregnancy	*630-678*	-	-	-	-	-	-	-	-	-	-
Skin, subcutaneous tissue	*680-709*	*3*	*6*	*4*	*1*	*2*	*3*	-	*1*	*9*	*11*
Musculoskeletal, connect. tissue	*710-738*	*3*	*4*	*3*	-	*1*	-	-	-	*7*	*4*
Arthritis, all forms	710-718	-	-	2	-	-	-	-	-	2	-
Congenital anomalies	*740-759*	*2*	-	-	-	*2*	-	-	*1*	*4*	*1*
Symptoms, ill-defined conditions	*780-796*	*3*	*5*	*17*	*2*	*5*	-	-	-	*25*	*7*
Accidents	*800-999*	*1*	-	*1*	-	-	-	-	-	*2*	-
Conditions, exams w/o sickness	*793, Y00-Y13*	-	-	-	-	-	-	-	-	-	-
Total all diagnoses (italics)		*42*	*40*	*66*	*6*	*22*	*7*	-	*3*	*130*	*56*
People examined		16	24	39	10	10	3	-	1	65	38

Adapted from Díaz et al. (1978) and Murillo et al. (1980).
- = 0
[1] Subjects 15 years of age and older

comparison. Since they are defined on the basis of clinical experiences at lower altitudes, they are not calculatedly self-serving insofar as observations at high-altitude are concerned. It warrants noting, however, that for individuals less than 15 years of age, even at sea level, these standards exceed the 90th percentile for ages 6 through 15 inclusive (Report of the 2nd Task Force on Blood Pressure Control in Children, 1987).

The diagnosis of anemia presents similar problems when inadequate nutrition is present. Here one of the conventional metrics is the amount of hemoglobin in the blood. Again, we took as our standards those values normally viewed as indicative of anemia at sea level, namely, less than 12 gms per cent of hemoglobin in males and less than 10 gms per cent in females. The hemoglobin was determined using a spectrophotometer and a heparinized venous blood specimen.

SPECIFIC DIAGNOSES

We present our clinical findings in Bolivia and Chile separately. We do so for the following reasons: in working in these communities, it was soon apparent that the Chilean altiplano is somewhat different from much of the altiplano in Bolivia. The former is generally higher, although possibly not significantly so from a physiological or adaptational point of view; it is also drier, and seemingly more inimical. Cereals do not do as well, potato cultivation is more limited, the bearing capacity of the land seems less, and in fact the population is sparser. Moreover, there are differences in settlement patterns and mobility that may influence behavior and ultimately disease and disability.

CHILE: Some 419 different ICDA (1968) codable diseases or 'symptoms and ill-defined conditions' listed in the International Classification of Diseases (ICDA, 1968) were encountered among the 2,096 persons examined. Most of these involved only a few individuals at most, making diagnosis-specific comparisons for different altitudes, sex, or age groups statistically meaningless. Accordingly, we have grouped our findings into broader diagnostic categories, but will in the paragraphs that follow call attention to the most frequently encountered problems in each category (in addition to those other specific diagnoses indicated in the tables).

BOLIVIA: Some 145 different ICDA codable diseases or symptoms and ill-defined conditions were encountered among the 429 individuals studied. Again, most of these involved no more than a few individuals, and as a consequence, we have grouped our findings into the same diagnostic categories used for Chile.

Infective and parasitic diseases

CHILE: The illnesses most commonly encountered in children were diarrhea, upper respiratory infection (including otitis media), tuberculosis, whooping cough, and bacterial infections of the skin. The illness most commonly observed in adults was tuberculosis. Stools were not routinely examined; it can be surmised from the work of others (Buck et al., 1968) that had they been, parasites, mostly worms, would undoubtedly have been encountered.

BOLIVIA: The most commonly seen infective disorders were tuberculosis (14 cases) and whooping cough (4 cases). This number of tuberculosis cases did not come as a surprise. Other studies (Omran et al., 1967) have obtained positive sputums from about 2 per cent of the individuals tested in altiplano communities, and have reported that by age 20 almost 90 per cent of the people will be tuberculin reactors. The most prevalent parasitic disorder was scabies (26 cases); however, no stool examinations were done, and experience gained elsewhere suggests that both Ascaris and Trichuris are common – indeed, they are present in some 30 percent of the people in this region of Bolivia (Omran et al., 1967, Table 44).

Neoplasms

CHILE: Only one malignancy was seen, and all of the benign tumors were essentially inconsequential as threats to health.

BOLIVIA: Two malignant tumors were recognized clinically (it was impracticable to obtain histologic confirmation). One of these involved a salivary gland and the other the skin.

Endocrine, nutritional, and metabolic disorders

Obesity and undernutrition were the most common disorders of these types, both in adults and children; an undernourished individual was defined as one who fell into the lowest one percentile of his or her age and sex class (based on Chilean standards.) We did not routinely test for blood sugar and cannot, therefore, estimate the prevalence of diabetes; however, one woman, in Bolivia, reported herself to be diabetic.

Diseases of the blood and blood-forming organs

CHILE: Anemia, generally thought to be nutritional in origin, was the most frequent disease, but some of the 'simple' anemias seen may have been due to causes other than iron deficiency or a more generalized malnutrition.

BOLIVIA: Anemia was the only disorder of the blood or blood forming organs that was recognized. Most individuals designated as anemic were women in the child-bearing years. As previously stated, the diagnosis of anemia was based solely on the observed hemoglobin concentration. We believe this diagnosis largely reflects an iron deficiency of nutritional origin.

Diseases of the nervous system and sense organs

CHILE: Otitis media was common in children; and cataracts, otitis media, otosclerosis, and hearing impairments were frequently observed in adults. It warrants reiteration that the examinations were conducted in the spring (October and November), a season during which otitis media and respiratory diseases were presumably at neither a maximum nor a minimum.

BOLIVIA: The most frequently observed nervous system disorders involved the eye, the ear, or both. Common among the ophthalmic problems were pterygium, conjunctivitis, and inflammation of the lacrimal tract. These complaints were common in the sierra and altiplano of Chile as well; they can be ascribed either to the dust and persistent wind that characterize these elevations, or to neglect. Otitis media was frequent, and impaired hearing was recorded in one or both ears of 33 individuals. Presumably, much of this impairment was secondary to chronic ear infections.

Diseases of the circulatory system

CHILE: Systemic hypertension in Aymará adults living permanently in the sierra or the altiplano was uncommon, but it occurred more frequently than the literature would suggest. Eight of 187 adults who had resided permanently in the sierra or the altiplano had systolic blood pressures equal to or greater than 160, or diastolic pressures equal to or greater than 95. Nineteen additional individuals had blood pressures equaling or exceeding 140/90 but less than 160/95. None of the 6 Aymará adults examined who were permanent coastal residents had blood pressures equaling or exceeding 160/95, and only 1 had a blood pressure between 140/90 and 160/95. Only 1 of 239 Aymará children living permanently in the sierra or altiplano had a blood pressure greater than 140/90, and none of those living permanently along the coast had elevated blood pressure.

Among the 155 Aymará adults who were residing in the sierra or altiplano at the time of these examinations and had acknowledged spending at least 10 percent of their lives elsewhere, 6 had systolic blood pressures over 160 or diastolic pressure above 95. An additional 16 individuals had blood pressures in the range of either 140-159 (systolic) or 90-94 (diastolic) or both. These frequencies are very similar to those observed among permanent residents at these altitudes, and lower than those found among the coastal Aymará. None of the 33 Aymará children who had spent only part of their lives in the sierra or altiplano had elevated systolic or diastolic pressures.

Peripheral vascular disease was common among the more elderly adults. Only one instance of a stroke was encountered, a mestizo male residing permanently in the sierra.

Cardiac auscultatory findings were of interest and surprising. The most common finding among adults was premature contractions, the vast majority of which were superventricular in origin.

Rheumatic fever is a significant health problem in many Central and South American countries, and it came as a surprise that none of the Aymará adults or children living at altitude or sea level had murmurs of mitral insufficiency, mitral stenosis, or aortic insufficiency that suggest previous attacks of rheumatic fever. It is unlikely that all hemolytic streptococcal infections in the Aymará are treated adequately. So it must be assumed that the hemolytic streptococcus is not a common pathogen among the Aymará, or else, for some reason, the Aymará either do not have acute rheumatic fever or are resistant to carditis. It is improbable that altitude itself is protective, since a 1964 survey in the United States showed high rates of rheumatic fever in the Rocky Mountain area (Marienfeld et al., 1964). The lack of crowding in the areas studied – both in the villages at altitude and the two valleys at sea level – could have been partially responsible for the apparent low incidence of rheumatic fever.

Virtually all of the murmurs were insignificant, being either soft ejection murmurs over the upper left sternal border or vibratory short systolic murmurs over the lower left sternal border. Significant murmurs were found in five patients with pulmonary stenosis, four with aortic stenosis, two with small ventricular septal defects, one with a common ventricle, and one with a partial atrioventricular canal. Although the occurrence of patent ductus arteriosus is reportedly more common (15 times) at high altitude (Marticorena et al., 1962), only one child yielded auscultatory findings of a patent ductus. It is unlikely that the examiner (an experienced pediatric cardiologist) would have overlooked the murmur of patent ductus arteriosus, particularly since it was expected that the incidence would be high. It is possible, but not probable, that most of the infants with patent ductus arteriosus had died.

BOLIVIA: Three of some 177 adults who claimed to have lived at no other elevation than that of the altiplano were hypertensive by conventional standards, and another nine had either systolic or diastolic pressures sufficiently high to be labeled borderline. These case frequencies are higher than has often been assumed, but they are only half as high as the frequencies encountered in the sierra and altiplano of Chile. The numbers are small, of course, and the differences between these frequencies and others observed are not statistically significant. If one considered the ages of the adults (119 were 30-69 years of age) and applied the age-specific frequencies of hypertension that prevail in the white population of the United States, however, one would have expected 14 hypertensive individuals.

Figures 1 and 2 show the distribution of systolic and diastolic blood pressures of males and females by age (Figure 1) and weight (Figure 2). Our measurements in the two communities have been pooled, since there was only a trivial difference in the means obtained for Turco and Toledo subjects. No clear dependence on age could be detected among either males or females; however, weight was clearly associated with blood pressure. Systolic pressure, in particular, increased linearly with weight, doing so almost equally among males and females. Indeed, weight alone accounted for about 22 per cent of the variation observed in the systolic pressures of different individuals. It warrants mention that weight here is virtually synonymous with lean body mass; few of the individuals examined fell within the upper twentieth percentile of the weight for height ratio based upon United States standards. In general, this blood pressure rise with increasing weight in Bolivia is in accord with what we have previously reported for Chile (Makela et al., 1978). Systolic pressure increased about 0.3

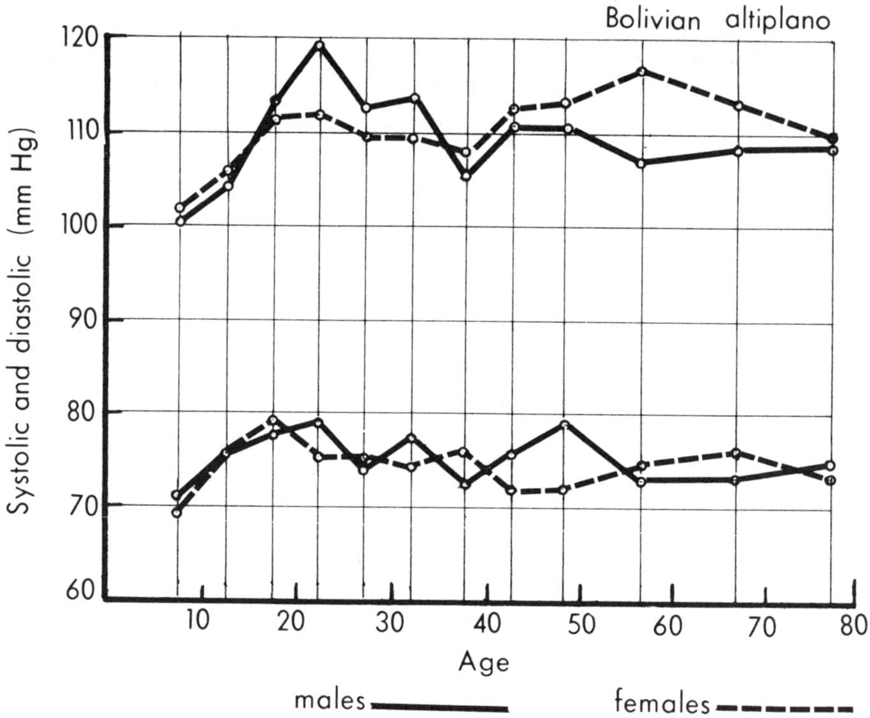

FIGURE 1. Distribution of systolic blood pressures (above) and diastolic blood pressures (below) among male and female residents of Turco and Toledo, by age at the time of examination. Murillo et al., 1980, Figure 1, p. 60. Reprinted with permission of the Pan American Health Organization, Washington, D.C.

mm/kg of weight in both sexes in Bolivia and about 0.4 mm/kg in Chile.

Among other cardiovascular problems, the most common were abnormalities of rhythm – ventricular contractions (8 cases), ventricular fibrillation (1 case), and right bundle branch block (2 cases). Right ventricular hypertrophy and right bundle branch block (complete or incomplete) are commonly seen among high-altitude indigenes (Rotta and López, 1958). Continuous cardiac monitoring in this population has revealed bradycardia to be even more frequent than has generally been surmised from clinical examinations (Barton et al., 1976).

Again, we observed none of the cardiac sequelae commonly associated with rheumatic fever.

Diseases of the respiratory system

Common cold, bronchitis, tonsillitis, and pneumonia were the more common diagnoses in this disease category among both adults and children. Auscultatory

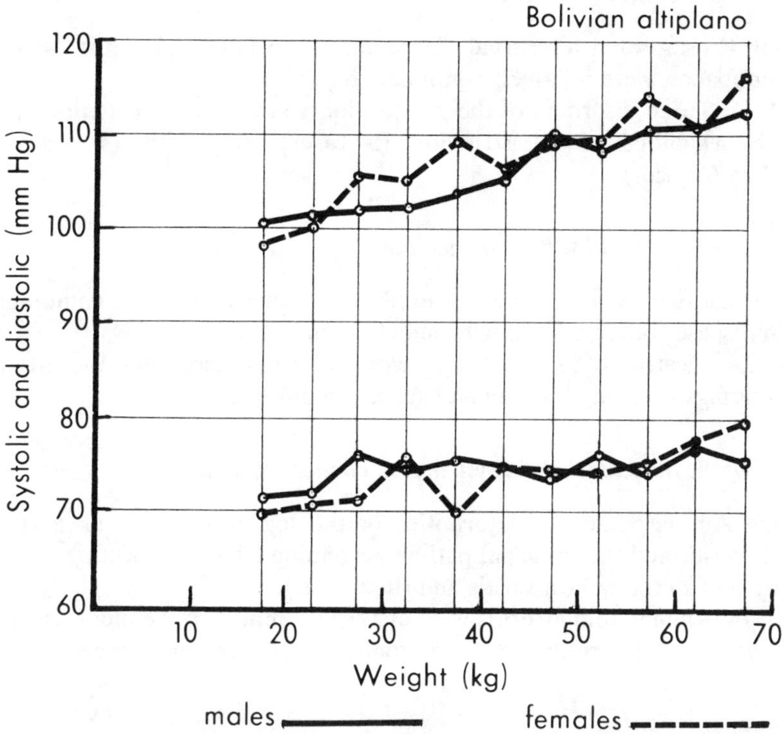

FIGURE 2. Distribution of systolic blood pressures (above) and diastolic blood pressures (below) among male and female residents of Turco and Toledo, by weight in kg at the time of examination. Murillo et al., 1980, Figure 1, p. 61. Reprinted with permission of the Pan American Health Organization, Washington, D.C.

findings suggesting asthma were not noted; but the older Aymará living at altitude commonly had symptoms and auscultatory findings suggesting pulmonary tuberculosis.

Diseases of the digestive system

CHILE: Severe dental caries and ill-defined gastrointestinal disorders constituted the bulk of adult problems; no single diagnosis stood out among children. Dental caries were often so severe that extraction was frequently necessary.

BOLIVIA: Widespread dental caries (Palomino, 1978), a non-specific gastritis, and inguinal hernia accounted for most of the digestive system problems found.

Diseases of the genitourinary system

CHILE: Prostate and menstrual disorders, in the latter case those associated with menopause, were relatively common.

BOLIVIA: Three disorders of the genitourinary system were prominent. These were abnormalities of menstruation (5 cases), salpingitis (4 cases), and leukorrhea (6 cases).

Diseases of the skin and subcutaneous tissue

CHILE: Cicatrix, keloids, and acquired keratoderma were the commonest of the skin diseases observed in adults and children.

BOLIVIA: Cicatrices (55 cases) and keloids (2 cases) accounted for virtually all of our findings involving the skin and subcutaneous tissue.

Diseases of the musculoskeletal system and connective tissue

CHILE: Among children, deformities of the leg, most often as a result of trauma, constituted the principal pathology; among adults, deformities were also common, but so too were arthritis and rheumatism.

BOLIVIA: Rheumatoid arthritis was relatively common in the older age groups, and kyphosis and deformities of the extremities were seen in subjects of all ages.

Congenital anomalies

CHILE: Ogival palate and deformities of the chest (pectus excavatum and pectus carinatum) predominated among the Aymará. The diagnosis of 14 congenital heart defect cases revealed an incidence among the Aymará similar to that found in the United States (7 per 1,000 population). Although of minor, if any, health importance, supernumerary nipples were far more common than we anticipated. Among 1,630 individuals in Chile, no less than 184 (11.3%) had one or more supernumerary nipples (66 persons had one or more additional nipples on the right, 90 on the left, and 28 had extra nipples on both sides of the chest). 466 individuals had been examined before we recognized the commonness of this minor abnormality and began to record its frequency systematically.

BOLIVIA: The most frequently observed congenital anomalies were undescended testis (5 cases), pigeon chest (pectus excavatum (6 cases)), and congenital dislocation of the hip (2 cases). It should be mentioned that we saw only one case of harelip (with or without cleft palate) during some 2,500 examinations performed in Bolivia and Chile; the affected child failed to survive a year. Interestingly, supernumerary nipples were not a particularly common finding; only eight cases (2.9%) were seen among 417 individuals (3 right only, 0 left only, and 5 bilateral).

Symptoms and ill-defined conditions

CHILE: Among children, enlarged lymph nodes and hemoptysis were the most frequent findings in this category; among adults, enlarged lymph nodes, hemoptysis, abdominal and/or joint pain, and senility were the predominant findings.

BOLIVIA: Palpation frequently revealed enlarged lymph glands (15 cases), and complaints referable to the genitourinary system (5 cases) and the upper gastrointestinal tract (5 cases) were common. The commonness of lymphadenopathy seen in both Bolivia and Chile could reflect the high frequency of parasitic infestations or chronic low-grade infections.

Accidents

Perforated eardrums, one or both, was the most common finding normally recorded in this category in both countries.

OPHTHALMIC DISEASE

Individuals unaccustomed to altitude can and frequently do experience a kind of psycho-physiological effect upon prolonged exposure to the hypoxia which prevails at high elevations. If oxygen deprivation is sufficiently profound, memory falters, the central visual field is impaired, and the individual may be appreciably and permanently handicapped (Buskirk, 1971; McFarland, 1969 and 1972). Ocular accommodation, convergence, and stereoacuity are all reported to be measurably degraded at altitudes as low as 4500 m (Ohlbaum, 1969). Still more subtle visual effects occur, the sensitivity of color perception, for example, decreases progressively and systematically as hypoxia becomes more severe and extends over longer periods (Kolbrick, 1970). Engorgement, with tortuosity, of the retinal vessels, an increase in venous and arterial diameters, and retinal hemorrhages are frequently observed in mountain climbers at altitudes as low as 3600 m (Frayser, Houston, Gray, Bryan and Rennie, 1971; Rennie and Morrissey, 1975; and Weidman, 1975) and a familial proclivity to their development may exist (Shults and Swan, 1975).

These risks and the discomfiture experienced by lowland visitors notwithstanding, more than 10 million individuals now live in the Andes at altitudes of 3000 m or more. Nonetheless, oxygen deprivation, extremely low humidity for most of the year, persistent wind, and high levels of ultraviolet radiation at these elevations can all be viewed as inimical to ophthalmic health.

Some of the adjustments associated with Andean peoples that promote oxygen transport and utilization may also have deleterious long-run ophthalmic consequences. Polycythemia can lead to retinal cyanosis, for example; it can also lead to retinal hemorrhages and papilledema that have been so gross on occasion as to result in blindness (Duke-Elder and Dobree, 1967). Furthermore, brain tissue is known to be sensitive to oxygen deprivation; and since the eye is developmentally and histologically an extension of the brain, more profound eye tissue damage might be expected at low oxygen levels than would characteristically occur in other tissues.

On the other hand, we are aware of few studies of a systematic nature that provide information on chronic as well as acute ophthalmic disease or disability among Andean peoples. Buck and his colleagues (Buck, Sasaki, and Anderson, 1968) have reported on the frequency of eye diseases and conditions encountered in epidemiologic studies of four Peruvian villages, one of which, Pusi, is in the altiplano. Some 240 inhabitants of this village, presumably of Quechua origin, were studied. All of the findings recorded involved the cornea, conjunctiva, or lids – which suggests that ophthalmoscopy was not done. The largest differences among the four villages were observed with regard to conjunctivitis and pterygium; in both instances data from the altiplano village were intermediate in value. A keratoconjunctival lesion allegedly restricted to individuals indigenous to high altitudes in Bolivia, said to resemble limbal vernal catarrh has been described (Solares, 1941). We failed to see this lesion at equally high altitudes in Chile. Rennie and Morrissey (1975) observed no retinal hemorrhages in a limited number of Sherpa at altitudes where one out of three American co-climbers were affected, and we likewise failed to find this phenomenon increased among the Aymará of the Chilean altiplano.

The ophthalmic examinations reported here were all conducted in Chile and included testing of visual acuity, color vision, and tonometry, as well as slip lamp microscopy, an external examination, and an ophthalmoscopic examination. The slit lamp microscopy was carried out with a Marco (model MT-304-JSM) slit lamp and the ophthalmoscopic examination was conducted with a conventional Welch-Allyn ophthalmoscope. Color vision tests were performed with AO H-R-R pseudoisochromatic plates. Visual acuity was determined with a Snellen Illiterate E chart at 20 feet, each eye tested separately.

After color vision and visual acuity examinations were completed, two drops of 1 percent mydriacil were instilled into the conjunctival sacs 20 to 25 minutes prior to fundoscopy, save where medically contraindicated, to enhance visualization of the posterior chamber, fundus, and retina. It was observed that dilation occurred less frequently than it normally does among non-Indian populations. Indeed, dilation failed to occur in some 21 (8.8%) of the 238 Aymará, in 17 (5.8%) of 292 mestizos, and 4 (2.8%) of 143 non-Aymará. For a variety of reasons, no effort was made to dilate the pupils of 33 individuals (11 Aymará, 19 mestizo, and 3 non-Aymará) who were otherwise examined ophthalmologically. A good view of the fundus is generally obtained 10 to 15 minutes after instillation, and at 20 minutes the average pupil diameter is about 7.5 mm; little change in pupillary diameter occurs in the succeeding hour or two (Nano, Gavarini, and Perez, 1960).

Two ophthalmic examinations were carried out – one by the physician who performed the general physical examination and the second by an ophthalmologist certified by the American Board of Ophthalmology (Goldsmith). The former examination was given each time a physical

Table 7a
Distribution of ophthalmic diseases and disorders among children[a] examined in the population of the Department of Arica, Chile by sex[b], ethnicity[c], and ecological niche

	Coast						Sierra						Altiplano						Total
	Aym.		Mes.		N-A		Aym.		Mes.		N-A		Aym.		Mes.		N-A		
Disease category	M	F	M	F	M	F	M	F	M	F	M	F	M	F	M	F	M	F	
Globes and adnexa:																			
Blepharitis	-	-	-	-	-	-	-	-	-	-	-	1	-	1	-	-	-	-	2
Cyst, meibomian	-	1	-	-	-	-	-	-	-	2	-	-	-	-	-	1	-	-	4
Exotropia	-	-	-	-	-	-	1	-	-	-	-	-	-	-	1	-	-	-	2
Hypertelorism	-	-	-	1	-	-	-	-	-	-	-	-	-	-	-	-	-	-	1
Lacrimal drainage system, inflammation of	-	-	-	-	-	-	-	-	-	-	1	-	-	-	-	-	-	-	1
Cornea, conjunctiva, choroid, and sclera:																			
Conjunctiva, hyperemia of	-	-	6	3	2	2	3	-	10	8	3	1	3	6	4	1	-	-	52
Conjunctivitis	-	-	-	-	-	-	-	-	-	2	-	-	-	-	-	-	-	-	2
Melanoma, conjunctiva	-	-	-	1	-	1	-	-	-	-	-	-	-	1	-	-	-	-	3
Opacity, corneal	-	-	-	-	-	-	1	-	-	2	-	-	1	1	-	-	1	-	6
Pseudopterygium	-	-	-	-	-	-	-	1	-	-	-	-	-	-	-	-	-	-	1
Subconjunctival hemorrhage, secondary to trauma	-	-	-	-	1	-	-	-	-	-	-	-	-	-	-	-	-	-	1
Anterior chamber, lens, and uveal tract:																			
Cataract, unspecified	-	-	-	-	1	-	-	-	-	-	-	-	-	-	-	-	-	-	1
Cyst, iris	-	-	1	-	-	-	-	-	-	-	-	-	-	-	-	-	-	-	1
Opacity, vitreous	-	-	-	-	-	-	-	-	1	-	-	-	-	-	-	-	-	-	1
Refractive error	-	-	1	2	-	-	-	1	2	5	-	1	4	2	2	3	1	-	24
Uveitis	-	-	-	-	1	-	-	-	-	-	-	-	-	-	-	-	-	-	1
Retina and optic nerve:																			
Retina, cicatrix	-	-	1	-	-	-	-	-	-	-	-	-	-	-	-	-	-	-	1
Retina, pigmentary deposits	-	-	-	-	-	1	-	-	-	-	-	-	-	-	-	-	-	-	1
Other data:																			
Other anomalies	2	-	7	10	1	-	8	2	11	11	-	1	5	3	2	1	-	-	64
'Normal' eye examinations	1	0	16	16	6	6	12	9	20	18	5	6	26	20	7	8	-	-	176
Total number of children	3	1	26	30	10	9	22	12	38	40	7	8	35	28	12	13	1	-	295

Goldsmith et al. (1979), Table 1, p. 61.
Reprinted with permission of Pan American Health Organization, Washington, D.C.
[a] Subjects less than 15 years of age
[b] M = males, F = females
[c] Aym. = Aymará, Mes. = Mestizo, N-A = Non-Aymará

examination occurred; the latter, the results of which we report here, involved slightly more than a third of the 2,096 individuals who were examined in the basic Chilean sample. The persons who had this more detailed ophthalmologic examination were all residents of three communities; Poconchile in the coast, Putre in the sierra, and Visviri in the altiplano. Each community is typical of the

Table 7b
Distribution of ophthalmic diseases and disorders among adults[a] examined in the population of the Department of Arica, Chile by sex[b], ethnicity[c], and ecological niche

	Coast						Sierra						Altiplano						Total
	Aym.		Mes.		N-A		Aym.		Mes.		N-A		Aym.		Mes.		N-A		
Disease category	M	F	M	F	M	F	M	F	M	F	M	F	M	F	M	F	M	F	
Globes and adnexa:																			
Burn, eye	-	-	-	-	-	-	-	-	-	-	1	-	-	-	-	-	-	-	1
Cyst, meibomian	2	-	-	-	1	-	1	1	1	-	1	-	2	3	-	-	-	-	12
Exotropia	1	-	-	-	-	-	1	-	-	-	-	-	-	-	-	-	-	-	2
Lacrimal drainage system, inflammation of	-	-	-	-	-	-	-	-	1	-	-	1	1	-	-	-	-	-	3
Melanoma, benign, eyelids	-	-	-	-	1	-	1	-	-	-	-	-	-	-	-	-	-	-	2
Neoplasm, benign, eyelids	-	-	-	-	1	1	-	-	1	-	-	-	-	-	-	-	-	-	3
Ptosis	-	-	-	-	-	-	-	-	-	-	-	1	-	-	-	-	-	-	1
Strabismus	-	-	-	-	1	-	-	-	-	-	-	-	-	-	-	-	-	-	1
Cornea, conjunctiva, choroid, and sclera:																			
Blindness, one eye	-	-	-	-	-	-	-	-	-	-	1	-	-	-	-	-	-	-	1
Conjunctiva, hyperemia of	5	-	8	2	5	6	9	8	11	10	8	3	15	9	3	1	6	-	109
Conjunctivitis	-	-	3	1	1	2	3	1	-	-	-	-	1	-	1	1	-	-	14
Embryotoxon	-	-	-	1	1	-	1	1	2	1	-	-	-	1	-	-	-	-	8
Eye inflammation (episcleritis)	-	-	-	-	-	-	-	-	-	-	-	-	1	-	-	-	-	-	1
Keratitis	-	-	1	-	-	-	-	1	-	-	-	-	1	-	-	-	-	-	3
Melanoma, benign conjunctiva	-	-	-	1	1	-	-	-	-	-	-	-	-	-	-	-	-	-	2
Nevi, choroid	-	-	-	-	-	-	-	-	1	-	-	-	-	-	1	-	-	-	2
Nevi, conjunctiva	-	-	-	-	-	-	-	-	1	-	-	-	-	-	-	-	-	-	1
Nevi, pigmented	-	-	-	1	-	-	-	-	-	1	1	-	1	1	1	-	-	-	6
Opacity, corneal	-	-	-	-	-	-	-	1	1	1	3	-	3	1	1	-	-	-	11
Pterygium	-	-	-	-	-	-	-	-	1	-	-	-	-	-	-	-	-	-	1
Trachoma	-	-	1	-	-	-	-	-	-	-	-	-	-	-	-	-	-	-	1

(continued)

Goldsmith et al. (1979), Table 2, p. 62.
Reprinted with permission of Pan American Health Organization, Washington, D.C.
[a] Subjects 15 years of age or older
[b] M = males, F = females
[c] Aym. = Aymará, Mes. = Mestizo, N-A = Non-Aymará

ecologic niche to which it belongs; among the 975 residents of these communities (some 70 per cent of the communities) who were seen in the basic study, 706 were examined ophthalmologically.

Table 7 provides data on the ophthalmic disorders seen in the children (7a) and adults (7b) examined in the course of this study. (For the purposes of the study, as previously stated children were arbitrarily defined as individuals less than 15 years of age at the time of examination). These findings are grouped according to each subject's ethnic background and area of residence (coast, sierra, or altiplano). For convenience, the discussion that follows aggregates

Table 7b (continued)
Distribution of ophthalmic diseases and disorders among adults[a] examined in the population of the Department of Arica, Chile by sex[b], ethnicity[c], and ecological niche

	Coast						Sierra						Altiplano						Total
	Aym.		Mes.		N-A		Aym.		Mes.		N-A		Aym.		Mes.		N-A		
Disease category	M	F	M	F	M	F	M	F	M	F	M	F	M	F	M	F	M	F	
Anterior chamber, lens, and uveal tract:																			
Blindness, one eye, cataract, traumatic	-	-	-	-	-	-	1	-	-	-	-	-	-	-	-	-	-	-	1
Cataract, congenital	-	-	-	1	-	-	-	-	-	-	-	-	-	-	-	-	-	-	1
Cataract, senile	-	1	2	2	3	3	1	2	3	4	-	1	4	3	-	-	1	1	31
Cataract, traumatic	-	-	-	-	-	-	1	-	-	-	-	-	-	-	-	-	-	-	1
Cataract, other	-	-	-	-	-	-	1	-	-	-	-	-	3	-	-	-	-	-	4
Lens, exfoliation of capsule	-	-	-	-	-	1	1	-	1	-	-	-	2	-	-	-	-	-	5
Refractive error	3	3	10	5	11	12	5	7	9	12	3	4	16	12	3	2	3	1	121
Uveal tract, scar	-	-	-	-	1	-	1	-	-	1	1	-	1	-	-	-	-	-	5
Uveitis	-	-	-	-	-	1	-	-	-	1	-	-	-	-	-	-	-	-	2
Retina and optic nerve:																			
Amblyopia	-	1	-	-	1	-	-	-	-	-	-	-	-	-	-	-	-	-	2
Blindness, both eyes, primary optic atrophy	-	-	-	-	-	-	-	1	-	-	-	-	-	-	-	-	-	-	1
Macula, degeneration of	-	-	2	2	1	1	-	1	-	-	-	-	1	2	-	-	-	-	10
Optic nerve, structural variants	-	-	-	-	-	-	1	2	-	-	-	-	-	-	-	-	-	-	3
Retina, cicatrix	-	-	-	1	-	-	-	-	-	-	-	-	-	-	-	-	-	-	1
Retina, vascular changes of	-	-	-	-	1	1	-	1	-	-	1	-	-	1	-	-	-	-	5
Retinopathy, arterio-sclerotic	-	1	-	1	3	-	2	1	3	2	-	-	2	2	1	-	-	-	18
Retinopathy, diabetic	-	-	-	-	1	-	-	-	-	-	-	-	-	-	-	-	-	-	1
Retinopathy, hypertensive	-	-	-	-	1	2	-	1	-	-	-	-	1	-	1	-	1	-	7
Veil, glial	-	-	-	-	-	-	-	-	1	-	-	-	1	-	-	-	-	-	2
Other data:																			
Normal' eye examinations	5	4	26	20	10	8	7	12	12	13	23	6	18	14	2	5	2	-	187
Total number examined	11	7	44	33	29	26	23	26	29	30	37	11	46	35	9	7	7	1	411

[a] Subjects 15 years of age or older
[b] M = males, F = females
[c] Aym. = Aymará, Mes. = Mestizo, N-A = Non-Aymará

these findings into those affecting (1) the globe and its adnexa; (2) the cornea, conjunctiva, choroid, and sclera; (3) the anterior chamber, lens and uveal tract; and (4) the retina and optic nerve. Normality in this context implies no loss of function; that is nothing was seen that would limit ocular activity. No biopsies were performed; clinically, the benign neoplasms reported appeared to be papillomata.

Disorders of the globe and its adnexa

Surprisingly few instances of strabismus or blindness were seen; and aside from epicanthus, which is to be expected in the Aymará, few congenital anomalies affecting the adnexa were noted. Indeed, much of the pathology involving the globes as a whole or their adnexa was of traumatic origin. We saw no clinical evidence of avitaminoses despite local government concern, particularly with respect to vitamin A deficiency; nor did we see evidence of ocular changes secondary to cardiovascular anomalies such as patent ductus arteriosus that are known to be more common at higher altitudes.

Disorders of the conjunctiva, cornea, choroid, and sclera

The most frequent disorders – actinic and keratoconjunctivitis, pterygium, and corneal scarring – can all be ascribed to either the increased ultraviolet radiation, the dust and persistent wind to which we have previously called attention, or to neglect. No professional medical attention was consistently available in the sierra and altiplano villages studies. Four villages were served by a practicante, a member of the Chilean police force (Carabineros) with paramedical training. Little of this training, however, appeared to be directed at alleviation of eye injuries, although clearly some skill in the use of pressure dressing and simple ophthalmic medications would be helpful.

Conjunctival and corneal pigmentation were common; in fact, the latter was recorded in 123 (49.4%) of 249 Aymará, 121 (38.9%) of 311 mestizos, and 11 (7.5%) of 146 non-Aymará. Conjunctival hyperemia was also frequent, but no significant differences were observed in its distribution among the three ethnic groups. Hyperemia was found in 58 of 249 Aymará, 67 of 311 mestizos, and 36 of 146 non-Aymará – that is, in 23.3%, 21.5% and 24.7% of the respective subjects. Increased corneal (or conjunctival) pigment would not seem to diminish the risk of conjunctival hyperemia. Only one case of trachoma was encountered and it was of long standing.

Disorders of the anterior chamber, lens and uveal tract

Here two diagnoses prevailed, namely, exfoliation of the lens and refractive errors. The former was variously reported among 3.5 to 8% of the subjects, rates higher than the rates usually thought to obtain in most populations (Duke-Elder, 1941). In general, exfoliation of the lens is most often seen in the 60 to 80 year age group, although it has been described as occurring earlier. In our study all of the cases seen occurred among subjects in the customary age group (ranging from 54 to 79 years of age).

Many of the refractive errors were presbyopic in nature; few people were encountered who regularly used glasses, though the number who had conspicuous errors of refraction but did not wear glasses was not notably high. Tonometry was routinely performed on subjects in the older age groups, or where otherwise indicated. Among 158 adults almost equally distributed among the three ethnic groups, not a single case of elevated intraocular pressure was seen.

Minor opacities of the lens were not considered cataracts; the latter term was used only to describe an opacity of the lens that decreased vision. Examination of the lens was always performed after dilation.

Disorders of the retina and optic nerve

Andean man and women are commonly reputed (a) to have lower systolic and diastolic blood pressures than most non-Andean populations, (b) to have blood pressures that fail to exhibit the usual age-dependence, and (c) to be free, or virtually free, of cardiovascular disease. Elsewhere we have presented data that support the belief that the blood pressures of Andean peoples are generally lower, but that failed to support a belief in either the absence of hypertension or the independence of blood pressure and age (Díaz et al., 1978). As previously noted, hypertension was encountered in all three ethnic groups, albeit more commonly in the non-Aymará than in either the mestizos or the Aymará.

As indicated in Table 7b, hypertensive retinopathy was seen on no less than seven occasions; these involved all three ethnic groups, as well as individuals residing in all three ecological niches. Of the 38 individuals examined ophthalmologically who were judged to have hypertension solely on the basis of blood pressure, eight were found to have retinal changes, either of an arteriosclerotic (two) or hypertensive (six) nature. One person whose blood pressure at the time of examination was 120/86 exhibited both arteriosclerotic and hypertensive changes of the retina; he claimed not to be on medications at the time, but he was a user of coca. Among the 25 subjects with retinal changes characteristic of circulatory disease, 10 were Aymará, 9 were mestizos and 7 were non-Aymará. The age ranges at diagnosis were similar, namely, 40-71 years among the Aymará, 43-67 among the mestizos, and 48-78 among the non-Aymará. From these data we can adduce no evidence of a difference among the three ethnic groups, regarding either the frequency of these retinopathies or their apparent distribution in different age groups. Clearly, cardiovascular disease does occur among the indigenous peoples of the interior of the Department of Arica, even at altitudes where these peoples had been thought free of such disorders.

Only one case of diabetic retinopathy was seen – in a somewhat obese (144 lbs, 64 inches) 36 year old non-Aymará male who resided in Arica's coastal zone.

As previously stated, no increase in frequency of retinal hemorrhage was seen among the Aymará of the altiplano, nor could we find evidence of retinal changes secondary to the polycythemia of altitude. To examine the latter issue, a careful study was made of the ophthalmic findings on 20 individuals with hemoglobins in excess of 19.5 gm at the time of their examination and hematocrits of 50% or higher. Approximately two-thirds of these hematocrits were in the 50-59% range, the remaining third being in the 60-69% range. None of these subjects had retinal changes worthy of comment, such as increased tortuosity or vascular engorgement.

Concluding remarks

How representative, now, are these findings – not only of disease and disability in these specific communities but of other towns and villages in western Bolivia and the interior of northern Chile? Elsewhere (Schull and Rothhammer, 1977) we have argued that these examinations – in the various villages within each ecological niche – were done on a broad enough base to make systematic biases in our evaluation of the prevalence of disease and disability unlikely. Intuitively, however, one tends to presume that the acutely ill, the blind, the deaf, and the halt are underrepresented (for they may have been physically unable to present themselves at the examination site), and afford a basis for bias, insofar as such disorders are altitude-dependent. While this presumption is difficult to challenge, it does fail to reckon with the importance ascribed to medical attention in areas where such attention is not routinely available. We suspect, but cannot clearly establish, that the handicapped and acutely ill that we did not see were few in number. Three lines of evidence support this notion. First, at the time of the examinations we routinely sought to determine from 'village elders' the names of individuals who might be physically unable to come to where the examinations were to take place. Invariably this inquiry revealed few if any such individuals. Second, the demography and socioeconomic characteristics of our community samples were always representative of the community as known to local authorities, save insofar as teen aged girls were concerned. Finally, our findings in Bolivia are very similar to those reported by the United States A.I.D. Mission to Bolivia (1975). We presume, therefore, that the burden of disease and disability revealed by our survey is similar to that prevailing in most of the sierran and altiplano villages.

We note that the prevalence of disease varied significantly for different regions and ethnic groupings, as well as for the same ethnic grouping in different regions. For example, taking all altitudes together, systemic hypertension was more commonly observed among adult non-Aymará (in 33 of 220 subjects) than among mestizos (28 of 405), and was more often found among mestizos than among the Aymará (17 of 396). It is also interesting to note that the frequency of hypertension increased with increasing altitude among adult non-Aymará, decreased among the Aymará, and remained more or less constant among the mestizos. This increase among the non-Aymará cannot be accounted for solely in terms of the transitory increase in blood pressure which frequently accompanies migration to high altitude during the acclimatization process.

Many of the other altitude-related diagnoses reflect differences in the rigors of life. Respiratory diseases increased with altitude, presumably because of colder temperatures and ill-heated homes; the rate of skin diseases reflecting the diminished moisture and increased cold was also elevated; and otitis media was more common. More evidence of past traumatic accidents was also seen at high altitudes; this must reflect in part the limited health care available to people in these regions. Fractures often went unset. However, we did not see increased rates of arthritic or rheumatoid disorders, gallbladder disease or other conditions possibly ascribable to differences in adaptation to altitude. We did not encounter clinically recognizable diabetes or obvious nutritional disorders. Obese as well as undernourished individuals were encountered in all groups and at all altitudes; however, obesity was rarer among the Aymará and undernourished individuals were somewhat more common.

Interesting contrasts were observed between permanent and non-permanent residents within given ethnic groups. Overall, migrants to a new region tended to experience the diseases and disorders associated with the region they entered rather than the one they left behind. But this statement requires immediate qualification. In particular, the result is heavily influenced by infectious and parasitic disorders, respiratory diseases, and the like which undoubtedly account for the bulk of the disability prevalent in any population such as the one under discussion. It is also true that the three broad ecological zones in the Departamento de Arica differ so markedly in temperature, humidity, and atmospheric pressure that diseases or conditions which relate directly to these physical parameters can and do differ – as in the case of the acquired keratoderma resulting from the chill and dessication which occur at high altitude. However, as we have pointed out in the case of hypertension, there are also real differences between migrants and non-migrants which suggest some more fundamental biological response to environmental stress. Unfortunately, rather than elucidating the nature of this stress response, our data merely serve to indicate its existence.

Viewed in terms of public health needs, some consolation may be obtained from this general observation, for it implies that public health authorities need not anticipate two totally different sets of health care requirements, one for immigrants and the other for permanent residents. Some acute problems will differ in frequency, however, and provisions must be made for their occurrence. Such provision must include an awareness by both professionals and the lay public of those disorders which may be virtually unique or which may occur with elevated frequency among immigrants.

Our observations suggest a need for other more specific public health activities. Steps should be taken to promote improved dental care, particularly preventive work, and – if needed – reconstructive work capable of obviating severe tooth loss. The current school health programs are obviously beneficial, but do not reach the older individuals requiring some reinforcement of earlier education. A program in the sierra and altiplano to improve skin hygiene would have immediate rewards. Continuation of the use of BCG in children is clearly indicated. And, finally, the routine use of chloramphenicol, largely by the practicantes, should be discouraged; penicillin involves significantly less risk, is less expensive, and is often more effective.

WILLIAM H. MUELLER, PATRICIA SOTO-HEIM, AND VICTORIA SCHULL

Chapter 10
HETEROZYGOSITY AND PHYSICAL GROWTH IN AN ANDEAN POPULATION

Introduction

Differences between lowland and highland peoples of the Andes in body size and shape have intrigued students of the hypoxia of altitude for a century or more (see, e.g., Forbes, 1870). Until recently, most of the studies of growth and adult size have, however, focused mainly on the variability of single measurements rather than the use of anthropometric indices or summary measures of multiple anthropometric observations, such as principal components, to assess body proportion or shape. Although not without some inconsistency, these studies have nonetheless described in considerable detail the effects of altitude on body size (for a review, see, Frisancho, 1978). Collectively, they suggest that the main effects are on size for age during growth, but altitude may also affect body proportions and in particular, chest dimensions suchwise as to enhance functional adaptation to the hypoxia of altitude (Frisancho and Greksa, 1989). Ethnicity, on the other hand, appears to have a greater effect on body proportions rather than size. The Aymará, for example, have relatively larger sitting heights, more prominent heads and bony diameters than non-Aymará when altitude is held constant (Palomino, Mueller, and Schull, 1979). However, as commonly used, ethnicity measures population genetic differences rather than actual heritability, and in comparisons between populations living at different altitudes or even within the same altitude, regional differences in environmental factors may be confounded with genetic effects to a greater or lesser extent. Little has been published on changes, if any, in the correlation between specific measurements within defined genetic relationships with changing altitude as, for example, the correlation between siblings born and reared at the same altitude as opposed to different altitudes. As a result, more statistically rigorous, direct efforts to separate the role of genetic and environmental factors in the changes seen in growth and adult size are few.

Genotypes responsible for quantitative or morphological variability, except in the case of rare conditions like chondrodystrophy or growth hormone deficiency, have consistently escaped detection. There tends to be a separation in this search between the approach of quantitative genetics that has relied on familial correlation analysis to infer genetic influences on measurements and the one locus models of the biochemical geneticist. Thus an intriguing question in the genetics of human physique and physical growth is the relationship between morphology and genetic markers. This is a particularly interesting question in studies of human adaptability to environmental stress, such as that at high

William J. Schull and Francisco Rothhammer (eds.), The Aymará: Strategies in Human Adaptation to a Rigorous Environment, 133-142.

altitude, where physical growth and physiological measurements, i.e., quantitative traits, have been widely used as possible measures of adaptation (see, e.g., Frisancho and Baker, 1970; Frisancho, Borkan, and Klayman, 1975; Stinson, 1980, 1982, and 1985).

One approach to this issue is to see whether anthropometric means differ by genotypic class for a single gene locus, a strategy that has been termed the measured genotype (Boerwinkle, Chakraborty, and Sing, 1986). Such differences could imply that the locus in question was one of many genes contributing to phenotypic variation, or that it is closely linked to such a gene. It is unlikely, however, that genetic markers in blood, particularly the antigenic properties of the red cell, so commonly used have a direct effect on a measurement like human stature, for example. A second approach is generally known as the theory of stability of development of heterozygotes (Waddington, 1942; Jinks and Mather, 1955; Lerner, 1954). Here one takes a series of loci, regards them as a sample of an individual's genome and hence a way to get at the degree that the individual in question is heterozygous. Each individual is scored as to the proportion of measured loci at which he or she is heterozygous. One can then examine whether anthropometric means and variances differ between groups of individuals: Those more heterozygous and those less heterozygous. In most studies of this kind carried out in non-humans (some in plants), the means of morphological classes seldom differ by degree of individual heterozygosity, but the variances often do (Soule, 1979; Mitton, 1978; and Singh and Zouros, 1978). There are only two informative possibilities: (1) either heterozygotes vary less than homozygotes or (2) they vary more. If heterozygotes vary less, this might suggest that they have a greater ability to withstand environmental changes (canalization). If, however, they vary more than homozygotes, this suggests that heterozygotes have a greater genetic flexibility (plasticity) presumably because of biochemical alternatives that homozygotes do not possess. In other words the heterozygotes can increase or decrease growth rate as favorable or unfavorable circumstances permit.

Livshits and Kobylianski (1984) have studied this problem in a genetically homogeneous group of young men from Israel. Their results suggest that for most principal components of anthropometry, heterozygotes have decreased morphological variance, yet for one component they have an increased variance. Thus a greater or lesser degree of variance may be associated with heterozygosity, depending on the morphological component chosen. We explore here the relationship between anthropometry in young and adult human subjects and heterozygosity, and the implications of this relationship for adaptability to high altitude.

The study

The number of subjects in the Chile and Bolivia studies by age and sex have been presented in Mueller et al. (1978a and 1980b). There are 356 male children, 297 female children, 477 male adults and 483 female adults for whom there was complete anthropometric data. However, some have missing data at some of the genetic loci. Thus, sample sizes will vary somewhat in the analyses that follow. The morphological variables considered are 22 anthropometrics of body size and composition, and chest and head morphology. For details of the anthropometric methodology see Mueller et al. (1978 a,b,c), Palomino et al. (1979), Mueller, et al. (1980b) and Mueller et al. (1981b). To reduce these 22 variables to a manageable few a principal components analysis of the anthropometrics was performed. Prior to this, all measurements were standardized on age by regression analysis (as in Mueller at al., 1978a). Both age and age^2 are included to account for the known non-linear trends of anthropometrics with age. For these regressions the data from all three altitude zones – coast, sierra and altiplano – were combined but they were done within sex and age group (child and adult). A total of 22 serum and/or red cell enzyme or protein genetic markers are available on each subject (see Chapter 15). Of these, 4 are polymorphic: red cell acid phosphatase (ACP), phosphoglucomutase (PGMI), esterase-D (ESD), and haptoglobin (HP) (Schull, Ferrell and Rothhammer, 1978). At each of these loci there are two common alleles, the least frequent of these has a frequency of about 0.2. At two loci there are in addition, electrophoretic variants. Such individuals are assumed to be heterozygotes. The allelic frequencies at these four loci do not vary significantly with altitude or between Chilean and Bolivian samples (Ferrell et al., 1978 and 1980). The 4 polymorphic loci were used to determine an individual's degree of heterozygosity, because the monomorphic loci would not add additional information. The degree of heterozygosity was defined as the percent of loci out of these 4, for which the individual is heterozygous.

Results

Varimax rotation was used to maximize the association of the least set of anthropometrics with each component; the results are given in Table 1. The first four components are shown and these account for over 60% of anthropometric variability. The first component correlates highly with chest measurements, weight and arm circumference. The second relates to skeletal length, particularly to body height and tibial length, and the third and fourth to head and facial measurements. All measurements but four, have significant and substantial correlations with one of the principal components in at least two of the age/sex groups. The four measurements which failed to relate to a component are: wrist and biacrominal breadths and sternal and nose lengths. Hence these three principal components appear to summarize most of the information contained in the anthropometric measurements. For components 3 and 4 in children and adult males, there are two separate components: one dealing with head and facial breadth, the second dealing with head length and facial height. In female adults only the head breadth component is evident as the third component, while the fourth is a hand width component. Because of this variability of the third and fourth components, we will focus on the head breadth component (the third in

TABLE 1
Principal components analysis with varimax rotation of 22 anthropometric variables in male and female children (Mc, Fc) and adults (Ma, Fa)*

	PC1				PC2				PC3				PC4			
Measurement**	Mc	Fc	Ma	Fa	Mc	Fc	Ma	Fa	Mc	Fc	Ma	Fa	Mc	Fc	Ma	Fa
Weight	73	75	84	86												
Height					78	88	89	91								
Sitting ht.					66	72	73	75								
Knee height					76	85	83	86								
Calf circ.	71	70	73	80												
Arm circ.	72	81	85	85												
Hand width					62											77
Hand length					73	82	74	74								
Wrist breadth						61										
Biacromial br.																
Max chest circ.	84	83	92	92												
Min chest circ.	85	84	92	93												
Transverse chest	75	77	84	85												
A-P chest	62	71	64	75												
Sternal length	60															
Head breadth									82	81		83			65	
Head length													66	76		
Nose length											67					
Nose width											60		60			
Face height											64			65		
Bizygo. breadth									79	75		72			71	
Bigonial breadth										64					66	
Eigenvalue	9	9	7	7	2	2	3	3	1	2	2	2	1	1	1	1
% variation	41	40	32	32	7	9	12	13	7	7	7	7	6	6	6	6

* Standardized principal component weights × 100. Only coeffients of 60 or greater are shown to emphasize pattern.
** Measurements were adjusted for age and sex prior to the analysis.

children and adult females and the fourth in adult males) as it occurs in all four age/sex groups. Thus we have three consistent components, the first is concerned with cross-sectional measurements and body mass, the second with linear (skeletal) size and the third with head size.

Rather than use the principal components themselves, we chose selected measurements representing each of the three major principal components. A moderate to high level of intercorrelation among anthropometric measures is implied when these appear on the same principal component. The associations, however, may be purely statistical and not necessarily functional. For example, it is with some surprise that measurements such as body weight, chest and arm circumferences should appear together on the same component; arm circumference may primarily reflect nutritional state and chest measures may reflect the underlying morphology of the chest, a character of importance in Andean high altitude studies. Weight, of course, may be a composite of both functions. For this reason weight, arm circumference and maximum chest circumferences were chosen to represent together the first component. Height

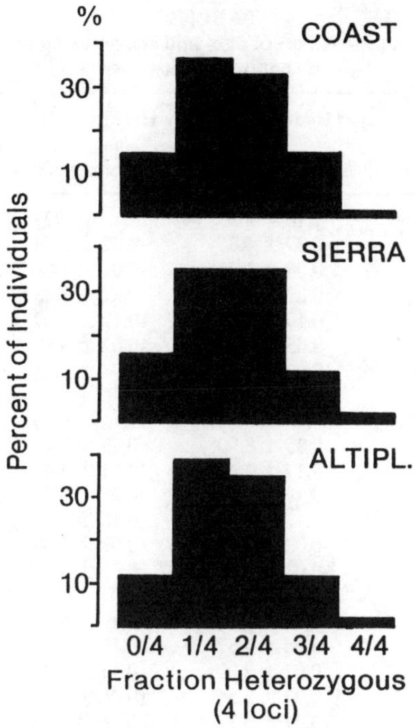

FIGURE 1. The distribution of heterozygosity by altitude

was chosen to represent the second component, as it has the consistently highest coefficients of the skeletal length measurements in Table 1. Finally, head and bizygomatic breadths were chosen to represent the last principal component, for cranial and facial development could functionally reflect slightly different aspects of development.

The distribution of heterozygosity is as follows: of 1,512 persons, 2% are heterozygous at all four loci, 13% at 3 loci, 34% at 2 loci, 37% at 1 locus and 14% at none (see Figure 1). There were no significant differences in the distribution of heterozygosity by altitude. We divided this distribution at the median: those 0-25% (none or one out of four loci heterozygous) heterozygous are termed 'homozygotes' for purposes of the analysis; those with 50% or more heterozygosity are termed 'heterozygotes'. We sought differences in means and variances of the anthropometric measurements most representative of the three principal components, which had been age and sex adjusted, between the two heterozygosity classes. The measurements were not adjusted for altitude, ethnicity or permanence of residence.

Means and standard deviations of sex and age adjusted anthropometric variables are shown by degree of heterozygosity and age group in Table 2. At the top of this table none of the means or variance differences reach a level of

TABLE 2
Means and standard deviations (s.d.) of age- and sex-adjusted anthropometric variables by heterozygosity class

Measurement	Homozygotes mean ± s.d.	Heterozygotes mean ± s.d.	P* Mean diff.	P* Variance diff.
Children	(n = 303)	(n = 297)		
Weight (kg)	0.39 ± 4.85	-0.32 ± 4.74	<0.10	n.s.
Arm circ. (cm)	0.08 ± 1.70	-0.01 ± 1.62	n.s.	n.s.
Max chest circ. (cm)	0.22 ± 4.09	-0.27 ± 3.85	n.s.	n.s.
Height (cm)	0.19 ± 5.60	-0.12 ± 6.07	n.s.	n.s.
Head breadth (cm)	0.05 ± 0.53	-0.02 ± 0.52	<0.10	n.s.
Bizygo. breadth (cm)	0.03 ± 0.47	-0.01 ± 0.53	n.s.	<0.10
Adults	(n = 465)	(n = 447)		
Weight (kg)	-0.35 ± 8.90	0.39 ± 8.46	n.s.	n.s.
Arm circ. (cm)	-0.17 ± 2.60	0.21 ± 2.68	<0.05	n.s.
Max. chest circ. (cm)	-0.17 ± 6.34	0.28 ± 5.88	n.s.	0.10
Height (cm)	-0.12 ± 4.96	0.18 ± 5.54	n.s.	<0.05
Head breadth (cm)	-0.02 ± 0.52	0.02 ± 0.50	n.s.	n.s.
Bizygo. breadth (cm)	-0.01 ± 0.49	0.01 ± 0.51	n.s.	n.s.
Total	(n = 768)	(n = 744)		
Weight (kg)	-0.06 ± 7.57	0.10 ± 7.21	n.s.	n.s.
Arm circ. (cm)	-0.07 ± 2.29	0.11 ± 2.31	n.s.	n.s.
Max chest circ. (cm)	-0.02 ± 5.56	0.06 ± 5.17	n.s.	<0.05
Height (cm)	0.01 ± 5.22	0.06 ± 5.76	n.s.	<0.01
Head breadth (cm)	0.01 ± 0.53	0.00 ± 0.51	n.s.	n.s.
Bizygo. breadth (cm)	0.01 ± 0.48	0.00 ± 0.51	n.s.	<0.10

* Significance of difference: for mean difference, F ratio of between to within mean squares, for variance difference, Cochran's C

statistical significance ($p < 0.05$) in preadults. However, measurements of the first component tend to be smaller and less variable in heterozygous children. For height, the measurement representing the second component, heterozygotes tend to be more variable than homozygotes. Among adults (middle of Table 2) one mean difference and one variance difference are statistically significant ($p < 0.05$). Heterozygotes have larger arm circumferences (1st component), on average, and are more variable in body height (2nd component), than homozygotes. In addition, heterozygotes tend to be less variable than homozygotes for maximum chest circumference although this trend is not quite significant ($p < 0.10$). In the total sample (bottom Table 2), there are no significant mean differences, yet the trends for maximum chest circumference (less variable in heterozygotes, $p < 0.05$) and height (more variable in heterozygotes, $p < 0.01$) seen in the top of the table are now statistically significant.

Are any of these trends influenced by altitude of residence (Table 3)? Although the trends in Table 2 are significant only in adults, they are of very similar magnitude and direction in children. Hence age groups are combined in

TABLE 3
Means and standard deviations (s.d.) of age- and sex-adjusted anthropometric variables by heterozygosity class and altitude of residence

Measurement	Homozygotes mean ± s.d.	Heterozygotes mean ± s.d.	P* Mean diff.	P* Variance diff.
Coast	(n = 194)	(n = 184)		
Weight (kg)	-1.48 ± 5.14	-0.81 ± 5.63	n.s.	n.s.
Arm circ. (cm)	-0.28 ± 1.80	-0.09 ± 1.77	n.s.	n.s.
Max chest circ. (cm)	-0.69 ± 4.12	-0.41 ± 4.17	n.s.	n.s.
Height (cm)	-0.29 ± 4.90	0.34 ± 5.24	n.s.	n.s.
Head breadth (cm)	0.01 ± 0.48	-0.01 ± 0.48	n.s.	n.s.
Bizygo. breadth (cm)	-0.02 ± 0.47	-0.08 ± 0.53	n.s.	0.10
Sierra	(n = 224)	(n = 215)		
Weight (kg)	0.38 ± 6.73	0.56 ± 6.44	n.s.	n.s.
Arm circ. (cm)	0.04 ± 2.27	0.13 ± 2.22	n.s.	n.s.
Max. chest circ. (cm)	0.05 ± 5.20	0.17 ± 4.71	n.s.	n.s.
Height (cm)	0.13 ± 4.97	0.16 ± 5.58	n.s.	<0.10
Head breadth (cm)	0.04 ± 0.54	-0.01 ± 0.51	n.s.	n.s.
Bizygo. breadth (cm)	0.01 ± 0.50	0.00 ± 0.49	n.s.	n.s.
Altiplano	(n = 350)	(n = 345)		
Weight (kg)	0.45 ± 8.99	0.31 ± 8.31	n.s.	n.s.
Arm circ. (cm)	-0.02 ± 2.54	0.22 ± 2.61	n.s.	n.s.
Max. chest circ. (cm)	0.32 ± 6.40	0.24 ± 5.86	n.s.	0.10
Height (cm)	0.09 ± 5.55	-0.15 ± 6.13	n.s.	<0.10
Head breadth (cm)	-0.02 ± 0.54	0.02 ± 0.52	n.s.	n.s.
Bizygo. breadth (cm)	0.02 ± 0.47	0.05 ± 0.51	n.s.	n.s.

* Significance of difference (see note at bottom of Table 2)

Table 3. There are no mean differences between heterozygosity classes at any altitude. Variance differences are more evident, yet none reach statistical significance ($p < 0.05$). The fact that heterozygotes tend to be more variable in height is evident at all altitudes, yet marked differences are apparent only at higher altitudes ($p < 0.10$). The height standard deviations are for example, 5.55 and 6.13 for homozygotes and heterozygotes, respectively in the altiplano. The corresponding values for the total sample (Table 2) were 5.22 and 5.76, a similar difference. Likewise the tendency for heterozygotes to be less variable in chest circumference is evident at all altitudes, but approaches a statistically significant level only in the altiplano ($p < 0.10$). There is a tendency for the variance to increase with altitude for all measurements of the first component. This is difficult to explain, as this was not evident in the sample in the separate age and sex groups (Mueller et al., 1978a). However, the variances of body weight and arm and chest circumferences in the altiplano are similar to those for the adult sample (Table 2). This could be an effect of the generally more elderly population at high altitude (Mueller et al., 1978a). It could also be due to the inclusion of all classes of residency in the present sample, whereas in earlier reports we included only permanent residents. At any rate the variances increase with altitude in both heterozygosity groups.

Finally, there is a slight tendency for bizygomatic diameter to be more variable in heterozygotes but only on the coast ($p < 0.10$). Bizygomatic breadth is one measurement that was consistently related to ethnicity (Palomino et al., 1979). This trend may simply reflect the greater variability in ethnicity on the coast than at higher altitudes (Mueller et al., 1978c).

Discussion

Some limitations of these data need to be pointed out before drawing hard and fast conclusions. First, we have included related individuals in the sample. The effect would be to under estimate the variance and overestimate the significance of differences. Secondly, one would like to have had the largest possible sample of loci to determine with greatest precision an individual's heterozygosity. We have four (4) loci. Chakraborty (1981) has studied this problem by simulation, taking the largest number of known polymorphic loci in humans (about 125) and correlating the individual heterozygosity obtained at 125 loci with the value obtained from smaller numbers of loci. For example, the correlation between heterozygosity obtained from 4 and from 125 loci is about 0.15. Thus heterozygosity from four loci is not, on average, a very sensitive index of individual heterozygosity. Given these limitations, what speculations can we make concerning these observations?

Studies in plants and non-human animals of this kind indicate a decrease or increase in morphological variance in heterozygotes but not an increase in some characters and a decrease in others in the same sample. These studies have not dealt with uncorrelated principal components, but have instead relied on a single measurement or correlated measurements. Our results show that the problem is more complex and may depend on the morphological component selected for study. In this respect, the study of Livshits and Kobylianski (1984) is in accord with our results. Out of ten anthropometric traits five (5) were significantly less variable and one was significantly more variable in heterozygotes than homozygotes, and four showed no significant variance difference by heterozygosity. The trait that is more variable (vertex pronasale) is so at a highly significant level ($p < 0.01$), indeed more significant than any of the other traits studied, hence it cannot be regarded as fortuitous.

A decrease in morphological variance in heterozygotes would support the idea of better 'canalization' of heterozygotes. The phenotype follows a predetermined genetic path better in heterozygotes. This could occur if there is natural selection for an intermediate optimum on the morphological variable, or stabilizing selection (Mueller, 1979; Mueller et al. 1981a). Stabilizing selection will lead to increased heterozygosity because intermediate morphological types are more likely to be heterozygous. We see a reduced variance in maximum chest circumference among heterozygotes, which seems consistent with the idea of natural selection for an optimal chest size in the population, presumably connected with efficiency of the oxygen transport system. If this is the case, the variance difference between heterozygotes and homozygotes should increase with altitude, i.e., with greater selection pressure, which it seems to do (Table 3). The trend should also be more evident in adults than children, because adults are a more selected group, and this does seem to occur too (Table 2). Here our results are again in accord with those of Livshits and Kobylianski (1984). They found chest circumference to be less variable with increasing heterozygosity. Of interest is the fact that this dimension also appeared on their first principal component.

Turning to the second component, represented by height, an increase in morphological variance of heterozygotes is seen. This supports the supposition that heterozygotes are better able to make phenotypic adjustments in varying environments. The high altitude environment may vary in several ways as examples, seasonal availability of foods, temperature and hypoxia as movement to lower or higher altitudes may occur. Such an effect in our study is more likely to occur at high altitude where there is potentially more environmental stress, which it seems to do (Table 3). It is also more likely to be evident in adults than children, as adults would have completed their adult size and would have been exposed to environmental pressures longer, and this also seems to be the case (Table 2). This amounts to arguing for a greater developmental plasticity for heterozygotes. Here our results differ from those of Livshits and Kobylianski (1984). For height (represented on their second principal component as it was on ours), the morphological variance is reduced in heterozygotes. Their sample of course differs from ours in many respects. They studied two hundred young adult Israeli males, all of whom were presumably well-nourished. We suggest that long bone growth is not under the same selection pressures at high altitude that components of chest size may be and that a good deal more developmental plasticity in body height is likely to be seen. In this case varying conditions at high altitude, possibly those connected with malnutrition, may be more reflected in height than chest size. For this reason a developmental flexibility of heterozygotes is more readily detectable in this population.

In the main our results are similar to those of Livshits and Kobylianski (1984) in that development may be more or less variable in heterozygotes depending on the morphological component studied. However, why height is more variable with increasing heterozygosity in our study, and less variable in the Israeli study remains a mystery, unless it is due to the environmental conditions which differ between the two studies. Livshits and Kobylianski (1984) have cogently discussed the mechanisms underlying the growth-heterozygosity relationship. We have assumed in our discussion up till now that the four gene loci represent a sample of the individual's heterozygosity level. Livshits and Kobylianski (1984) reject the notion that this is the mechanism, on the basis that heterozygosity at the four blood group loci they studied showed no relationship to heterozygosities at other loci in the Israeli subjects. The lack of such a correlation is expected, however, given the small number of loci and the low expected correlation between these and total heterozygosity in the individual. For example, they could have found the very same relationships with four other loci, even though the individuals in each of the morphological classes would not have been strictly the same.

The mechanism of the heterozygosity-morphology relationship they suggest is that blood group loci modify the intracellular environment and thereby morphological development. In this respect, our four loci are red cell and serum enzymes and protein polymorphisms. We used different loci which could have modifying effects different from those of red cell surface antigens. But then why would these 'modifiers' produce the same result in the two studies for chest circumference, but not for height? Also there is no direct evidence that blood group loci affect development. Blood groups have been linked to protection from infection, but it appears to be null alleles (homozygosity) that are related to disease resistance (Livingstone, 1984).

One wonders whether choosing traits on the basis of principal components has not created some statistical artifact. Mueller and Reid (1979) noted that principal components were linearly uncorrelated due to their statistical structure, yet they found significant non-linear correlations between the first and other principal components of morphology. This possibility should be explored further because of the puzzling shift in the direction of the heterozygosity – morphology relationship in different principal components in both studies.

In another way our results and those of the Israeli study are consistent: Those components that show statistically significant associations with heterozygosity are measurements of probably high levels of heritability, namely traits of the skeletal system (Mueller, 1983, 1986). For example, in the Israel study the diminished variability in heterozygotes was evident in measurements of low heritability, such as arm circumference and weight/height2, but not significantly so. Likewise in our study, the morphological variance of measurements of presumed lower heritability (arm circumference and weight) were insignificantly related to heterozygosity, even though they resided on the same principal component as chest circumference, which was significantly related to heterozygosity in the total sample. This gives us greater confidence that the relationships seen in both studies are due to genetic mechanisms and not the confounding effects of socioeconomic or cultural factors.

There are no doubt other possible explanations for the observations; our speculations will remain just that till further work in this area is done. We can for example, examine the reproductive success of individuals for the various anthropometrics to determine whether there is a strong stabilizing selection at high altitude for chest size. Elsewhere we have presented evidence for lack of change in genetic variance of body height with altitude in this population which seems consistent with the maintenance of genetic variance by stabilizing selection (Mueller et al., 1980a).

JULIA K. BAILEY AND BETSY WEIDMAN

Chapter 11
HEARING AND HYPOXIA AMONG THE AYMARA

Effects of high altitude on hearing have been observed both in members of expeditions to mountainous regions and in local residents of these areas. Barcroft (1925), for example, reported that some of the members of his expedition suffered from auditory disturbances at Cerro de Pasco, Perú, situated at an altitude of 4300 meters. Richter also noticed alterations in hearing on an expedition to the Himalayas (cited from Van Liere and Stickney, 1963). Raffo (1934), who studied 14 residents at Casapalca, Perú, in the Andes at 4000 meters, found their auditory sensitivity was decreased when compared with members of Raffo's scientific expedition. McFarland (1937a, b, c) published the findings of several extensive investigations of hearing he had conducted in Perú and Chile. First, he studied the effects of rapid ascents by airplane from Lima to Morococha, Perú at 4500 meters (1937a). He made audiometric measurements of the members of his expedition, and found that the auditory thresholds were increased after rapid ascents to high altitude. The differences were more noticeable at the higher frequencies, and the impairment was relatively greater for rapid ascents than during gradual ones to similar altitudes.

Secondly, McFarland (1937b) investigated auditory responses after gradual acclimatization of ten members of an expedition to Chile. The measurements were made near the Bolivian border beginning at Antofagasta (sea level) and climbing, in several stages, to 6000 meters at Punta de Cerro. Not all of the subjects were tested at the highest altitude. He found 'The thresholds observed at Quilcha (17,500 feet) compared with sea level for the 4 highest frequencies for each ear were significantly decreased.'

Finally, McFarland (1937c) measured the hearing of Andean residents in Chile at 5300 meters and 4500 meters, and workers of similar race living at sea level. Eight frequencies were assessed: 64, 128, 256, 512, 1024, 2048, 4096 and 8192 Hz. He also compared these results to the auditory measurements of the ten members of the expedition to Chile when they were at 5300 meters. A summary of the subjects is presented in Table 1. One can observe from this table that only young men were tested. The sample sizes were not large and neither ethnicity nor residence were carefully assessed. These tests were conducted in 1937 so the audiometer and the way it was calibrated were not refined when compared with modern technology. McFarland (1937c) stated 'the thresholds for the miners at 17,500 feet and for the yareta (llareta) gatherers at 15,500 feet were approximately 6 to 8 decibels higher than for the workmen at sea level at each of the eight frequencies.' He also concluded 'The increase in the thresholds for both groups [at high altitude] was considerably greater for the three highest frequencies.' The members of the expedition, at 5300 meters, had more acute

William J. Schull and Francisco Rothhammer (eds.), The Aymará: Strategies in Human Adaptation to a Rigorous Environment, 143-165.

TABLE 1
A summary of the subjects in McFarland's survey in Chile

Subjects (all male)	Mean age (yrs.)	Residence (altitude) (feet)	Ethnicity	Description
35 sulphur miners	29.7	17,500 (worked in mines at 19,000)	Mixture of native Quechua and Spanish	'For the most part they had always lived at high altitudes and they were well acclimatized.'
10 llareta gathers (nomads who herded llama and gathered llareta)	26	15,500	Native Quechua	'... none of them had ever been to sea level having lived their entire lifetime above 12 to 14,000 feet.'
35 workmen (heavy manual laborers on a railroad)	30.5	Sea level	'Same racial stock' as sulphur miners	Lived and worked at sea level
10 members of the scientific expedition		17,500 (altitude at which hearing was tested)		

Cited from McFarland, 1937c.

auditory sensitivity, especially in the lower frequencies, than the Andean residents at 5300 and 4500 meters.

Von Ruedi, in 1944, conducted experiments in Berne, Switzerland, at 500 meters and on the Jungfrau-Joch at 3100 meters above sea level. Eight subjects were measured for auditory sensitivity at both altitudes. Three participants were healthy men aged 30 to 60 years while five were women who suffered from aural disorders. Three of the women had otosclerosis, one had an inherited progressive loss of hearing in the inner ear, and one had loss of hearing due to meningitis. It was noted that of the three women with otosclerosis, two had increased tinnitus at high altitude. Otherwise, no differences in hearing were found between low and high altitude. The significance of these findings is unclear for the results of this investigation are confounded by the illnesses of the subjects.

Singh et al. (1976) studied the effects of high altitude on hearing in India. These investigators compared the auditory thresholds at eight frequencies in residents at low (200 meters) and high altitude (3400 meters). The ethnicity of these subjects was not investigated and their sex and age are not stated. Because the nature of the sample of residents at low and high altitude is ambiguous, the results of this study are difficult to interpret. However, the investigators state 'The threshold of hearing was found to be consistently better in local residents of high altitude than in the subjects of the same age group resident at low altitude. This could perhaps be attributable to the absence of the noises of civilization at high altitude.' Fifty-four soldiers aged 17 to 30 years were also tested for hearing at both of the aforementioned altitudes. This acclimatization study indicated that the 'Pure tone audiogram showed both low tone and high tone loss on arrival at high altitude. The hearing loss was reversible and came back to the original level by about the fourth day of stay at high altitude.'

These studies notwithstanding, we can find no evidence of an epidemiological study of the effects of hypoxia on hearing, a truly population-based investigation that examines both sexes and all age groups among individuals who reside permanently at altitudes above 3000 meters. It is moot, therefore, what the actual effects of hypoxia may be upon the hearing of individuals who live continuously at altitudes with partial oxygen pressures two-thirds (or less) those to which coastal dwellers are accustomed.

The present study

The audiometric tests described here were conducted using a battery-powered Zenith Portable Audiometer, ISO-1964, Model ZA-110T, Serial Number 15496, and were conducted according to the ISO-1964 Standard for audiometric zero, the hearing threshold level setting on an audiometer identified as 0 dB. This setting is different for each frequency. In 1964, the International Standards Organization (ISO) released its standard for audiometric zero. These levels, known as the ISO-1964, are based on 15 separate studies of the hearing of young adults, carried out in five different countries after 1946 (Davis, 1965). The examination itself involved several stages. First, any unusual physical findings in each ear were noted. Then, hearing levels were recorded at seven frequencies: 500, 1000, 2000, 3000, 4000, 6000 and 8000 Hz. Any reasons for decreased auditory sensitivity were included as 'comments.' Tests were not performed on children under three years of age or elderly persons not able to understand the procedure.

Due to the remoteness of the examination sites, the audiometric appraisals were less controlled than one would find in optimal circumstances. The testing was not done in sound treated or attentuated rooms although the tester and subject were isolated as much as possible. It is felt that these compromises were justified because of the uniqueness of the population and its problems. All of the tests were done under similar conditions, in isolated corners of large assembly halls or schools.

An introductory test was performed in order to familiarize the subject with the examination. The subject was told, in Spanish, to listen for the sound in the earphone and to raise a hand in response. The right ear was tested first and the frequency was set at 2000 Hertz. The decibel level was raised rapidly until the

TABLE 2
Ear problems by ICDA code

No. cases	ICDA code (8th Edition)	
14	380	Otitis externa
1	381	Otitis media without mention of mastoiditis
3	381.0	Acute otitis media without mention of mastoiditis
2	381.1	Chronic otitis media without mention of mastoiditis
49	381.9	Unspecified otitis media without mention of mastoiditis
	382	Otitis media with mastoiditis
	382.0	Acute otitis media with mastoiditis
	382.1	Chronic otitis media with mastoiditis
	382.9	Unspecified otitis media with mastoiditis
	383	Mastoiditis without metion of otitis media
	383.0	Acute mastoiditis without mention of otitis media
	383.1	Chronic masoiditis without mention of otitis media
	383.9	Unspecified mastoiditis without mention of otitis media
	384	Other inflammatory diseases of the ear
1	384.0	Labyrinthitis
3	384.99	Other inflammatory diseases of the ear and unspecified
	385	Meniere's disease
9	385	Otosclerosis
	387	Other diseases of the ear and mastoid process
	387.0	Cholesteatoma of the ear
169	387.1	Wax in the ear - cerumen (accumulation, impacted)
18	387.2	Perforation of tympanic membrane, nontraumatic
5	387.9	Other diseases of the ear
	388	Deaf mutism
1	389	Other deafness - includes: both acquired and congenital
8	389.0	Deafness, both ears
1	389.1	Deafness, one ear, and partial deafness in the other
4	389.2	Deafness, one ear
10	389.9	Impairment of hearing, one or both ears

Note: 12 cases had two diagnostic impressions for the ear

subject responded, indicating he (she) knew what to be listening for. This introductory test was then repeated for the left ear.

The machine was reset for the actual examination. The right ear was tested first. The Hertz level was set at 500 and the intensity of the sound was gradually increased from 0 decibels until there was a positive response. This procedure was then performed for the remaining six of the seven frequencies previously cited. The left ear was tested in the same way. Two factors determined whether the test was repeated for one or both ears. First, retesting occurred if the reactions of the subject suggested he (she) did not understand the examination. This was apparent if the subject responded when the sound level was very low or did not indicate hearing the tone at any decibel level. Secondly, the examination was repeated if distracting background noise was higher than usual.

The results

For the purpose of analysis, the data were divided into nine categories by ethnicity and residence (see Chapter 1 for definitions of these categories). Three age groups were chosen to optimize the understanding of these hearing data. The youngest group includes all children and young adults, aged 3 to 25 years. The rationale for grouping these ages together is that hearing loss due to age (presbyacusis) begins around 30 years of age. Thus individuals 25 years of age or younger are not affected by this process. The category containing those age 26 to 50 encompasses all middle-aged subjects, or those with slight presbyacusis. Most presbyacusis occurs after the age of 50, so this was chosen as the beginning point for the third group.

Exclusion of subjects

If a subject did not receive an audiometric exam, obviously he or she was excluded from analysis. These cases mainly involved children under the age of three and some elderly people unable to understand the examination procedure. In all, 412 of the original subjects (2096) were not tested. All individuals (286) with ear problems diagnosed by examining physicians at the testing site were also excluded. A list of these ear conditions can be found in Table 2, and the number of cases in each category is shown in Table 3. These numbers were not analyzed statistically because there were so few individuals in each category. Otitis externa, otosclerosis, perforation of the ear drum, and deafness were diagnosed most often in the sierra, and diagnoses of otitis media and accumulated earwax occurred most frequently among the Aymará who lived in the altiplano. But these numbers are not really indicative of trends because the sample sizes are not equal. There are, for example, many more Aymará in the altiplano (406) than non-Aymará (19).

After the exclusions identified in the previous paragraph, data were available for analysis on 1444 individuals (see Table 4). Approximately 30 per cent of the cases were eliminated as a result of ear problems or the absence of test data.

Exclusion of measurements

Left ear measurements were excluded since retrospectively it is clear that the audiometer was not calibrated correctly for this ear. It appears too that the background room noise present in the test surroundings masked the threshold measurements at 500 Hz. Therefore, the values for hearing loss at this frequency have not been analyzed. Finally, the decibel levels for 6000 Hz were excluded because they were not consistent with the rest of the frequency measurements. The higher frequencies, 6000 and 8000 Hz, are difficult to calibrate well in audiometers, particularly in portable ones, because the wavelengths at these frequencies are very close to the length of the ear and standing waves may occur. The values at 8000 Hz appeared to be more consistent than those levels recorded

TABLE 3
Distribution of ear conditions

Ethnicity	Age	Coast Males	Coast Females	Coast Total	Sierra Males	Sierra Females	Sierra Total	Altiplano Males	Altiplano Females	Altiplano Total
				Otitis externa - 14 cases						
Aymará	0-25							1		1
	26-50				1	1	2			
	51-99					2	2			
	Total				1	3	4	1		1
Mestizo	0-25					3	3			
	26-50					1	1			
	51-99				1		1			
	Total				1	4	5			
Non-Aymará	0-25		1	1						
	26-50	1		1						
	51-99	2		2						
	Total	3	1	4						
				Otosclerosis - 9 cases						
Aymará	0-25									
	26-50									
	51-99				2	2	4			
	Total				2	2	4			
Mestizo	0-25									
	26-50									
	51-99				1		1			
	Total				1		1			
Non-Aymará	0-25									
	26-50				1		1			
	51-99				2	1	3			
	Total				3	1	4			
				Perforation of tympanic membrane - 18 cases						
Aymará	0-25					1	1	1		1
	26-50				2		2			
	51-99		1	1	1	2	3			
	Total		1	1	3	3	6	1		1
Mestizo	0-25	1	1	2	1	1	2			
	26-50		2	2						
	51-99				1		1			
	Total	1	3	4	2	1	3			
Non-Aymará	0-25									
	26-50									
	51-99		1	1	1	1	2			
	Total		1	1	1	1	2			

TABLE 3 (continued)
Distribution of ear conditions

Ethnicity	Age	Coast Males	Coast Females	Coast Total	Sierra Males	Sierra Females	Sierra Total	Altiplano Males	Altiplano Females	Altiplano Total
				Otitis Media - 55 cases						
Aymará	0-25				2		2	4	1	5
	26-50							4	2	6
	51-99				1		1	5	2	7
	Total				3	1	4	13	5	18
Mestizo	0-25	3	1	4	6	4	10	1	3	4
	26-50	1	1	2	1	1	2	1	1	2
	51-99				1	1	2	1	1	2
	Total	4	2	6	8	6	14	3	5	8
Non-Aymará	0-25		1	1						
	26-50	1		1	1		1			
	51-99							1	1	2
	Total	1	1	2	1		1	1	1	2
				Wax in the ear - 169 cases						
Aymará	0-25	4	1	5	5	2	7	13	21	34
	26-50	1		1	3	4	7	2	3	5
	51-99	1		1	5	1	6	3	6	9
	Total	6	1	7	13	7	30	18	30	48
Mesitzo	0-25	14	11	25	17	5	22	4	6	10
	26-50	2		2	2	2	4	1	1	2
	51-99		2	2	2	1	3			
	Total	16	13	29	21	8	29	5	7	12
Non-Aymará	0-25	6	4	10	1	1	2			
	26-50	2	1	3	2	1	3	1		1
	51-99	1	1	2	2	1	3			
	Total	9	6	15	5	3	8	1		1

at 6000 Hz, and as a result, we have excluded only the latter. In summary, this analysis includes right ear auditory threshold values at 1000, 2000, 3000, 4000 and 8000 Hz.

Visual representation of the data

The data are plotted by residence and ethnicity in Figure 1. The three age groups are compared in each of the nine ethnicity-altitude categories. The graphs show that there is a masking effect at 1000 Hz presumably due to room noise at the testing site, and this is seen as a depression in each audiogram at 1000 Hz. The aging effect is evident in Figure 1 where subjects aged 51 and above show a

TABLE 4
Distribution of the cases available for study by age, sex, ethnicity and altitude of residence

Ethnicity	Age	Coast Male	Coast Female	Coast Total	Sierra Male	Sierra Female	Sierra Total	Altiplano Male	Altiplano Female	Altiplano Total
					Number of Cases					
Aymará	0-25	12	13	25	44	28	72	74	74	148
	26-50	15	11	26	24	44	68	48	44	92
	51-99	3	4	7	22	22	44	21	13	34
	Total	30	28	58	90	94	184	143	131	274
Mestizo	0-25	72	65	137	107	94	201	36	47	83
	26-50	39	39	78	36	33	69	24	17	41
	51-99	12	6	18	17	27	44	9	8	17
	Total	123	110	233	160	154	314	69	72	141
Non-Aymará	0-25	22	43	65	22	8	30	4	0	4
	26-50	34	34	68	17	7	24	3	2	5
	51-99	11	16	27	9	2	11	5	1	6
	Total	67	93	160	48	17	65	12	3	15
					Percent of all of the original subjects in the stated age-sex-ethnicity-residence category					
Aymará	0-25	70.6	72.2	71.4	65.7	57.1	62.1	61.2	56.5	58.7
	26-50	93.8	100.0	96.3	72.7	86.3	81.0	88.9	89.8	89.3
	51-99	75.0	80.0	77.8	62.9	59.5	61.1	70.0	61.9	66.7
	Total	81.1	82.4	81.7	66.7	68.6	67.6	69.8	65.2	67.5
Mestizo	0-25	54.5	57.0	55.7	69.0	61.0	65.0	48.0	53.4	50.9
	26-50	90.7	90.8	90.7	87.8	86.8	87.3	92.3	85.0	89.1
	51-99	85.7	75.0	81.8	65.4	81.8	74.6	90.0	88.9	89.5
	Total	65.1	66.7	65.8	72.1	68.4	70.2	62.2	61.5	61.8
Non-Aymará	0-25	55.0	69.4	63.7	95.7	66.7	85.7	100.0	0.0	80.0
	26-50	87.2	91.9	89.5	81.0	87.5	82.8	75.0	100.0	83.3
	51-99	83.3	84.2	79.4	52.9	33.3	47.8	83.3	50.0	75.0
	Total	71.3	78.8	75.5	78.7	65.4	74.7	85.7	60.0	78.9

marked increase in hearing loss when compared to the younger two age groups. This is especially noticeable in the higher frequencies 3000, 4000 and 8000 Hz. It is of note that in the non-Aymará residing in the altiplano, the subjects aged 26 to 50 years hear better than the younger group aged 3 to 25 years. However, the sample sizes are very small in these two groups (5 and 4, respectively) so this observation is probably not significant.

Hearing levels in the group aged 3 to 25 years are depicted in Figures 2 and 3. This age group has better hearing at 8000 Hz than at the lower frequencies. The variation in these data appears to be quite uniform (Figure 2). No marked differences are seen across altitude or ethnicity (Figure 3). Figures 4 and 5 show auditory thresholds in the age group 26 to 50 years. No differences between the ethnicity-altitude groups are evident. On the average, the decibel loss in this age

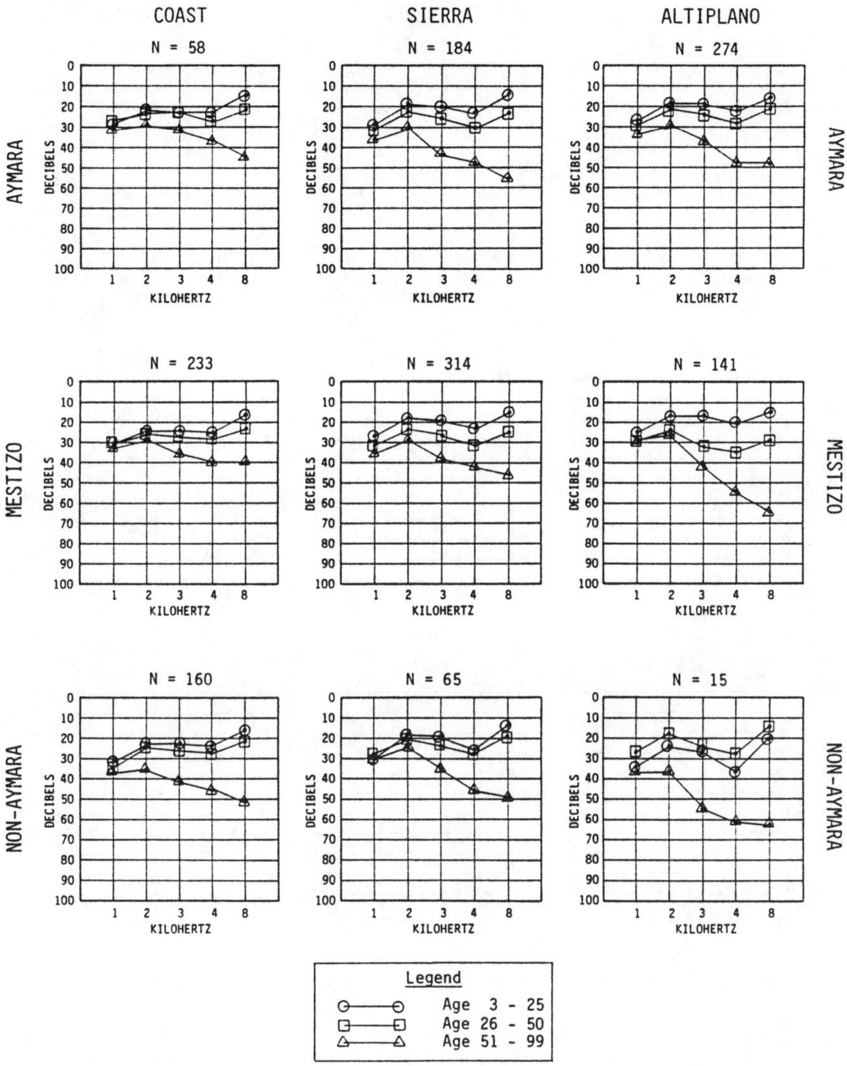

FIGURE 1. All age groups, plotted by residence and ethnicity (n = 1444)

category is slightly greater than that for the subjects aged 3 to 25 years, and the variation, measured by one standard deviation, is also greater. The age group 51 and over shows the typical 'ski-slope' shaped audiogram common in aging populations (Figures 6 and 7). As frequency increases, hearing loss increases. The variation in the data for this age group, indicated by one standard deviation, is greater than that for the two younger age categories.

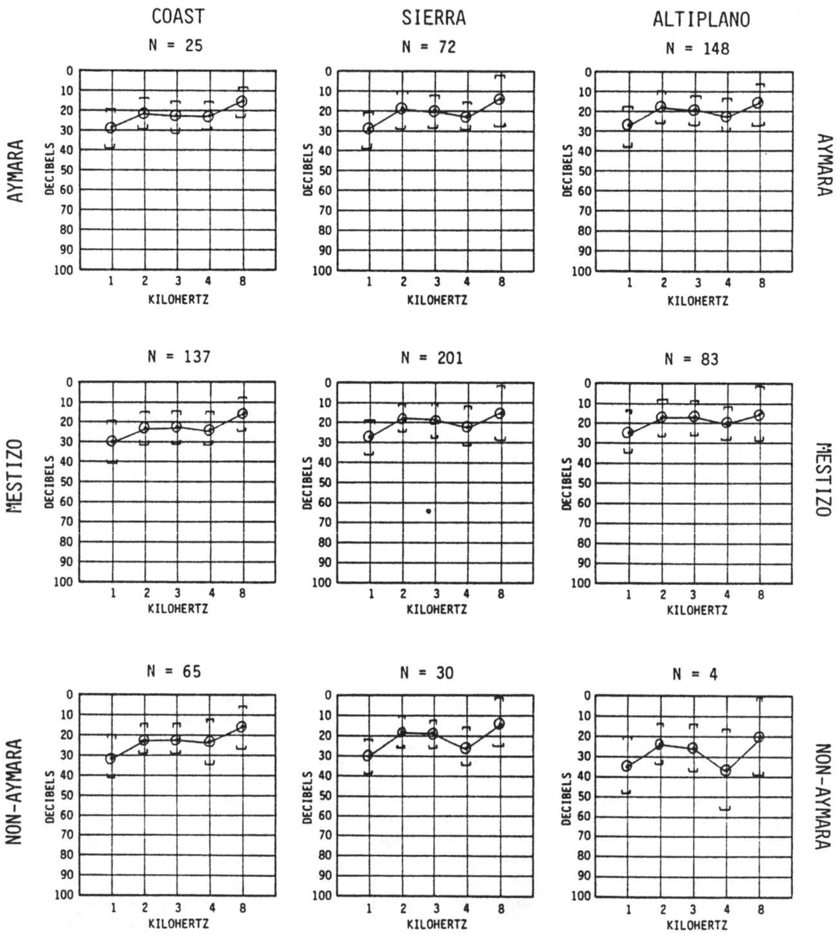

FIGURE 2. Age group 3 to 25: Showing variation by one standard deviation

Determination of significant factors

It is well known that hearing loss increases with age, particularly at the higher frequencies. However, there has been debate as to whether hearing loss in decibels as a function of age is an exponential or linear function. Glorig and Nixon (1962) stated that the log of hearing level in decibels is a linear function of the log of age. However, Hinchcliffe (1962) demonstrated that '... a linear relationship [of hearing loss with age] seems to hold for frequencies 250 cps to 4000 cps inclusive.' The basis for this latter finding is that decibels are in themselves a logarithmic function.

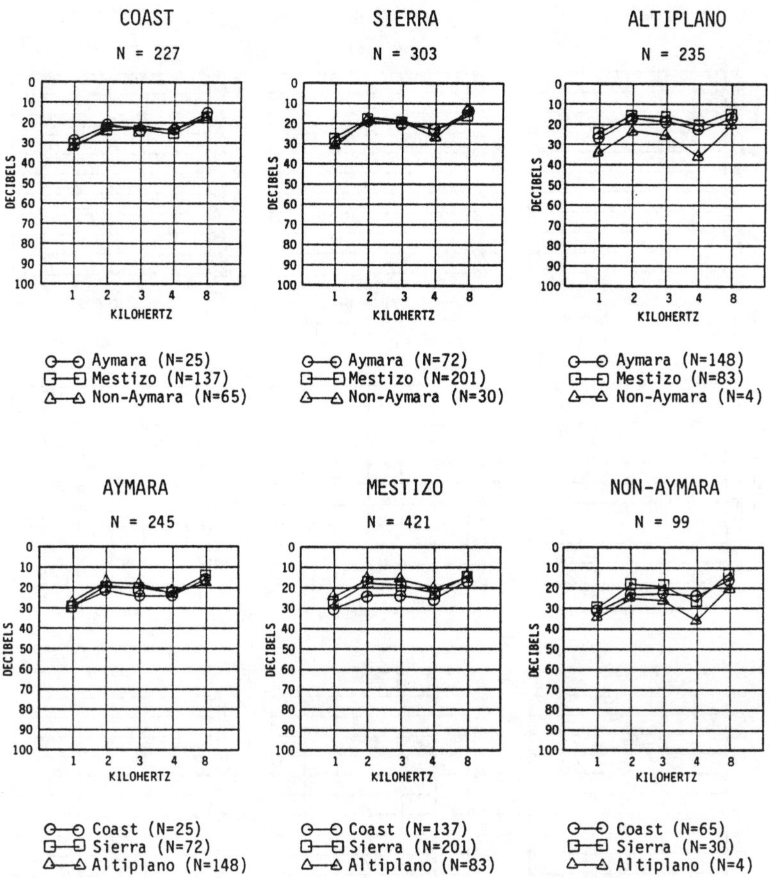

FIGURE 3. Age group 3 to 25: Comparisons by residence and ethnicity

Figure 8 depicts mean hearing loss plotted against age for the three altitudes and the five frequencies 1000, 2000, 3000, 4000 and 8000 Hz. The standard error of the mean is indicated on these graphs and a linear relationship of hearing loss with age is postulated. To provide some insight into possible changes in the variance in hearing levels with age, mean hearing levels with their standard deviations are depicted by age in Figure 9.

These graphs (Figures 8 and 9) must be viewed with the consideration that presbyacusis is not evident before the age of 30. It should be noted too that the standard errors for the groups at the midpoints 70 and 80 years are large, and thus it is difficult to identify positively a linear trend in the data by inspection alone. These figures also indicate that auditory thresholds are much greater in the older age groups, especially in those aged 65 to 85 years. However, these subjects have a slower response to the test and their measured auditory levels

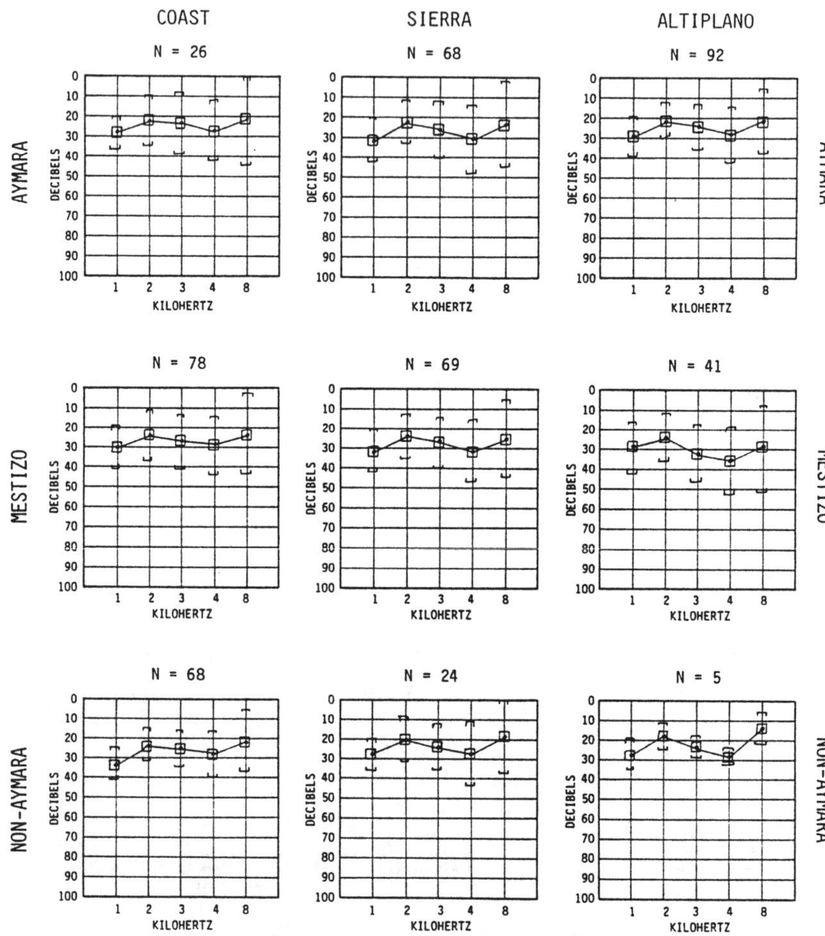

FIGURE 4. Age group 26 to 50: Showing variation by one standard deviation

could be greater than their actual hearing loss. As was previously stated, each subject was asked to raise a hand when hearing the tone from the audiometer, and for older subjects, the reaction time for this physical action is much longer than it is for younger people. (See Maurer and Rupp (1979) for a more detailed explanation of this.)

A priori it was moot whether to use a multivariate or a univariate method of analysis to determine the significance of altitude and ethnicity; accordingly, the data were subdivided into groups of age and altitude, and cross-correlations of hearing levels for the different frequencies were calculated (Table 5). The results of these calculations indicate that the correlation values are higher for neighboring frequency values than for widely separated ones. For example, the

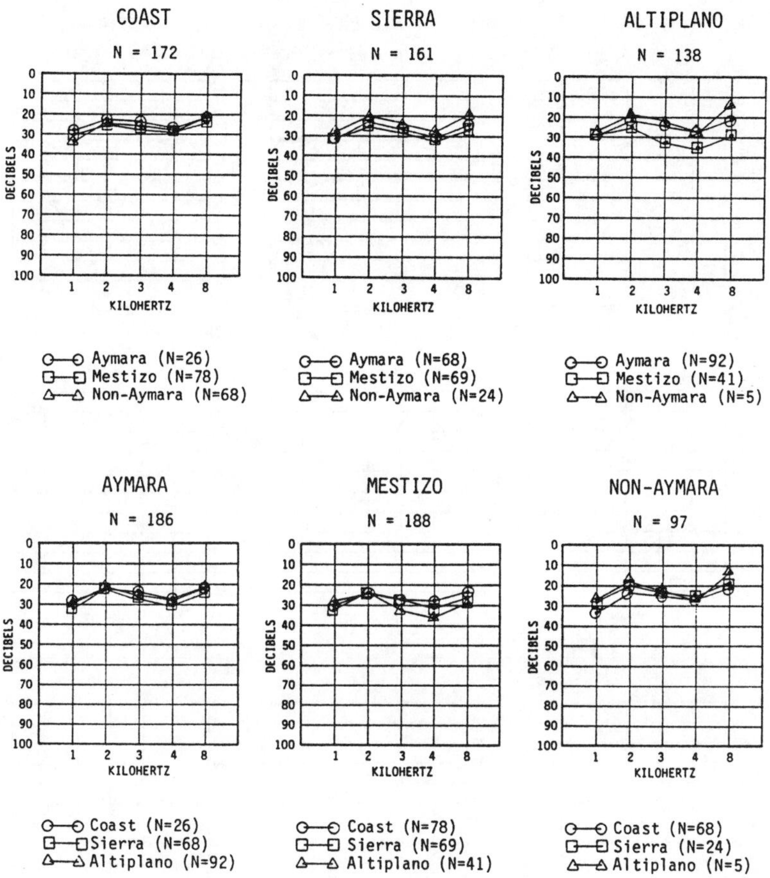

FIGURE 5. Age group 26 to 50: Comparisons by residence and ethnicity

values at a frequency of 8000 Hz are highly correlated with those at 4000 Hz but not at 1000 Hz. Therefore, a univariate analysis was used for it did not appear that analyzing the five frequencies together in a multivariate analysis would yield a different result.

An unbalanced two-way analysis of variance to test the statistical significance of the effects of altitude and ethnicity was performed on the entire data set with age as a linear covariate. The data were divided into nine ethnicity-altitude cells. Since the number of observations in the various cells were neither equal nor proportional, an unbalanced classical design was used. In these calculations, the sums of squares are obtained by regression after adjustment for the effects of the covariables, in this instance, age. This method is useful for detecting a combined effect of altitude and ethnicity that might not otherwise be evident. The results of

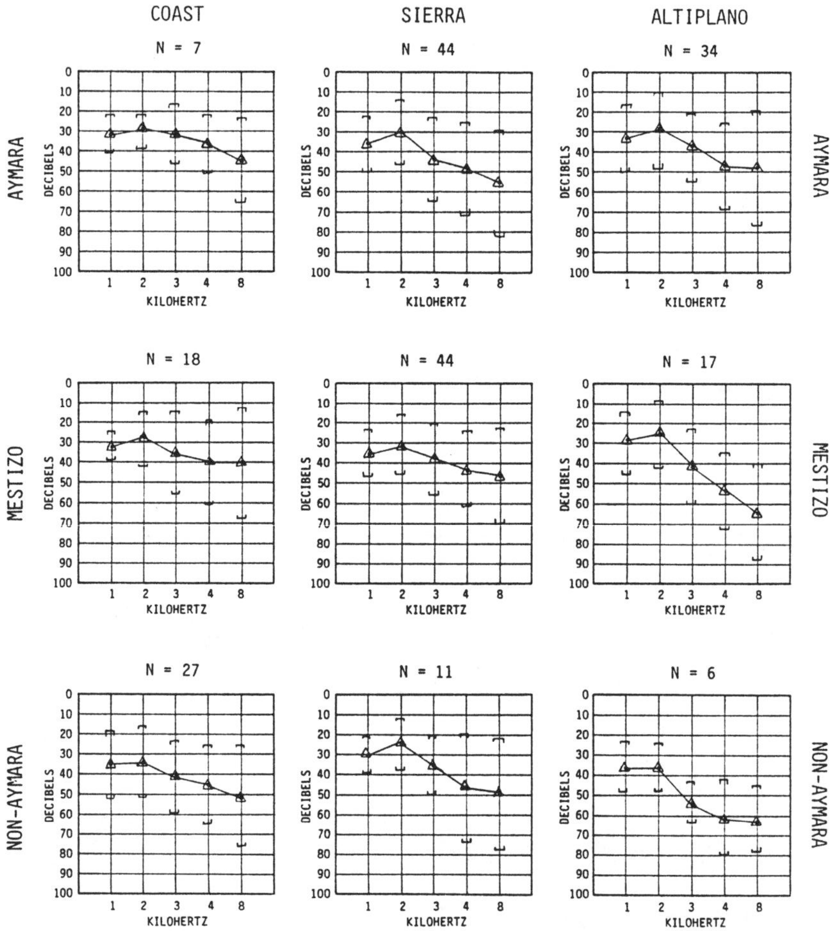

FIGURE 6. Age group 51 to 99: Showing variation by one standard deviation

this unbalanced covariance analysis are presented in Table 6. At 1000 and 2000 Hz, age, main effects, altitude and the explained variance are all significant at the 0.001 level. At 3000 Hz, age, the altitude-ethnicity interaction, and the explained variance are significant at the 0.001, 0.016, and 0.001 probability level, respectively. It should be noted that since an interaction of altitude and ethnicity exists and since the sample sizes are unequal, the tests of the effects of altitude and ethnicity in Table 6 confound one another, and are, therefore, uncertain guides to the effects of these variables considered singly. The effects of altitude and ethnicity are not significant at 4000 and 8000 Hz.

To confirm that a linear model provides the best descriptor of these data, both the log hearing level versus log age model (as in Glorig and Nixon, 1962) and the

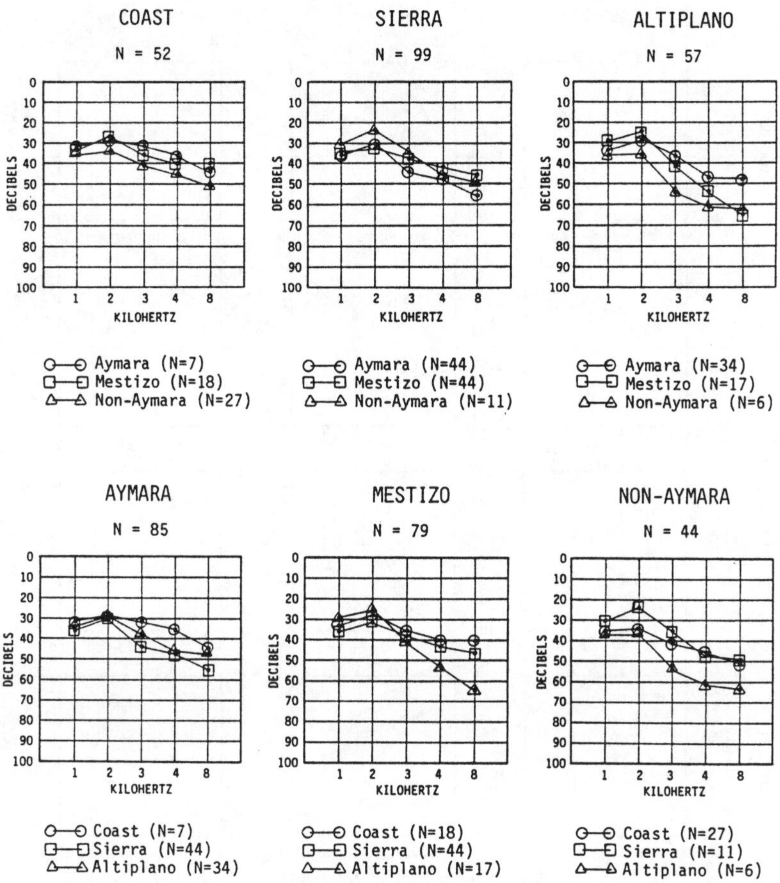

FIGURE 7. Age group 51 to 99: Comparisons by residence and ethnicity

linear hearing level versus linear age model (as in Hinchcliffe) were fitted. However, the variance explained by the log-log model was consistently less (results not shown) than for the linear model and thus the latter is the better fit.

In order to indicate trends in the data, Table 7 shows hearing levels by altitude and age. The coefficients were obtained by linear regression as a function of the continuous variable age and two categorical variables for altitude. Hearing at the altiplano is significantly better than that at the lower altitudes for the frequencies 1000, 2000 and 3000 Hz. At 2000 Hz, hearing in the sierra is significantly different than that at the coast. It is also evident that altiplano subjects have higher auditory thresholds at 8000 Hz than their coastal and sierran peers. This analysis shows that the effect of altitude within these data is internally consistent. At high altitudes, population hearing degrades as frequency increases when compared with auditory thresholds of coastal residents. This table also indicates

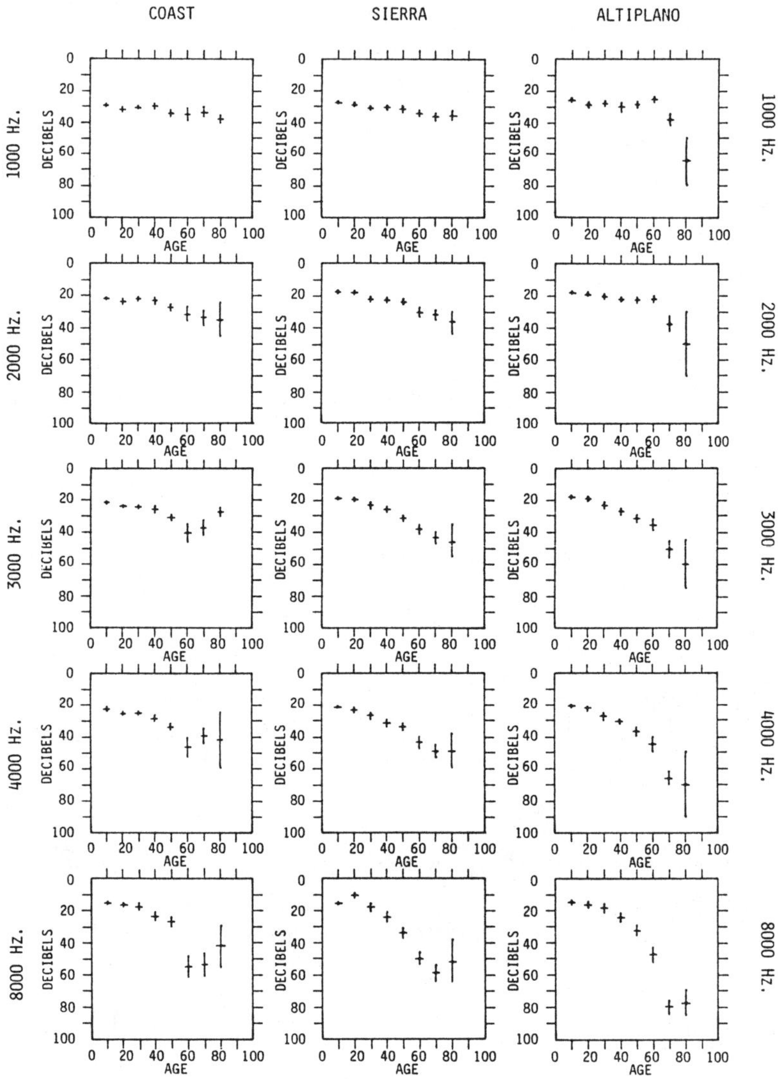

FIGURE 8. Mean hearing loss plotted versus age, showing variation by one standard error and compared by residence

the increasing importance of age as frequency increases. Thus age and altitude are significant factors influencing hearing levels but ethnicity appears to have no effect.

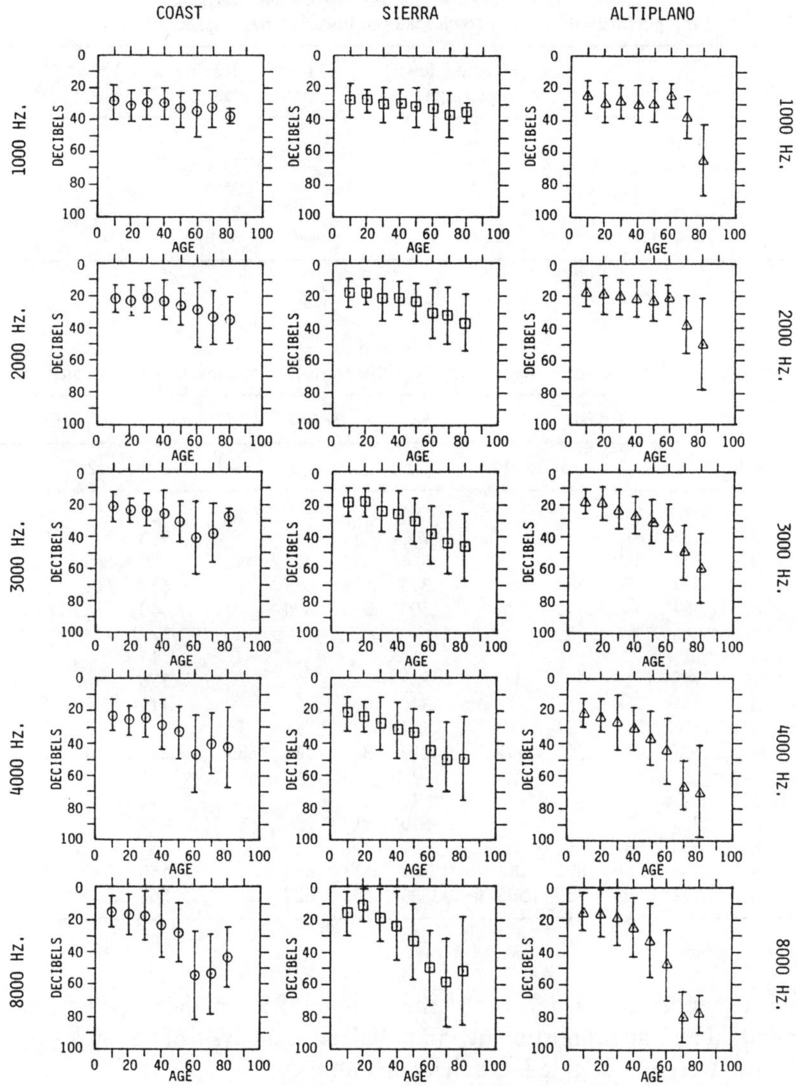

FIGURE 9. Mean hearing loss plotted versus age, showing variation by one standard deviation and compared by residence

Analysis of the three age groups

To determine exactly in which age groups the effects of altitude are evident, the entire data set was again divided into the three age and nine ethnicity-altitude

TABLE 5
R-squared values (%) for the regression analysis performed in order to choose the linear or log-log model

	Log (Hearing level) *vs* Log (Age)	Linear (Hearing level) *vs* Linear (Age)
1000 Hz	3.4	4.0
2000 Hz	8.4	11.1
3000 Hz	20.5	25.0
4000 Hz	19.8	26.5
8000 Hz	16.6	31.0

TABLE 6
Cross-correlations between hearing levels at different frequencies, by age and altitude

		Coast				Sierra				Altiplano			
Age	kHz	1	2	3	4	1	2	3	4	1	2	3	4
3-25	1	1				1				1			
	2	.723	1			.700	1			.713	1		
	3	.574	.617	1		.514	.671	1		.729	.807	1	
	4	.547	.530	.680	1	.376	.502	.695	1	.642	.608	.746	1
	8	.384	.480	.495	.528	.300	.375	.396	.440	.440	.581	.611	.579
26-50	1	1				1				1			
	2	.745	1			.582	1			.576	1		
	3	.531	.758	1		.344	.695	1		.415	.639	1	
	4	.406	.567	.734	1	.234	.585	.781	1	.353	.533	.771	1
	8	.375	.481	.563	.661	.217	.386	.520	.685	.274	.461	.555	.675
51-99	1	1				1				1			
	2	.760	1			.650	1			.819	1		
	3	.536	.803	1		.431	.713	1		.565	.771	1	
	4	.436	.763	.891	1	.362	.618	.843	1	.560	.712	.886	1
	8	.252	.483	.566	.593	.338	.456	.627	.742	.564	.623	.704	.834

categories mentioned earlier. Since the sample sizes in these latter nine cells were unequal and disproportionate, an unbalanced analysis of variance was used. Two factors were investigated: ethnicity and altitude.

Table 8 displays the results for the age group 3 to 25 years for the five frequencies investigated. At 1000, 2000 and 3000 Hz, main effects or joint effects and the altitude factor are significant at the 0.001 probability level. In addition, at these three frequencies the explained variance is significant at the 0.001 level. At 4000 Hz, the main effects and the altitude-ethnicity interaction are significant at the 0.039 and 0.007 levels, respectively. Again, note that since an altitude-ethnicity interaction exists and since the sample sizes are unequal (and disproportionate) the test of altitude confounds the effect of ethnicity and vice versa. The explained variance is significant at 0.002, and thus altitude is

TABLE 7
Covariate unbalanced analysis of variance

	Source of Variation	Sum of Squares	Degrees of freedom	Mean Square	F	Significance of F
1 kHz	Covariate:age	6800.5	1	6800.5	61.040	.001
	Main effects	2371.1	4	592.7	5.321	.001
	Altitude	1930.2	2	965.1	8.663	.001
	Ethnicity	341.6	2	170.8	1.533	.216
	Alt x Eth[a]	881.4	4	220.3	1.978	.096
	Explained	10053.2	9	1117.0	10.026	.001
	Residual	159096.2	1428	111.4	-	-
	Total	169149.4	1437	117.7	-	-
2 kHz	Covariate:age	20243.8	1	20243.8	181.264	.001
	Main effects	2567.5	4	641.8	5.748	.001
	Altitude	2116.1	2	1058.0	9.474	.001
	Ethnicity	161.5	2	80.7	0.723	.485
	Alt x Eth[a]	599.4	4	149.8	1.342	.252
	Explained	23410.9	9	2601.2	23.291	.001
	Residual	159481.6	1428	111.6	-	-
	Total	182892.5	1437	127.2	-	-
3 kHz	Covariate:age	64012.4	1	64012.4	482.524	.001
	Main effects	1146.5	4	286.6	2.161	.071
	Altitude	449.0	2	224.5	1.693	.185
	Ethnicity	412.4	2	206.2	1.554	.212
	Alt x Eth[a]	1633.0	4	408.2	3.077	.016
	Explained	66792.0	9	7421.3	55.942	.001
	Residual	189440.9	1428	132.6	-	-
	Total	256232.9	1437	178.3	-	-
4 kHz	Covariate:age	90711.6	1	90711.6	519.295	.001
	Main effects	537.1	4	134.2	0.769	.546
	Altitude	394.7	2	197.3	1.130	.323
	Ethnicity	318.1	2	159.0	0.911	.403
	Alt x Eth[a]	1612.9	4	403.2	2.308	.056
	Explained	92861.7	9	10317.9	59.067	.001
	Residual	249446.1	1428	174.6	-	-
	Total	342307.9	1437	238.2	-	-
8 kHz	Covariate:age	190672.8	1	190672.8	646.730	.001
	Main effects	2428.9	4	607.2	2.060	.084
	Altitude	1014.5	2	507.2	1.721	.179
	Ethnicity	1441.2	2	720.6	2.444	.087
	Alt x Eth[a]	1405.8	4	351.4	1.192	.313
	Explained	194507.6	9	21611.9	73.304	.001
	Residual	421011.3	1428	294.8	-	-
	Total	615519.0	1437	428.3	-	-

[a] This denotes Altitude-Ethnicity interaction effect

important in explaining the variance among the means in this age group. Further analysis of the three lowest frequencies revealed a significant difference between the coastal and higher altitude (sierra and altiplano) residents. There were no significant comparisons between sierra and altiplano inhabitants.

TABLE 8
Unbalanced analysis of variance: Age group 3 to 25 years

	Source of Variation	Sum of Squares	Degrees of freedom	Mean Square	F	Significance of F
1 kHz	Main effects	2385.3	4	596.3	5.987	.001
	Altitude	1712.2	2	856.1	8.595	.001
	Ethnicity	572.3	2	286.1	2.873	.057
	Alt x Eth[a]	523.2	4	130.8	1.313	.263
	Explained	2908.6	8	363.5	3.650	.001
	Residual	75103.0	754	99.6	-	-
	Total	78011.6	762	102.3	-	-
2 kHz	Main effects	2871.0	4	717.7	9.427	.001
	Altitude	2673.5	2	1336.7	17.556	.001
	Ethnicity	55.8	2	27.9	0.367	.693
	Alt x Eth[a]	213.2	4	53.3	0.700	.592
	Explained	3084.2	8	385.5	5.063	.001
	Residual	57411.0	754	76.1	-	-
	Total	60495.2	762	79.3	-	-
3 kHz	Main effects	2739.4	4	684.8	10.224	.001
	Altitude	2413.0	2	1206.5	18.012	.001
	Ethnicity	55.9	2	27.9	0.418	.659
	Alt x Eth[a]	328.7	4	82.1	1.227	.298
	Explained	3068.2	8	383.5	5.726	.001
	Residual	50506.4	754	66.9	-	-
	Total	53574.7	762	70.3	-	-
4 kHz	Main effects	863.0	4	215.7	2.533	.039
	Altitude	343.3	2	171.6	2.015	.134
	Ethnicity	225.6	2	112.8	1.324	.267
	Alt x Eth[a]	1200.3	4	300.0	3.522	.007
	Explained	2063.4	8	257.9	3.028	.002
	Residual	64236.1	754	85.1	-	-
	Total	66299.5	762	87.0	-	-
8 kHz	Main effects	313.9	4	78.4	0.556	.694
	Altitude	300.3	2	150.1	1.065	.345
	Ethnicity	39.7	2	19.8	0.141	.869
	Alt x Eth[a]	224.8	4	56.2	0.399	.810
	Explained	538.7	8	67.3	0.478	.873
	Residual	106341.8	754	141.0	-	-
	Total	106880.6	762	140.2	-	-

[a] This denotes Altitude-Ethnicity interaction effect

The subjects aged 26 to 50 years are compared in Table 9. The results of this analysis revealed an ethnicity effect at 3000 Hz, significant at the 0.012 level. Further analysis in this frequency group showed a significant difference between the mestizos and non-Aymará. This result seems to be dependent on the high number of mestizos compared to the Aymará and non-Aymará. No significant effects of altitude or ethnicity were detected in the oldest age category, 51 years

TABLE 9
Unbalanced analysis of variance: Age group 26 to 50 years

	Source of Variation	Sum of Squares	Degrees of freedom	Mean Square	F	Significance of F
1 kHz	Main effects	339.1	4	84.7	0.780	.539
	Altitude	216.3	2	108.1	0.995	.370
	Ethnicity	35.8	2	17.9	0.165	.848
	Alt x Eth[a]	658.2	4	164.5	1.514	.197
	Explained	997.3	8	124.6	1.147	.330
	Residual	50104.1	461	108.6	-	-
	Total	51101.5	469	108.9	-	-
2 kHz	Main effects	658.2	4	164.5	1.406	.231
	Altitude	174.7	2	87.3	0.746	.475
	Ethnicity	385.2	2	192.6	1.646	.194
	Alt x Eth[a]	257.9	4	64.4	0.551	.699
	Explained	916.1	8	114.5	0.978	.452
	Residual	53967.9	461	117.0	-	-
	Total	54884.0	469	117.0	-	-
3 kHz	Main effects	1441.0	4	360.2	2.304	.058
	Altitude	149.4	2	74.7	0.478	.620
	Ethnicity	1394.7	2	697.3	4.460	.012
	Alt x Eth[a]	890.7	4	222.6	1.424	.225
	Explained	2331.8	8	291.4	1.864	.064
	Residual	72083.1	461	156.3	-	-
	Total	74414.9	469	158.6	-	-
4 kHz	Main effects	952.0	4	238.0	1.103	.355
	Altitude	584.5	2	292.2	1.354	.259
	Ethnicity	454.4	2	227.2	1.053	.350
	Alt x Eth[a]	1309.1	4	327.2	1.516	.196
	Explained	2261.1	8	282.6	1.309	.236
	Residual	99516.6	461	215.8	-	-
	Total	10177.8	469	217.0	-	-
8 kHz	Main effects	1923.8	4	480.9	1.325	.259
	Altitude	233.2	2	166.6	0.321	.725
	Ethnicity	1634.1	2	817.0	2.252	.106
	Alt x Eth[a]	1104.0	4	276.0	0.761	.551
	Explained	3027.8	8	378.4	1.043	.403
	Residual	167281.5	461	362.8	-	-
	Total	170309.3	469	363.1	-	-

[a] This denotes Altitude-Ethnicity interaction effect

of age or older, nor was there evidence of an altitude-ethnicity interaction (data not shown). These results may confound aging, however.

Comparisons of each age group by residence (coast, sierra, and altiplano) failed to disclose significant differences. However, at face value, in the age category 3 to 25 years, the altiplano and sierra residents hear slightly better than the coastal inhabitants and in the oldest age group, it appears that the coastal residents hear slightly better than the population of the altiplano and sierra.

Discussion

Previous adaptation studies of hearing at high altitude have been conducted by McFarland (1937c) and Singh et al. (1976). In 1937, McFarland compared the hearing of high altitude Andean residents at 4700 and 5800 meters with that of a coastal population of approximately the same race, and found that those individuals living at high altitude had poorer hearing at all frequencies tested but especially so at the higher ones. As previously noted, the subjects in this study were young men, and their ethnicity was not carefully assessed. Singh and his colleagues (1976) conducted a survey in India, and discovered that residents at high altitude (3800 meters) had better hearing than low altitude groups (200 meters). This finding was attributed to the absence of the noises of civilization at high altitude. The age, sex, and ethnicity of the populations in Singh's investigation were not assessed.

Thus, the extensive knowledge obtained about the ethnicity and residence of each subject in this survey makes this project unique. In addition, the population surveyed encompasses both sexes and all ages. But this investigation has its own limitations, notably the fact that the tests were not conducted in controlled surroundings such as a sound treated room. The actual values are not, therefore, comparable to those of other populations. However, the background noise was similar for all examinations, so that comparisons within the data should be valid even if the values themselves cannot be used for normative purposes.

The results of the covariate unbalanced analysis of variance, which adjusts for the age factor, show a statistically significant effect of altitude on hearing for the lower frequencies 1000 and 2000 Hz (Table 6). The interaction effect seen at 3000 Hz could indicate the influence of altitude; however, the non-significance of the main effects at this frequency is difficult to interpret. At all five frequencies, ethnicity is not a factor in determining the observed differences in hearing. To confirm and further analyze the altitude effect found in the covariate unbalanced analysis, the data were analyzed separately in each of three age groups. It appears there is a difference in auditory thresholds in the lower frequencies with respect to altitude, but this difference is detectable only in the younger subjects (ages 3 to 25 years) in the population. In this age group, residents at high altitudes, in the sierra and altiplano, hear better than those individuals who live at sea level. This trend is reversed in the oldest age category, since at higher frequencies the coastal residents hear better than their counterparts in the sierra and altiplano. These altitude effects are confirmed in Table 7. At frequencies of 1000, 2000 and 3000 Hz, the trend is toward better hearing as altitude increases. For 4000 and 8000 Hz, hearing becomes more acute as altitude decreases. The auditory thresholds at these latter two frequencies are greatly affected by age.

These apparent altitude effects are particularly interesting in the light of the socio-cultural differences between the residents in the three areas studied. The majority of the high altitude dwellers are Aymará as opposed to mestizo or non-Aymará. One would expect that the Aymará, who are less proficient in Spanish than those participants of Spanish extraction, would have difficulty in understanding the test procedure. Therefore, the finding that ethnicity is not a significant factor in influencing auditory threshold values takes on added meaning. It appears that long-term exposure over many generations to high altitude hypoxia has no effect on hearing. The Aymará, who are native to this region, have the same level of hearing as the non-Aymará and mestizos. This is true at all altitudes tested. The altitude differences that were detected are certainly not due to hypoxia, since the young residents at higher altitudes hear better than their age counterparts on the coast. Rather, it seems that, like the observation of Singh et al. (1976), the absence of loud noises at higher elevations promotes better hearing, but this promotion may be compromised by the poor medical care available, as testified by the higher frequency of otitis media, with some depression in the mean hearing thresholds at the higher altitudes expected if health care were better. Olmsted et al. (1964) reported: 'It has been stated that persistent loss of hearing may follow acute infection of the middle ear in childhood. It has also been suggested that this complication has increased frequency as a result of inadequate treatment of acute otitis media.' The effect of chronic middle ear infections is long term and may account for the trend toward poorer hearing at higher frequencies in the older altiplano residents.

In conclusion, the results of this analysis differ from the findings of McFarland (1937c) at the lower frequencies, since the residents at high altitude in this survey heard better than those on the coast at 1000, 2000, and 3000 Hz. However, at the higher frequencies, this study supports McFarland's findings since the high altitude population was found to have greater auditory thresholds than the sea level inhabitants. With regard to Singh et al. (1976), our results match their findings in the lower frequencies but do not agree at the higher ones. There appear to be other factors, such as otitis media and reduced noise pollution, influencing auditory thresholds in the mountainous regions. Perhaps future investigations will be able to assess the effects of these variables.

WILLIAM H. WEIDMAN, SARA ANN BARTON, AND VIVIAN LUNNY LENART

Chapter 12

ALTITUDE AND CARDIOPULMONARY RELATIONSHIPS

Pulmonary circulation

Pulmonary artery pressures of adults living at altitude are higher than in adults living at sea level (Peñaloza et al., 1963), and studies of small groups of their children have shown the same increase (Sime et al., 1963). This elevation appears to be a response to chronic hypoxia with changes in the pulmonary vasculature resulting in muscularization of the terminal portions of the pulmonary arteries and in an increase in pulmonary vascular resistance (Arias-Stella and Saldana, 1963). The degree of pulmonary hypertension in children living at high altitude is the same as that found in newborn infants at sea level in whom there is a normal increase in thickness of the pulmonary arteriole musculature.

There is considerable difference among species in the response of the pulmonary vascular bed to altitude; dogs and sheep show little response, whereas cattle, chickens and pigs are very responsive (Tucker et al., 1975). Von Tschudi (1847) commented on these differences; he noted: 'I have already described the effect of the Puna climate on beasts of burden. Its influence on some of the domestic animals is no less severe than on the human race. To cats, it is very fatal, and at the elevation of 3900 meters above the sea those animals cannot live. Numerous trials have been made to rear them in the villages of the upper mountains, but without effect; for after a few days' abode in those regions, the animals die in frightful convulsions; but when in this state they do not attempt to bite. ... Dogs are also liable to it, but it visits them less severely than cats, and with care they may be recovered.'

Studies of the response of the pulmonary vasculature in cattle have shown that offspring of 'hyper-responders' to altitude were also 'hyper-responders,' and offspring of cattle resistant to the hypoxic effect of altitude had a lesser increase in pulmonary vasculature resistance at altitude (Weir et al., 1974). Moreover, animals presumably evolutionarily adapted to the hypoxia of altitude, such as the viscacha, have a thin-walled pulmonary vasculature unlike that either of the domesticated animals to which we have referred or to the indigenous Indians themselves (Heath et al., 1981b). This suggests that not only is there a species difference in the response of the pulmonary vascular bed to altitude, but that there is an intra-species difference that is likely to be genetic in origin. Pathologic studies of pulmonary arteries from individuals living at high altitude have shown individual differences in the amount of muscular hypertrophy – suggesting that there are differences in response to hypoxia in the human with some individuals being hyper-responders and others hypo-responders

William J. Schull and Francisco Rothhammer (eds.), The Aymará: Strategies in Human Adaptation to a Rigorous Environment, 167-181. ©1990 *by Kluwer Academic Publishers.*

TABLE 1
Frequency of right ventricular hypertrophy by age and altitude of residence

Altitude of Residence		Age (yrs.) < 1	1-4	5-9	10-14	15-19	20-39	40-69	≥70
CHILE									
Coast	No.*	2	42	67	111	48	163	112	10
	%	0.0	4.8	4.5	7.2	6.3	4.9	3.6	0.0
Sierra	No.	13	66	138	134	54	138	197	39
	%	0.0	6.1	15.9	7.5	1.9	3.6	6.1	2.6
Altiplano	No.	3	56	96	121	42	122	129	13
	%	0.0	23.2	25.0	20.7	23.8	9.8	10.1	7.7
BOLIVIA									
Altiplano	No.	6	68	77	57	14	118	69	13
	%	0.0	5.9	10.4	3.5	7.1	3.4	4.3	7.7

* Number of subjects differs slightly between variables because it was not possible to measure all variables on all persons

(Wagenvoort and Wagenvoort, 1973; Heath and Williams, 1981). Heath and his coworkers (Heath et al., 1981a) have reported a distal extension of the vascular smooth muscle into pulmonary arterioles as small as 20 microns in diameter in natives of La Paz that is not seen in lowlanders. Finally, populations who have lived at altitude for centuries (such as the Aymará) have lower pulmonary artery pressures than do the shorter term Coloradans living at the same or nearly the same altitude (Vogel et al., 1962). This suggests that, in addition to species and intra-species differences, there are ethnic differences.

Most of the observations of the effect of high altitude on the human have been made on a limited number of adolescent and adult males. Much of our past knowledge on hemodynamic changes with altitude has rested on studies of groups of persons, largely male and occupationally selected (miners or soldiers), whose representativeness of high altitude populations is open to challenge. None of the investigators of the effect of the hypoxia of altitude on the pulmonary vascular bed have had an opportunity to examine large numbers of persons, children and adults, male and female, residing at high altitude and at sea level, and to appraise the contribution of genetic variability to the response of the pulmonary vascular bed to the hypoxia of high altitude. Our study presented the opportunity to extend the data to other age groups and to women, and is one of the largest epidemiologic studies covering the widest range of ages available on a high altitude population.

Since it is not practicable to conduct a large epidemiologic study, using conventional hemodynamic measurements, we chose to use the electrocardiogram as an indirect indicator of the level of pulmonary artery pressure. In the absence of auscultatory evidence of right ventricular outflow obstruction, right ventricular hypertrophy on the electrocardiogram indicates an

TABLE 2
QRS axis range and mean by age and altitude of residence

Altitude of Residence		1-4	5-9	10-14	15-19	20-39	40-69	≥70
CHILE								
Coast	range	-150-150	-39-150	-49-170	-76-115	-38-150	-60-110	-53-90
	mean	44.0	45.8	51.1	61.4	48.9	31.6	18.6
	no.	41	66	111	48	162	112	10
Sierra	range	-120-180	-136-180	-150-176	-125-130	-104-210	-90-150	-63-82
	mean	58.2	57.7	61.5	55.4	52.4	44.5	37.2
	no.	66	137	134	54	137	197	39
Alti-	range	-127-200	-164-200	-150-190	-150-150	-150-220	-150-180	-64-110
plano	mean	80.6	80.2	68.6	57.8	58.1	38.8	26.0
	no.	55	93	120	41	121	127	13
BOLIVIA								
Alti-	range	-210-180	-120-175	-125-210	-104-169	-90-210	-120-164	-90-138
plano	mean	63.6	65.7	62.2	62.2	66.1	54.6	34.5
	no.	68	76	57	14	116	69	13

Age (years) spans columns 1-4 through ≥70.

elevation of pulmonary artery pressure. The presence or absence of right ventricular hypertrophy correlated significantly with measured pulmonary artery pressure in the Natural History Study of Aortic Stenosis, Pulmonary Stenosis and Ventricular Septal Defect (Nadas, Ellison and Weidman, 1977). Finally, Vogel found that electrocardiographic findings in adolescents living in Leadville, Colorado (3000 meters) correlated with pulmonary artery pressure measured during right heart catheterization (Vogel et al., 1962; Vogel, Pryor and Blount, 1964).

The electrocardiograms in our study were taken by the same examiner (S.A.B.) and interpreted in the Laboratory of Physiologic Hygiene at the University of Minnesota. The readers had no knowledge of the residence of the subjects on whom the electrocardiograms were recorded. Age-specific electrocardiographic criteria for right ventricular hypertrophy, left ventricular hypertrophy or low left ventricular voltages were used. These measures were estimated from two percentiles and the 'normal' data by Ziegler (1951, see also Simonson, 1961).

Including all age groups, 2,096 persons were examined in Chile and 429 in Bolivia. Because of the small number of the very young or the truly aged, and the difficulty in establishing criteria for right and left ventricular voltages at these ages, only subjects who were 1 to 69 years old (Chile 1,837 and Bolivia 403) are included in this analysis. The subjects were more-or-less uniformly distributed between the sexes and the three altitudinal niches – altiplano, sierra and sea coast. And the age distribution is approximately evenly distributed, except more children between 10 and 14 years of age and persons more than 50 years of age

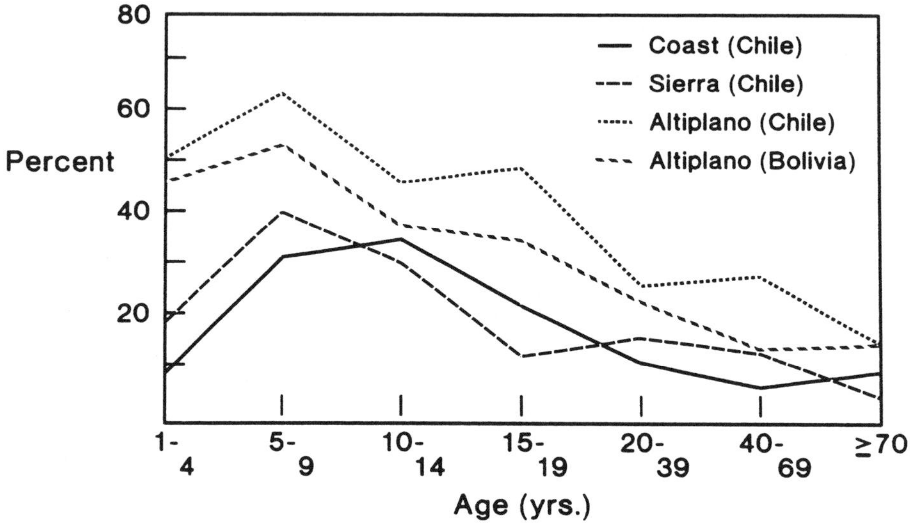

FIGURE 1. Frequency of right ventricular hypertrophy by age and altitude of residence

were seen than expected. In Bolivia, the age group 15 to 19 years was under represented (Table 1).

Electrocardiography

The mean QRS axis was directed more to the right in persons living in high altitude than in coastal dwellers (Table 2); however, the differences were greatest for those persons less than 15 years of age at the time of examination and were least for those more than 39 years of age.

Right ventricular hypertrophy clearly varied with age and all altitudinal niches, including Bolivia, but only in the latter country was the trend possibly linear. In Chile, at all altitudes, a non-linear dependence of the frequency of right ventricular hypertrophy on age existed (Figure 1). The frequency of right ventricular hypertrophy was successively higher in the sierra (22.3%) and altiplano (42.2%) than on the coast (19.1%).

The increase is not linear with altitude; the difference in frequency between the coast and 3000 meters is only modest; however, the next 1200 meters almost doubles the frequency, and the ages of the examinees are very similar. This increase is most definite in the age group 5 to 14 years. The trend of right ventricular hypertrophy in the Bolivian altiplano population was similar, but somewhat lower in all groups than in the Chilean population who lived in the altiplano; however, the Chilean altiplano was 300 meters higher and somewhat colder and drier. Whether these differences can account for the difference between the countries is uncertain.

Cardiac examination

None of the subjects exhibited pulmonary valve or infundibular stenosis on auscultation so that the electrocardiographic evidence of right ventricular hypertrophy can be assumed to reflect elevation of pulmonary artery pressure. Most individuals with right ventricular hypertrophy had an increased intensity of the pulmonary valve closure sound.

Electrocardiographic evidence of right ventricular hypertrophy occurred most frequently in the Aymará living at 4200 meters. The presence of right ventricular hypertrophy decreased with age, with the decrease occurring later in life than in persons living at 3000 meters and on the coast. It can be assumed that the right ventricular hypertrophy on the electrocardiogram is the result of an increase in pulmonary vascular resistance and an elevation of pulmonary artery pressure. Our study, involving persons of both sexes, of all ages from 1 to 69 years, and of various occupations, suggests that the hemodynamic changes previously reported only in male miners, soldiers and small groups of children are representative of the entire high altitude population. These hemodynamic changes are not, to a major degree, confounded by either sex or occupation.

The age in persons living at high altitude at which the electrocardiogram did not show right ventricular hypertrophy varied – and presumably the pulmonary vascular resistance had begun to decrease with a resulting decrease in pulmonary artery pressure toward coastal levels. In some children, our observations suggested that pulmonary artery pressure was normal before five years of age, whereas some adults who were more than 40 years old at the time of examination continued to have elevated pulmonary artery pressures. Yabek (1989) has noted that even in Albuquerque, New Mexico, at an elevation (1500 m) substantially lower than that in the sierra or altiplano, among children with the commonly occurring congenital heart defects, the high pulmonary vascular resistance present at birth persists more frequently, and that these children tend to develop pulmonary vascular obstructive diseases at an earlier age.

These observations support those of Peñaloza (Peñaloza et al., 1961; Peñaloza et al., 1959) that right ventricular hypertrophy, and presumably pulmonary hypertension, is less common in adults than children living at altitude. The greater than expected variability in response of the pulmonary vascular bed to chronic hypoxia is probably related to genetically determined variability and functional adaptation to hypoxia, reflected in modifications in oxygen transport and tissue utilization of oxygen. This interpretation is supported by other studies that have demonstrated that not only are there differences between species in the response to altitude, but that there are significant intra-species differences.

TABLE 3
The frequency of hypertension by sex and altitude of residence

Niche	Sex	Number Examined	Hypertensive	Proportion
Coast	Males	122	4	0.03
	Females	125	11	0.09
Sierra	Males	101	2	0.02
	Females	109	5	0.05
Altiplano	Males	146	6	0.04
	Females	156	2	0.01

Systemic circulation

Whereas hypoxia has a vasoconstrictive effect on the pulmonary arterial circulation, hypoxia, with a resultant lower systemic arterial oxygen saturation, has a vasodilating effect on systemic arteries with, presumably, a lowering of systemic blood pressure. High altitude residents do have lower systemic arterial pressures than do age-matched individuals living at sea level (Marticorena, Severino and Chaves, 1967; Comstock, 1957; Chaves, 1965). In addition, the rise in systolic blood pressure with aging that usually occurs in adults at sea level is not seen in most adults living in the Andes at high altitude (Marticorena, Severino and Chaves, 1967). Thus, there is apparently a protective effect on blood pressure in Andean residents. American adolescents, living at high altitude, have lower systolic, but not diastolic pressures than adolescents living at a lower level (Appleton, 1967).

Using a definition, in the adult, of hypertension as a systolic blood pressure greater than 160 mm of mercury and/or a diastolic blood pressure greater than 95 mm of mercury, the prevalence of systolic hypertension is more than 10 times greater at sea level than at altitude; the same is true of diastolic hypertension, but to a lesser degree (Ruiz and Peñaloza, 1977).

Another interesting observation is that, although in the adult living at high altitude there is less right ventricular hypertrophy on the electrocardiogram than in children at the same altitude, the usual increase in left ventricular forces seen in adults at sea level does not occur in adults at altitude (Peñaloza et al., 1961). This could, in part, reflect the lower systemic blood pressure in the adult living at high altitude.

As previously stated, 2,096 individuals were examined during the multidisciplinary study of the Aymará Indians. Of these, 759 had blood pressure, height and weight measurements and had spent less than one year of their lives at a different altitude from the one in which they resided at the time of examination. The range in age was from 3 to 84 years, and the subjects were evenly distributed between the sexes and altitudes (122, 125 coastal; 101, 109

TABLE 4
Comparison of mean blood pressure in Rochester, MN and altiplano children

Age (years)	Sex	Rochester Systolic	Rochester Diastolic	Altiplano Systolic	Altiplano Diastolic
6	Males	105	66	90	56
	Females	101	65	90	55
12	Males	118	71	104	68
	Females	118	72	104	68
15	Males	123	72	112	68
	Females	120	71	110	72
18	Males	133	77	120	78
	Females	119	72	118	73

sierra and 146, 156 altiplano; males and females, respectively). Two blood pressure measurements were recorded from the right arm, resting at the level of the heart, with the subject seated. A cuff was chosen that was at least two-thirds the length of the upper arm without obstructing the axilla or elbow. The fourth Korotkoff sound was used for diastolic pressure in the children and the fifth in the adults. The second blood pressure recording was almost always lower than the first and the second blood pressure was used in the data analysis.

Subjects with hypertension (systolic pressure greater than 160 and/or diastolic greater than 95 mm of mercury) were excluded from the present study. All were adults. Of the 247 subjects living on the coast, 15 (6%) were hypertensive, of the 210 living in the sierra, 7 (3.3%) were hypertensive, and 8 of 302 (2.6%) living in the altiplano were hypertensive (see Table 3). These frequencies are significantly less than the 20 to 25 per cent frequency of hypertension estimated in North American adults, and also differ somewhat from the altitude-related frequencies reported by Ruiz and Peñaloza (1977). They describe substantially more hypertension in the coastal communities they studied in Perú than we observed in the Azapa and Lluta valleys and slightly less hypertension in the altiplano. However, their values are presented as age-adjusted rates whereas ours are the crude frequencies, and it is not clear whether our population may have been somewhat older.

Both systolic and diastolic blood pressures increased from 6 to 20 years of age in males and females. For both systolic and diastolic blood pressures, coastal values tended to be higher at all ages than those seen in the altiplano or sierra (see Figures 2 through 5). This increase in blood pressure throughout childhood and adolescence has been observed in the United States among blacks, whites, Hispanics and Orientals (Harris et al., 1981; Cornoni-Huntley, Harlan and Leaverton, 1979). In comparing blood pressure measurements in Rochester, Minnesota, children and adolescents with age-matched Aymará Indians in the altiplano, systolic blood pressure was higher at age 6 in the North Americans and

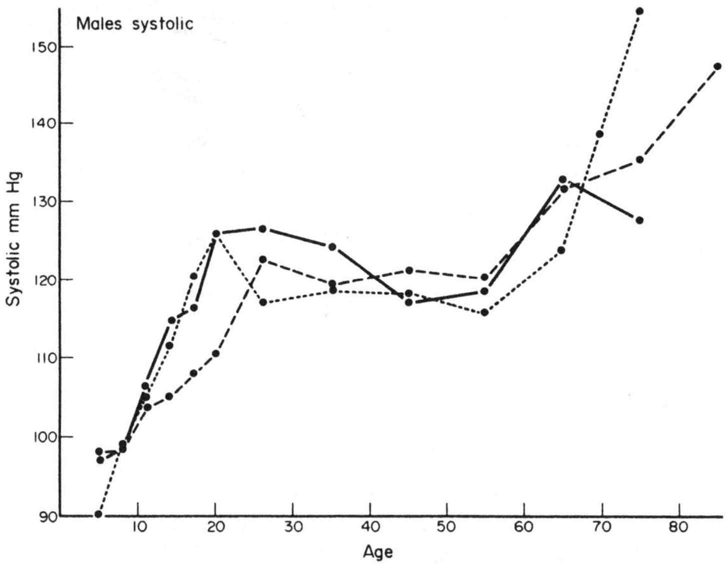

FIGURE 2. Distribution of blood pressure in mm Hg. as a function of age in years:
Males systolic (— Coast, --- Sierra, ··· Altiplano)
Makela, Barton, Schull, Weidman, and Rothhammer, 1978, Fig. 1a, p. 591.
Reprinted with permission of Pergamon Press Ltd, Great Britain

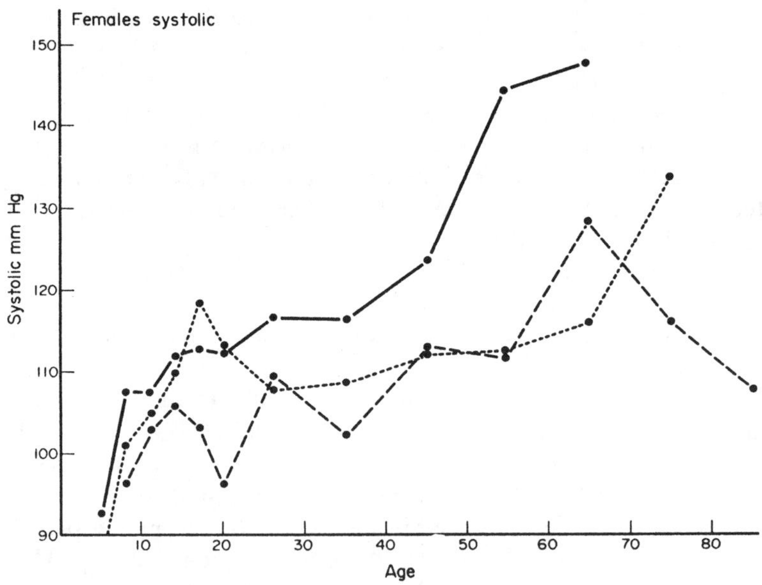

FIGURE 3. Distribution of blood pressure in mm Hg. as a function of age in years:
Females systolic (— Coast, --- Sierra, ··· Altiplano)
Makela, Barton, Schull, Weidman, and Rothhammer, 1978, Fig. 1b, p. 592.
Reprinted with permission of Pergamon Press Ltd, Great Britain

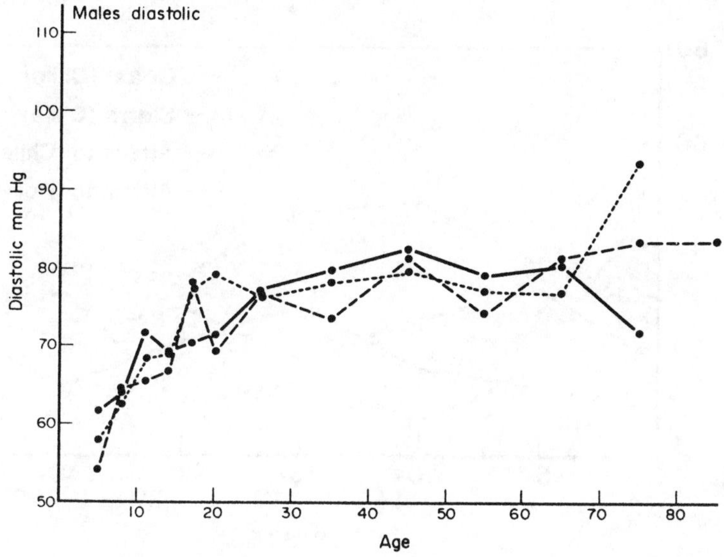

FIGURE 4. Distribution of blood pressure in mm Hg. as a function of age in years: Males diastolic (— Coast, --- Sierra, ··· Altiplano)
Makela, Barton, Schull, Weidman, and Rothhammer, 1978, Fig. 2a, p. 592.
Reprinted with permission of Pergamon Press Ltd, Great Britain

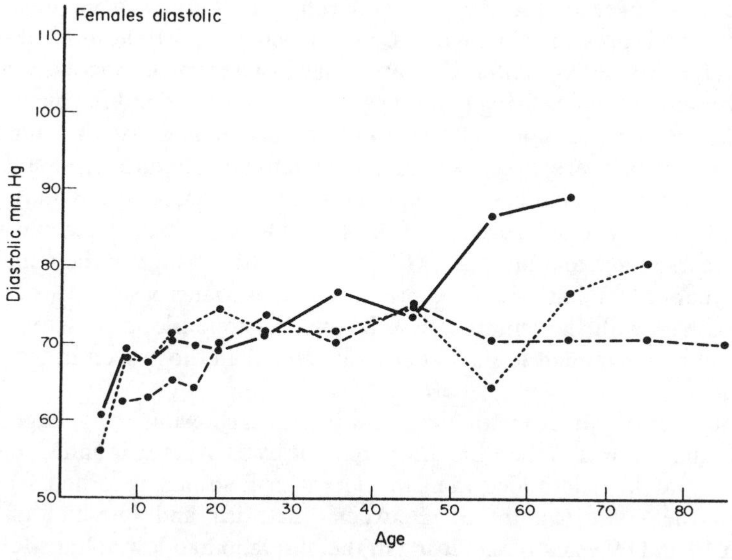

FIGURE 5. Distribution of blood pressure in mm Hg. as a function of age in years: Females diastolic (— Coast, --- Sierra, ··· Altiplano)
Makela, Barton, Schull, Weidman, and Rothhammer, 1978, Fig. 2b, p. 593.
Reprinted with permission of Pergamon Press Ltd, Great Britain

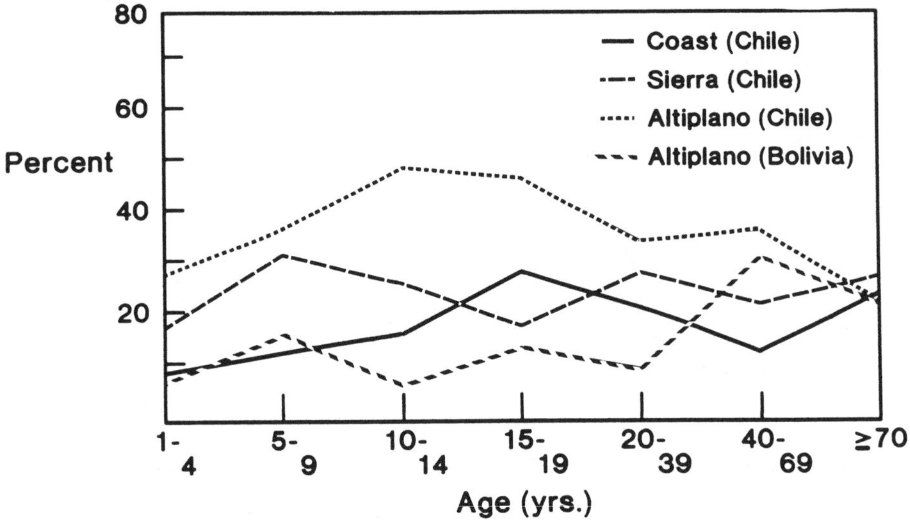

FIGURE 6. Frequency of low voltage left ventricle by age and altitude of residence

increased more steeply through 18 years of age (see Table 4). Diastolic blood pressure was lower in the Aymará children, but there was no difference in diastolic blood pressure in Aymará and Rochester, Minnesota, 18-year-old subjects (DHEW, 1978). After 20 years of age, there was no increase in systolic blood pressure, in males living in all three niches, until late in life (Figure 2).

The latter increase may reflect sampling variations since the numbers on which these means are based are small. In females (Figure 3), systolic blood pressure continues to increase throughout life, most conspicuously in the coastal females. Figures 4 and 5 reveal that diastolic blood pressures plateau in males after 20 years of age and up to later life; there is little change in the females from 20 to 45 years when diastolic blood pressure begins to increase.

As was true with the children, systolic and diastolic blood pressure values in the coastal adults tended to be higher at all ages than those seen in the altiplano or sierra.

The number of persons with electrocardiograms showing low-voltage R-waves in V-6 (equal to or less than the 5th percentile) was greater in individuals, at all ages, living at high altitudes than in electrocardiograms recorded from those living on the coast (Figure 6). Between one-third and one-half of persons between 10 and 69 years of age living in the altiplano had low voltage R and V-6. This supports previously published observations that high altitude residents do not develop the preponderance of left ventricular forces seen in residents at sea

TABLE 5
Frequency of low left ventricular forces by age and altitude of residence

Altitude of Residence		Age (yrs.) < 1	1-4	5-9	10-14	15-19	20-39	40-69	≥70
CHILE									
Coast	No.*	2	42	67	111	48	163	112	10
	%	0.0	9.5	13.4	17.1	29.2	22.1	13.4	30.0
Sierra	No.	13	66	138	134	54	138	197	39
	%	15.4	18.2	32.6	26.9	18.5	29.0	22.8	28.2
Altiplano	No.	3	56	96	121	42	122	129	13
	%	0.0	28.6	37.5	49.6	47.6	35.2	37.2	23.1
BOLIVIA									
Altiplano	No.	6	68	77	57	14	118	69	13
	%	0.0	7.4	16.9	7.0	14.3	10.2	31.9	23.1

* Number of subjects differs slightly between variables because it was not possible to measure all variables on all persons

TABLE 6
Obesity in Rochester, MN and Chilean altiplano children

Age (Yrs.)	Sex	Rochester Mean Wt	Mean Ht	Mean kg/m^2	Altiplano Mean Wt	Mean Ht	Mean kg/m^2
6	Males	23	121	16	20	111	16
	Females	21	124	14	19	110	16
12	Males	44	153	19	36	142	18
	Females	46	157	19	38	142	19
15	Males	62	173	21	45	154	19
	Females	55	164	20	46	149	21
18	Males	69	176	22	57	165	21
	Females	58	164	22	50	148	23

level with aging, and, in part, reflects the lower systemic blood pressures in the adult living at high altitude (see Table 5).

When systolic (Figure 7 and 8) and diastolic blood pressures (Figures 9 and 10) are distributed as a function of weight, both increase as weight increases at all altitudes. The increase in systolic and diastolic blood pressure is nearly the same in both sexes for the same weight increase. The children had systolic and diastolic blood pressures that correlated consistently well with age, height and weight (males higher than females). The correlations in these data are similar to those seen in the SCOR (Specialized Centers of Research) blood pressure study of Rochester, Minnesota, children (Cornoni-Huntley, Harlan and Leaverton,

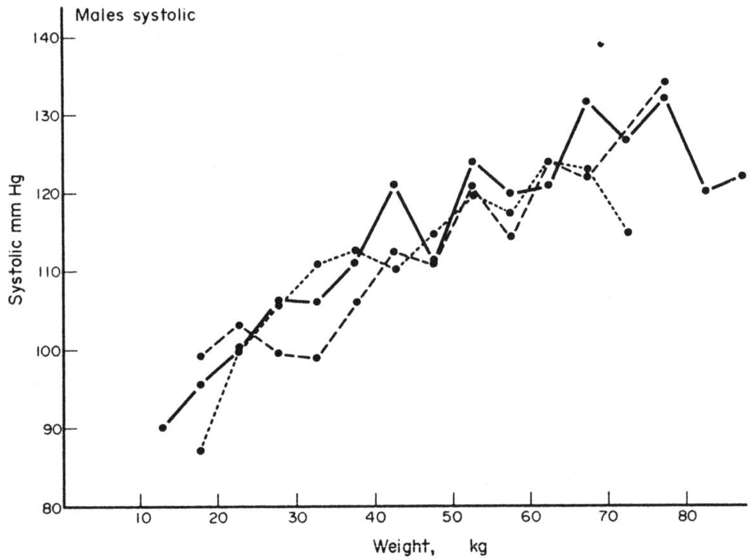

FIGURE 7. Distribution of blood pressure in mm Hg. as a function of weight (in kilograms): Males systolic (— Coast, --- Sierra, ··· Altiplano)
Makela, Barton, Schull, Weidman, and Rothhammer, 1978, Fig. 3a, p. 593.
Reprinted with permission of Pergamon Press Ltd, Great Britain

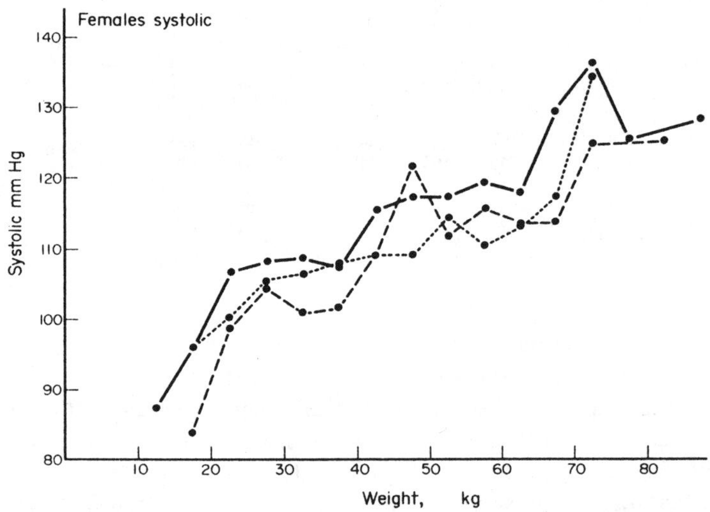

FIGURE 8. Distribution of blood pressure in mm Hg. as a function of weight (in kilograms): Females systolic (— Coast, --- Sierra, ··· Altiplano)
Makela, Barton, Schull, Weidman, and Rothhammer, 1978, Fig. 3b, p. 594.
Reprinted with permission of Pergamon Press Ltd, Great Britain

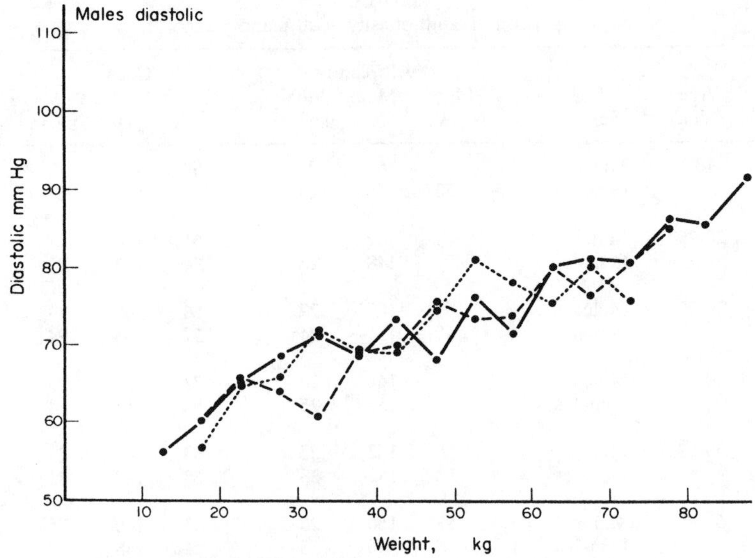

FIGURE 9. Distribution of blood pressure in mm Hg. as a function of weight (in kilograms): Males diastolic (— Coast, --- Sierra, ··· Altiplano)
Makela, Barton, Schull, Weidman, and Rothhammer, 1978, Fig. 4a, p. 594.
Reprinted with permission of Pergamon Press Ltd, Great Britain

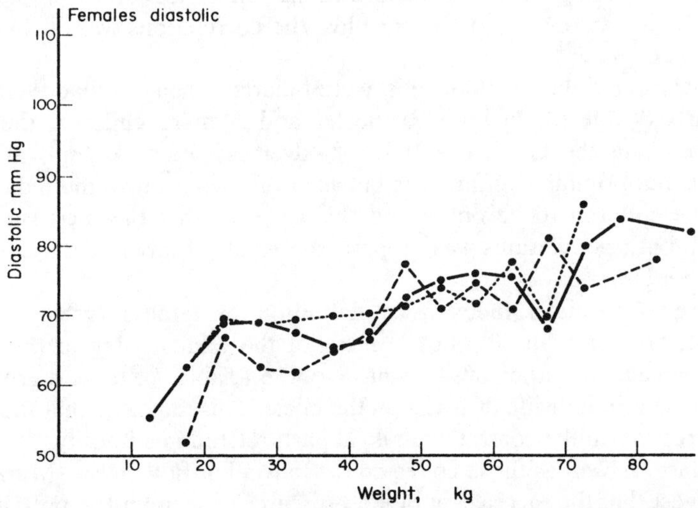

FIGURE 10. Distribution of blood pressure in mm Hg. as a function of weight (in kilograms): Females diastolic (— Coast, --- Sierra, ··· Altiplano)
Makela, Barton, Schull, Weidman, and Rothhammer, 1978, Fig. 4b, p. 594.
Reprinted with permission of Pergamon Press Ltd, Great Britain

TABLE 7
Comparison of adult obesity in altiplano and coast

Age (Yrs.)	Sex	Altiplano Mean Wt	Altiplano Mean Ht	Altiplano Mean kg/m2	Coast Mean Wt	Coast Mean Ht	Coast Mean kg/m2
18	Males	57	165	21	58	163	22
	Females	50	148	23	53	152	23
20-29	Males	61	162	23	61	166	22
	Females	51	148	23	54	153	23
30-39	Males	61	165	22	64	165	24
	Females	55	151	24	57	153	24
40-49	Males	64	164	24	72	167	26
	Females	57	152	25	56	154	24
50-59	Males	60	162	23	63	161	24
	Females	53	152	23	68	149	31
60+	Males	59	160	23	63	160	25
	Females	48	146	23	61	148	28

1979). In Rochester, in 6 to 11 year old children, the correlations between systolic blood pressure and diastolic blood pressure and weight were 0.43 and 0.33, respectively, in males, and 0.51 and 0.37 in females. In 12 to 14 year old children, these correlations were 0.50 and 0.27 in males, and 0.40 and 0.29 in females. Finally, among 15 to 18 year olds, the correlations were 0.49 and 0.32, and 0.36 and 0.23.

The Rochester children, at all ages, were taller and heavier than their Aymará counterparts (Table 6). In both Rochester and Aymará children, there was a slight increase in the Quetelet's Index (body mass index, kg/m^2) as children grew older, but no major differences between the two groups; the indices reveal none of the children to be obese and this suggests that the increase in blood pressure in both populations was, in part, the result of an increase in lean body mass and not fatness.

Using the Quetelet's Index as a definition of fatness (greater than 25, overweight; greater than 30, obese), none of the adults living in the altiplano would be considered either overweight or obese (Table 7). Indices greater than 25 were present in individuals living on the coast. This indicates that the increase in blood pressure in the coastal adult is, in part, related in adiposity.

These data, as well as those collected in Bolivia but not shown (Murillo et al., 1980), suggest that the increase in blood pressure throughout the pre-adult years is the result of an increase in lean body mass and that the absence of a continual increase in blood pressure in the adult years in the Aymará living at high altitude is, in part, because the adults do not gain weight. Finally, altitude differences in blood pressure most probably reflect systematic differences in body weight at different altitudes (high altitude dwellers being thinner than coastal dwellers) rather than a direct effect of the hypoxia of high altitude.

HERNAN PALOMINO

Chapter 13
ORAL CHARACTERISTICS OF THE AYMARA

Caries has commonly been regarded as the major dental disease throughout the world, but periodontal disease and malocclusion are also present in almost all human populations although the frequency of their occurrence and severity varies greatly. Several studies have attempted to describe the prevalence of these various pathological conditions in different ethnic groups and among people living in primitive circumstances, and to evaluate the environmental and genetic contributions to their etiology (Ramfjord, 1959; Krogman, 1960; Waerhang, 1966; Chung et al., 1970; Palomino and Pereira, 1971; Niswander, 1975; and Palomino, 1978). These investigations suggest that dental caries and periodontal disease are caused mainly by local influences, e.g., water, minerals, sweet fruits, candies, or sugar consumption (Suomi, 1978; Glass, 1982; Bowen et al., 1977; Niswander, 1967; Waerhang, 1966; Heloe and Hangejorden, 1981; Bibby, 1970; and Liu, 1977). It has been argued, largely on the basis of comparison with primitive populations where a lower frequency of caries is seen, that such differences in prevalence are attributable to the type of food ingested, especially carbohydrates and the method of food preparation, raw versus cooked (Bibby, 1970). The same occurs in periodontal disease, where supragingival plaque is known to cause gingival inflammation (Loe et al., 1965), and the role of specific Gram-negative bacteria in the etiology and pathogenesis of destructive forms of periodontal disease is well established (Slots and Genco, 1984). Juvenile periodontal disease, however, is of clear genetic origin. The prevalence of juvenile periodontitis is generally low in most populations, although it is higher among Negroes than Caucasians or Orientals (Rao and Tewani, 1968; Saxon, 1980; Melnick et al., 1976).

In malocclusion, genetic factors seem to be more important than environmental ones. Proper dental occlusion requires the harmonious development of several body components involving tooth size and shape, tooth position, timing and sequence of eruption as well as dental arch size, shape, and pattern of craniofacial growth. Variability in occlusion results also from the interplay of genetic and environmental factors that affect both prenatal development and postnatal modification. Racial variation in tooth and dental arch size and shape also exists (Graber, 1972; Palomino et al., 1977 and 1978; Bailit et al., 1970; Bailit, 1975; Brown et al., 1965; Sofaer et al., 1972). Undoubtedly, complex hereditary factors are involved and it has not as yet been possible to ascertain the reason for the differences between populations. On the other hand, there are differences among populations in body size and shape and in the rate of growth in children. For example, the populations living in northern Chile, at different levels of altitude, show variation in several anthropometrical

William J. Schull and Francisco Rothhammer (eds.), The Aymará: Strategies in Human Adaptation to a Rigorous Environment, 183-191. *©1990 by Kluwer Academic Publishers.*

measurements including craniofacial ones (Mueller et al., 1978a; Palomino et al., 1979).

Growth in the craniofacial complex has a different pattern according to these variables (genetic and environmental) and these different patterns may explain the differences in the prevalence of malocclusion. It has been postulated that the observed variability in malocclusion is a consequence of population admixture and inbreeding (Niswander, 1975; Chung et al., 1971; Schull and Neel, 1965; and Stockard, 1941) or relaxed natural selection pressures affecting secular trends (Wolpoff, 1969). Bass (1982) suggests that genetic programming of the development of the dental arches lies mainly in the underlying skeletal elements, in the patterns of activity of the soft tissue elements, and in the sequence and spatial position of the erupting teeth. The establishment of harmonious occlusion involves an interaction between the eruptive forces and the shape and force of elements surrounding the teeth, as well as the forces arising from the contact between opposing cusps.

Malocclusion may also result, in part at least, from the lack of forward growth of the maxilla and the mandible associated with nasal stenosis, a soft diet, and postural habits (Schulhof, 1978; Mew, 1981). Beecher and Corruccini (1981) state, 'The reduction of chewing resistance and related growth stimulation provided by 'civilized' man's refined diet may be the strongest causal factor in developmental malocclusions'. King (1983) summarizes the evidence on the various factors thought to be associated with the etiology of malocclusion: racial admixture, inbreeding, relaxed selection, and diet.

The populations of northern Chile and western Bolivia provide an excellent opportunity to study the variables contributing to the variation in impact of environmental and ethnic influences on different pathological oral conditions, including dental caries, periodontal disease and malocclusion. The specific population studied here lives either in the altiplano of western Bolivia, or in Chile, in an altitudinal gradient from sea level to over 4,500 meters of altitude. The people living at these different altitudes have different growth rates (Mueller, 1978a), different foods, and environmental conditions, all of which can affect the prevalence of these pathologies.

Materials and methods

Subjects of this review are the individuals residing in the 14 different villages or locales previously described (Chapter 1) who presented themselves for examinations either in Bolivia or Chile in the course of the study of the health status of the Aymará. Oral and dental examinations were completed on 1,685 individuals ages six years and older residing in Chile, and on 337 individuals in western Bolivia. Included in the examination were an assessment of dental caries, periodontal status, oral hygiene, dental arch measurement, and craniofacial measurements and occlusion. Dental caries were assessed in permanent teeth using the conventional decayed, missing, and filled teeth index (DMF), excluding congenitally missing teeth. Periodontal disease was ascertained using Russell's (1956) periodontal index (PI), and oral hygiene was evaluated using Greene and Vermillion's (1964) simplified oral hygiene index (OHI-S).

All individuals were coded as Aymará, mestizo or non-Aymará, according to the classification previously described (see Chapter 1) using paternal and maternal surnames (Díaz et al., 1978; Schull and Rothhammer, 1977). Residence was taken to be the place where individuals habitually lived – coastal, sierran or altiplano zones.

RESULTS AND DISCUSSION

For purposes of discussion we focus, first, on the findings in Chile, for these alone allow an altitudinal comparison, and second, upon contrasts involving two age classes: children (6 to 14 years of age) and adults (15 years of age and older). It should be noted that growth of the head and face is essentially completed by 14 years of age.

Occlusion

As previously stated, dental occlusion varies among individuals according to the shape of their teeth, the size and position of the latter, arch shape, and the pattern of craniofacial growth (Graber, 1972). Normal occlusion also varies among populations according to their racial origins. Among the Aymará, for example, an harmonious occlusion involves shorter and broader arches with upper incisors positioned almost in a straight line. The anterior incisor relationship exhibits slightly less overjet than the one described for the normal Caucasian pattern. There is a greater tendency for a bis-a-bis relationship (lower and upper teeth are more parallel and exhibit an almost vertical axis with a greater angle between upper and lower incisors) in the Aymará than in Caucasian populations (Dempster et al., 1963; Palomino, 1978).

Various epidemiological studies have shown the diversity among populations in malocclusion to be very large (Chung et al., 1971; Graber, 1972; Krogman, 1960; King, 1983). The significant differences that are seen in the various malocclusive traits emphasize the broad diversity of categories of malocclusion. For example, the Danes show the deepest overbite, the most frequent Class II pattern of occlusion, and the greatest frequency of occlusal anomalies in the incisor region; whereas the Japanese exhibit more maxillary incisor protrusion (Graber, 1972; Bjork and Helm, 1961; Mills, 1966). Overall, primitive populations show the lowest prevalences (Lavelle et al., 1971).

The frequencies of normal and abnormal occlusion in the Aymará population, by age and sex group, are presented in Table 1. The only individuals considered were those for whom the relationship between the upper and lower first molars could be evaluated. Neutral occlusion was found in 84% of the boys, 77.5% of the girls, 82.1% of the adult males and 86.4% of the adult females. No differences were observed between male children and adults; however, adult

TABLE 1
Posterior and anterior dental arch relationships by sex and age

Posterior	Normal No.	Normal %	Openbite No.	Openbite %	Overbite No.	Overbite %	Crowded No.	Crowded %	Overjet No.	Overjet %	Underjet No.	Underjet %	No exam No.	Total No.	Total %
Male children															
Neutral	169		9		13		26		8		5		40	230	84.0
Distal	0		3		7		3		16		0		5	29	10.6
Mesial	1		0		4		0		0		10		0	15	5.5
Total	170	62.2	12	4.4	24	8.7	29	10.6	24	8.8	15	5.5	45	274	100.0
Female children															
Neutral	162		9		9		28		2		4		28	214	77.5
Distal	0		7		5		1		32		0		1	45	16.2
Mesial	0		0		2		2		0		13		0	17	6.2
Total	162	58.7	16	5.8	16	5.8	31	11.2	34	10.6	17	6.2	29	276	100.0
Male adults															
Neutral	245		1		54		33		2		3		37	338	82.1
Distal	1		8		8		6		13		0		6	36	8.8
Mesial	0		0		20		0		0		18		0	38	9.2
Total	246	59.7	9	2.2	82	19.9	39	9.5	15	3.6	21	5.1	42	412	100.0
Female adults															
Neutral	247		4		26		22		5		1		22	305	86.4
Distal	2		2		7		0		17		0		5	28	7.9
Mesial	1		0		6		2		0		11		0	20	5.7
Total	250	70.8	6	1.7	39	11.1	24	6.8	22	6.2	12	3.4	27	353	100.0
Total Children and Adults															
Males	416	60.6	21	3.1	106	15.1	68	9.9	39	5.7	36	5.2		686	100.0
Females	412	65.5	22	3.5	55	8.7	55	8.7	56	8.9	29	4.6		629	100.0

Significance:

Posterior relationships:

- Males between children and adults by posterior relationships — $\chi^2 = 3.66$; df = 2; n.s.
- Females between children and adults by posterior relationship — $\chi^2 = 10.90$; df = 2; $P < 0.01$
- Between sexes by posterior relationship — $\chi^2 = 3.75$; df = 2; n.s.

Anterior relationships:

- Males between children and adults by anterior relationship — $\chi^2 = 23.80$; df = 5; $P < 0.001$
- Females between children and adults by anterior relationship — $\chi^2 = 28.28$; df = 5; $P < 0.001$
- Between sexes by anterior relationship — $\chi^2 = 18.93$; df = 5; $P < 0.01$

females have a significantly higher frequency of neutral occlusion than girls. Given that there is a decrease in the percentage of distal occlusion and an increase in the percentage of neutral occlusion in adult females, these latter differences are partially associated with growth patterns. Mesial occlusion may increase in adults because of the forward displacement of the mandible through the cusp abrasion related to the chewing of coca, a common occurrence in the Aymará male.

Frequencies of normal and abnormal occlusion, according to Angle's classification, in children and adults, are exhibited in Tables 2 and 3 by sex, ethnicity, and altitude. Normal occlusion increases in adults in each subgroup of

TABLE 2
Angle's classification by age group, altitude of residence and sex

	Normal		Malocclusion Class I		Class II Division 1		Class II Division 2		Class III		Total
	No.	%	No.	%	No.	%	No.	%	No.	%	
Children											
Coast											
Males	56	64.4	19	21.8	8	9.2	1	1.4	3	3.4	87
Females	60	65.9	16	17.6	12	13.2	1	1.1	2	2.2	91
Sierra											
Males	78	58.6	34	25.6	11	8.3	5	3.8	5	3.8	133
Females	52	49.5	27	25.7	21	20.0	1	1.0	4	3.8	105
Altiplano											
Males	60	60.6	24	24.2	3	3.0	6	6.1	6	6.1	99
Females	59	54.1	27	24.8	8	7.4	4	3.7	11	10.1	109
Adults											
Coast											
Males	89	57.4	32	20.6	15	9.7	7	4.5	12	7.7	155
Females	89	76.1	15	12.8	7	6.0	2	1.7	4	3.4	117
Sierra											
Males	117	66.9	36	20.6	9	5.1	3	1.7	10	5.7	175
Females	95	69.9	26	19.1	8	5.9	3	2.2	4	2.9	136
Altiplano											
Males	56	44.8	45	36.0	5	4.0	3	2.4	16	12.8	125
Females	67	52.8	35	27.6	8	6.3	5	3.9	12	9.4	127
Total											
Males	456	58.9	189	24.4	51	6.6	25	3.2	53	6.8	774
Females	422	61.6	146	21.3	64	9.3	16	2.3	37	5.4	685

the studied population (58.5% in children and 61.4% in adults); however, these differences are evident only in individuals living in the sierra. It is possible that in the sierra there exists a greater number of children with larger occlusal discrepancies because of racial admixture. The adults have less admixture than the children. Adults from the coast and altiplano residents have less normality, because of increasing mesial and distal occlusal relationships with a closed bite in the coast, and mesial and neutral occlusion with crowding in the altiplano. Mesial occlusion is not necessarily reflected in a true prognathism; moreover, it can be a genetic defect, like the 'true' or hereditary prognathism (an autosomal dominant trait). However, as earlier noted, mesial occlusion in the Aymará population may reflect a mandibular forward displacement as a consequence of crown abrasion. Aymará adults who exhibit higher frequencies of mesial occlusion also have more abrasion and attrition. Corruccini et al., (1983), reporting on their study of occlusal variables and arch measurement among the Pima, found younger individuals, raised on more refined commercial foods (soft

TABLE 3
Angle's classification by age group, ethnicity and sex

	Normal No.	Normal %	Malocclusion Class I No.	Malocclusion Class I %	Class II Division 1 No.	Class II Division 1 %	Class II Division 2 No.	Class II Division 2 %	Class III No.	Class III %	Total
Children											
Aymará											
Males	60	58.3	27	26.2	6	5.8	3	2.9	7	6.8	103
Females	46	51.1	24	26.7	11	12.2	2	2.2	7	7.8	90
Mestizo											
Males	117	61.9	43	22.8	15	7.9	7	3.7	7	3.7	189
Females	105	56.8	40	21.6	27	14.6	3	1.6	10	5.4	185
Non-Aymará											
Males	17	63.0	6	22.2	1	3.7	2	7.4	1	3.7	27
Females	20	66.7	6	20.0	3	10.0	1	3.3	0	0.0	30
Adults											
Aymará											
Males	92	53.2	50	28.9	8	4.6	3	1.7	20	11.6	173
Females	97	57.8	42	25.0	8	4.8	7	4.2	14	8.3	168
Mestizo											
Males	107	55.4	55	28.5	12	6.2	6	3.1	13	6.7	193
Females	115	74.7	25	16.2	10	6.5	1	0.6	3	1.9	154
Non-Aymará											
Males	63	70.8	8	9.0	9	10.1	4	4.5	5	5.6	89
Females	39	67.2	9	15.5	5	8.6	2	3.4	3	5.2	58
Total											
Males	456		189		51		25		53		774
Females	422		146		64		16		37		685

diets), have more variable permanent normal dental occlusion than older persons raised on the traditional diet.

In summary, in northern Chile, individuals of all ages and both sexes present relatively low frequencies of malocclusion as compared with other populations. This holds true also for the villages examined in western Bolivia (see Palomino, 1978). Some of these malocclusions may be spontaneously corrected during normal growth periods, especially mesial occlusion and open bite. No altitude influence is detected, although non-Aymará individuals have higher frequencies of normal occlusive relationships. The main occlusal abnormalities seen among the Aymará correspond to an anterior position of the mandible, and in most cases is probably due to cusp abrasion.

Caries and periodontal disease

As previously noted, substantial variation exists between populations in the frequency of dental caries and periodontal disease. Although the importance of

TABLE 4
DMF, periodontal (PI), and oral hygiene (OHI-S) indexes and number of caries-free individuals by sex, age group, altitude of residence and ethnic group: Males

	DMF			PI			OHI-S			Caries-free	
	No.	mean	s.d.	No.	mean	s.d.	No.	mean	s.d.	No.	%
						Children					
Coast											
Aymará	8	1.1	1.8	7	0.29	0.42	7	0.33	0.36	5	62.5
Mestizo	62	1.0	1.4	51	0.20	0.31	50	0.26	0.38	35	56.5
Non-Aymará	18	0.6	1.1	11	0.18	0.33	11	0.25	0.40	13	72.2
Sierra											
Aymará	44	1.1	1.6	40	0.35	0.49	40	0.31	0.39	25	56.8
Mestizo	108	1.4	2.1	99	0.45	0.53	99	0.46	0.54	58	53.7
Non-Aymará	8	1.4	1.8	8	0.25	0.35	8	0.19	0.22	4	50.0
Altiplano											
Aymará	61	1.3	1.8	40	0.31	0.45	40	0.35	0.41	33	54.1
Mestizo	38	0.9	1.6	22	0.51	0.87	22	0.42	0.41	24	63.2
						Adults					
Coast											
Aymará	31	7.0	7.1	30	1.11	1.27	30	0.69	0.56	3	9.7
Mestizo	86	7.2	6.5	83	0.97	1.40	82	0.63	0.84	13	15.1
Non-Aymará	63	14.2	8.8	57	1.64	2.04	53	0.89	0.93	2	3.2
Sierra											
Aymará	86	9.3	7.6	81	2.40	1.84	80	1.27	0.87	4	4.7
Mestizo	94	10.0	6.8	90	1.93	1.55	89	1.09	0.72	3	3.2
Non-Aymará	51	12.2	7.6	48	2.14	1.83	47	1.10	0.82	2	3.9
Altiplano											
Aymará	104	9.0	8.3	92	1.61	1.70	91	0.94	0.63	7	6.7
Mestizo	45	8.7	6.7	38	1.22	1.65	38	0.70	0.59	2	4.4
Non-Aymará	12	14.8	6.6	10	1.83	2.30	10	0.74	0.71	0	0.0

environmental influences – especially carbohydrate consumption and water containing fluoride on dental caries (Heloe and Hangejorden, 1981) and bacterial infection on periodontal disease (Loe et al., 1965; Slots and Genco, 1984) – is evident, various authors have discussed the importance of race and the tendency of various racial groups to exhibit different incidences of these characteristics (Chung et al., 1970 and Niswander, 1975). Tables 4 and 5 provide the DMF, PI and OHI-S indexes and the percentage of caries-free individuals by sex. The mean DMF values are relatively low for the total population in the present study and are similar to our findings in the Bolivian Aymará population (Palomino, 1978) as well as those reported in primitive populations elsewhere (Niswander, 1967); 23.7% of the individuals are caries free. Higher DMF values were found in females of both age groups. The means are as follows, boys 1.19, girls 1.67, adult males 9.79 and females 12.92). Similar findings are described in the literature. The effect is much more pronounced among adult women and

TABLE 5
DMF, periodontal (PI), and oral hygiene (OHI-S) indexes and number of caries-free individuals by sex, age group, altitude of residence and ethnic group: Females

	DMF			PI			OHI-S			Caries-free	
	No.	mean	s.d.	No.	mean	s.d.	No.	mean	s.d.	No.	%
						Children					
Coast											
Aymará	9	1.0	1.7	8	0.03	0.05	8	0.08	0.14	5	55.6
Mestizo	60	1.6	2.2	49	0.14	0.34	49	0.11	0.25	31	51.7
Non-Aymará	26	1.8	2.3	26	0.08	0.23	26	0.11	0.27	12	46.2
Sierra											
Aymará	28	1.3	2.0	28	0.34	0.54	28	0.28	0.37	16	57.1
Mestizo	104	2.0	2.8	99	0.33	0.53	100	0.32	0.39	50	48.1
Non-Aymará	10	0.9	1.7	10	0.31	0.67	10	0.26	0.57	7	70.0
Altiplano											
Aymará	58	1.9	1.9	45	0.35	0.56	45	0.37	0.49	21	36.2
Mestizo	52	1.2	1.9	33	0.16	0.37	33	0.24	0.38	28	53.8
						Adults					
Coast											
Aymará	23	13.0	9.0	23	1.82	2.17	23	0.70	0.68	1	4.3
Mestizo	69	12.8	8.8	69	0.94	1.65	69	0.46	0.63	3	4.3
Non-Aymará	77	18.0	9.0	77	1.50	2.11	77	0.85	1.14	2	2.6
Sierra											
Aymará	93	13.6	7.6	93	2.47	1.91	93	1.08	0.82	2	2.2
Mestizo	98	12.7	8.0	98	2.19	1.99	98	1.11	0.97	2	2.0
Non-Aymará	17	13.8	6.4	17	2.25	1.75	17	0.97	1.00	0	0.0
Altiplano											
Aymará	102	9.9	7.9	102	1.45	1.65	102	0.91	0.66	8	7.8
Mestizo	45	9.2	7.5	45	1.18	1.45	45	0.68	0.49	4	8.9
Non-Aymará	5	19.8	11.5	5	2.70	3.54	5	1.14	0.64	0	0.0

Adult females: altiplano vs sierra: $t = 3.73$; $df = 358$; $P < 0.01$
altiplano vs coastal: $t = 5.44$; $df = 319$; $P < 0.01$
sierra vs coastal: $t = 2.28$; $df = 375$; $P < 0.01$

could be pregnancy related. However, there is also a higher frequency of DMF among nonpregnant women in Araucanian populations (Palomino and Pereira, 1971). U.S. white females, ages 1 to 74 years, also have a higher DMF score (14.0) than males (12.9) of the same age and ethnic group (Kelly, 1979). When comparing males and females according to ethnicity, the DMF index reveals that the non-Aymará exhibit significantly higher indices in comparison to mestizos or Aymará, regardless of the altitude in which they live. No differences were detected between Aymará and mestizos. These two latter groups have not only biological affinities, but also cultural ones that set them apart from the non-Aymará (Ferrell et al., 1980). Generally the non-Aymará have more resources, a better economical situation, and the ability to purchase more sugar, candies, soda water, and prepared foods. They do not eat charqui and consume fewer hard or raw foods than the Aymará. In the altiplano, for example, in the different villages where data were obtained, the highest DMF index was found in Visviri, which is on the railroad between Arica and La Paz, the capital of Bolivia, and has access to refined food products not commonly found in the other high altitude villages. Although Visviri has the highest DMF in both adults and children, the difference between Aymará and non-Aymará was maintained.

In most population studies, where comparisons of caries prevalence have been possible, an association has been found between caries and the amount of sugar consumed in the diet (Bibby, 1970). However, several studies have shown that differences in the quantity and quality of foods available may be the cause of the observed differences with respect to the numbers of caries-free individuals. The mineral and trace metal content of drinking water may also contribute to the differences in caries prevalence that are seen (Suomi, 1978; Bowen et al., 1977 and Heloe and Hangejorden, 1981). This was true in our study of two groups of Aymará residing in different areas in the Bolivian altiplano. The constituents of the water in the two communities were quite different and so too were the caries rates (Palomino, 1978). Preliminary reports have found high fluoride levels in some waters in northern Chile. This may relate to the observed caries-free frequencies. However we do not have fluoride levels for all villages where examinations were conducted.

A significantly lower frequency of caries obtains among Chilean altiplano females when compared to their same sex counterparts in the sierra and coastal areas. The inhabitants of the altiplano live in a very dry, cold environment and consume rather dry foods and raw vegetables, especially when herding and farming. These factors undoubtedly contribute to the development of fewer caries but more abrasion than occurs in the sierra or coast.

Gingivitis and periodontal disease are also more frequent in the altiplano as a consequence of the diet, which implies the use of a stronger force to accomplish normal mastication, and poorer dental hygiene. In adults, as time passes these lesions will degenerate into complete bone and radicular atrophy together with severe crown abrasion and attrition.

FRANCISCO ROTHHAMMER, RANAJIT CHAKRABORTY, AND ROBERT E. FERRELL

Chapter 14
INTRATRIBAL GENETIC DIFFERENTIATION AS ASSESSED THROUGH ELECTROPHORESIS

In the late sixties, the significance and maintenance of genetic variability in populations were considered to be central problems in human genetics (Neel and Schull, 1968). The strategies advocated to address these issues included the analysis of marker gene variation in relatively untouched groups of 'contemporary ancestors' living in remote regions of America, Africa or Australia. Neel (1978a), who developed the most extensive efforts to apply various methodological approaches to the analysis of 'primitive' population structure, concludes that the genetic microdifferentiation of South American tropical forest village inhabitants is largely the consequence of the 'fission-fusion' of villages and a 'lineal effect' produced by dissident polygynous Indian leaders. Chance, he furthermore deduces, 'has been highly disruptive to the action of natural selection'. More recently, Smouse (1984), after completing the latest reanalysis of the Yanomama gene frequency data, comes to essentially similar conclusions.

It can be argued that tropical forest villagers are exposed to different environmental influences resulting from diet or slight altitudinal differences, but definitely their natural milieu is much more homogeneous than that of Andean highlanders (see Chapters 1 and 3). In fact, few regions on earth appear more challenging of man's physiologic adaptability than the Andes. Under these circumstances, it is conceivable that natural selection not only eliminated disadvantageous genetic variation but, perhaps, also favored a few mutant genes which conferred on their carriers unusually favorable physiological characteristics in this peculiar environment.

Furthermore, the location of tropical forest villages is frequently changed as a consequence of social structure and of the agricultural technology practiced by their inhabitants (Neel, 1978a; Smouse, 1984). Andean Indians, however, live in geographically fixed, permanent villages, which are only temporarily abandoned for herding llamas or exchanging agricultural products.

In a previous chapter (Chapter 4) we discussed the origin of the Aymará and will examine their biological affinities to other aboriginal populations in Chapter 15, in this one we shall study their pattern of intratribal genetic variation and contrast it with previous results obtained in tropical forest tribes. This procedure is thought to serve two objectives, first, to establish if in a very hostile, heterogeneous environment most of the genetic variation encountered is also attributable to chance and, second, to evaluate the impact of different social and consequently population structures on the distribution of genetic variation.

William J. Schull and Francisco Rothhammer (eds.), The Aymará: Strategies in Human Adaptation to a Rigorous Environment, 193-201.

The quantification of genetic variation

Clearly the amount of genetic variation encountered within a population will depend on the traits employed to measure it. This seems an obvious assertion; however, after the manipulation of blood group gene frequencies, researchers have frequently commented on the unexpected magnitude of variation they observed without considering that the marker systems used were discovered initially because they had the peculiarity of being highly variable. A less biased estimate of the amount of genetic variation at the protein level may be obtained through electrophoresis of erythrocyte and (or) leukocyte enzymes and serum proteins, despite the well known fact that this technique fails to detect variation in regulatory genes, 'silent' amino-acid substitutions and mutations leading to quantitative variation other than gross deficiency.

Methods for statistics to measure genetic variation

Methodologically interested geneticists have justified the use of a variety of statistics to measure genetic variation within and between populations (see, Nei 1977, for the details on some of these). All of these measures are functions of gene and genotype frequencies, and consequently, are closely related. Many differ in names only. Such is the case of the standardized gene frequency or Wahlund's variance, σ^2/pq, which is identical to Wright's F_{ST} (Wright, 1965), Malecot's a (Malecot, 1969) and, if the locus of interest has only two alleles, Nei's G_{ST} (Nei, 1977). This last quantity, in the two allele case, when multiplied by the number of genes sampled, turns out to be identical to the chi-square value of the heterogeneity test proposed by Snedecor and Irwin (1933).

In what follows we shall quantify, by various statistics, the genetic variability present among the Aymará and then compare it with the pattern of variation encountered among tropical forest Indian villages and Central and South American tribes.

During the years 1973-1975 twelve Chilean and two Bolivian Aymará villages were visited as part of the Multinational Andean Health Program. The geographic locations and altitudes of the villages are given elsewhere (Chapter 1). Extensive genealogical information allowed us to confirm the genetic nature of unusual phenotypes. Blood samples were available on 1,695 individuals. The methods of blood collection, preservation, and electrophoretic analysis have been reported elsewhere (Ferrell et al., 1978). The following genetic loci were examined for variation: acid phosphatase (ACPI), esterase D (ESD), phosphoglucomutase I and II (PGMI and PGMII), haptoglobin (HP), adenosine deaminase (ADA), adenylate kinase 1 (AKI), peptidases A, B, and C (PEPA, PEPB, and PEPC), glucosephosphate isomerase (GPI), lactate dehydrogenase A and B (LDHA and LDHB), 6-phosphogluconate dehydrogenase (PGD), malate dehydrogenase (MDHI), isocitrate dehydrogenase (IDHI), glucose-6-phosphate dehydrogenase (G6PD), carbonic anhydrase I and II (CAI and CAII), hexokinase (HK), phosphofructokinase (PFK), pyruvate kinase (PK), aldolase

(AL), glyceraldehyde-3 phosphate dehydrogenase (GPD), phosphoglycerate kinase (PGK), 2,3-diphosphoglycerate mutase (2,3-DPGM), hemoglobin A and B (HBA and HBB), ceruloplasmin (CP), albumin (ALB) and transferrin (TF).

Invariant loci

The Aymará were totally homozygous for the common electrophoretic type at the IDHI, MDHI, PGMII, PEPC, CAI, CAII, HK, PFK, PK, AL, GPD, LDHB, ALB, PGK, 2,3-DPGM, CP, TF, HBA and HBB loci (Ferrell et al., 1980 and 1981). According to Neel (1978a), the frequency of variants per 1000 typings at these loci (IDHI, MDHI, PGMII, CAII, CP and TF) in 21 Amerindian tribes is, respectively, 1.4, 0.2, 4.8, 10.1, 10.7, and 0.2. Accordingly, not all invariant loci in the Aymará are also homozygous among South and Central American Indians. Included among the invariant loci are some ten glycolytic enzymes that are directly involved in red cell metabolism (Ferrell et al., 1981).

Rare alleles

Altogether 10 rare variants were found in the Aymará. These include six (one each at the ADA, AKI, PEPA, PEPB, PGD, and G6PD loci) that (a) are electrophoretically similar to those produced by genes that are polymorphic in non-Indian populations and may be present at a low frequency in the Aymará because of genetic admixture, and 4 (one each at the GPI and PGD loci and two at the LDHA locus) that (b) appear to be unique to the Aymará. Ferrell et al. (1978 and 1980) described the biochemical characteristics of these variants in detail.

Estimation of mutation rates

Various authors have tried to estimate the frequency of mutations using the number of rare phenotypic variants of erythrocyte and serum proteins (Neel, 1973; Nei, 1977; Neel and Rothman, 1978; Chakraborty and Roychoudhury, 1978; Tchen et al., 1978; Bhatia et al., 1979; Bhatia et al., 1981). Neel and Rothman (1978) estimated a mutation rate of 1.61×10^{-5} for tropical forest Amerindians averaging the results obtained by three different methods. If we restrict our attention to the Chilean Aymará and assume that (1) the rare variants encountered are selectively neutral, (2) the Chilean Aymará constitute a reproductive unit, (3) population size has remained relatively constant during the last centuries and, finally (4) the variants originated in the Aymará population and were not introduced by gene flow, it is possible to generate an estimate of mutation rates. Kimura and Ohta (1969) suggest estimating the mutation rate (μ) from

$$\mu = \frac{K}{2N_e} \times \frac{1}{\bar{t}_0} , \qquad [1]$$

where K is the average number of variants per locus, N_e the effective population size and $\bar{t}_0$ the average survival time of a mutant in generations. The parameter $\bar{t}_0$ can be estimated using

$$\bar{t}_0 = 2(N_e/N) \log_e(2N), \qquad [2]$$

where N is the actual population size (generally larger than N_e by a factor of almost three to four). If we take N to be 2810 and the effective population size (N_e) to be 36% of the population size, $\bar{t}_0$ is 6.22 generations. Substituting these values in equation [1] and considering that four unique Aymará variants were found at 31 loci, we compute the mutation rate to be 1.0×10^{-5} which is quite close to Neel and Rothman's (1978) estimate. Nei (1977) uses

$$\mu = \frac{I}{2N_e} \times \frac{1}{2 \log_e(2nq)} \qquad [3]$$

where I is the frequency of variants per locus not exceeding a frequency of 1%, n is the sample size, and q is 0.01. Substituting the corresponding quantities into formula [3] we obtain 1.1×10^{-5}, which is almost identical to the estimate derived above.

On the basis of anamnestic information we did not observe significant differences between the mean number of offspring of carriers of variants who had completed their reproduction and the mean number of offspring of the inhabitants of the village to which they belonged. Furthermore, migrational information allows us to consider the Chilean Aymará as a reproductive unit despite the fact that the population receives some migrants from Bolivia. Population size has remained relatively stable during the last 230 years as shown previously (see Chapter 4) and, finally we excluded from the analysis the variants introduced by gene flow. Consequently, we feel that the basic assumptions underlying the formulae are reasonably well met by our data.

Variable loci

Turning now to the polymorphic loci, we note that there are only four of these, namely, ACPI, ESD, PGMI, and HP.

Inspection of Table 1, which is a tabulation of gene frequencies by village, reveals no altitudinal clines. Gene frequencies seem to vary heterogeneously within as well as between altitudes. Variation for the four loci is statistically significant. The chi-square values, computed according to Snedecor and Irwin (1933), are shown in Table 2, as well as the Wahlund variances and heterozygosity estimates. ESD is the most variable locus (based on Wahlund variance), followed by PGMI, HP and ACPI.

The Aymará exhibit gene frequencies of ACPI that are in agreement with those reported for Peruvian Aymará (Yen, 1972), Cayapo from Brazil (Salzano et al., 1972) and finally Noanama, Cofan and Ingano from Colombia (Kirk et al.,

TABLE 1
Frequencies of the common allele for diallelic, polymorphic erythrocyte enzymes and plasma proteins in Aymará Indians

Village	No.	ACPI*B	No.	ESD*1	No.	PGMI*1	No.	HP*1	% of total population sampled
Azapa	204	.770 (.753)	202	.785 (.789)	204	.773 (.769)	202	.641 (.633)	.34
Lluta	215	.765 (.770)	214	.799 (.794)	214	.797 (.806)	206	.585 (.603)	.60
Putre	190	.736 (.732)	189	.743 (.750)	185	.809 (.794)	204	.615 (.616)	.49
Socoroma	22	.864 (.843)	22	.783 (.825)	22	.659 (.676)	22	.614 (.623)	.16
Murmuntani	19	.737 (.621)	19	.789 (.733)	19	.895 (.889)	19	.711 (.690)	.25
Chapiquiña	83	.765 (.742)	83	.819 (.782)	81	.654 (.633)	66	.727 (.708)	.69
Belén	73	.788 (.784)	73	.760 (.722)	73	.788 (.808)	69	.725 (.720)	.66
Tignamar	102	.789 (.771)	102	.809 (.793)	102	.789 (.830)	95	.626 (.613)	.45
Visviri	225	.757 (.750)	225	.717 (.730)	225	.804 (.782)	224	.640 (.621)	.63
Caquena	111	.680 (.672)	111	.752 (.768)	111	.725 (.715)	96	.740 (.740)	.62
Parinacota	71	.732 (.754)	71	.655 (.691)	71	.775 (.737)	67	.672 (.651)	.53
Guallatiri	63	.833 (.833)	63	.889 (.860)	63	.921 (.901)	56	.705 (.702)	.53
Turco	222	.651 (.680)	222	.653 (.656)	222	.833 (.833)	196	.650 (.642)	.71
Toledo	94	.745 (.764)	94	.750 (.779)	94	.830 (.843)	90	.800 (.773)	.01

Note: Gene frequencies corrected for inclusion of relatives in parenthesis.

TABLE 2
Various measures of electrophoretic variability among 14 Aymará villages

Locus	df	Chi-square	Wahlund variance	Heterozygosity
ACPI	13	40.64 (31.03)**	0.0119 (0.0091)	0.3807 (0.3820)
ESD	13	62.91 (47.40)**	0.0185 (0.0139)	0.3725 (0.3712)
PGMI	13	53.36 (61.33)**	0.0158 (0.0181)	0.3277 (0.3320)
HP	13	44.58 (34.89)**	0.0139 (0.0108)	0.4509 (0.4549)
Total*	312	201.49 (174.65)	0.0025 (0.0021)	0.0638 (0.0641)

Note values corrected for inclusion of relatives in parentheses.
* 24 loci
** $P < 0.01$

1974). The Yanomama, the Makiritare and the Macushi from Venezuela and Brazil exhibit lower frequencies for the A allele (Tanis et al., 1973).

The ESD gene frequencies of the Aymará are similar to those estimated in the Makiritare, the Yanomama and the Mapuche (Mestriner et al., 1976). The Parakanan, the Gorotire, and the Kraho from Brazil show lower frequencies of the ESD*1 allele, whereas the Moro from Paraguay are fixed for the ESD*1 allele. PGMI frequencies are similar to those reported for the Makiritare (Tanis et al., 1973), Cayapo (Salzano et al., 1972) and Nonama, Cofan and Ingano (Kirk et al., 1974). The Yanomama exhibit lower frequencies for the PGM*1 allele (Tanis et al., 1973). Haptoglobin gene frequencies are in agreement with previous results obtained in the same population (Rothhammer and Spielman,

1972), in the Bolivian Aymará (Matson et al., 1966a; Quilici, 1973), Peruvian Aymará (Matson et al., 1966b), and Quechua from Perú and Ecuador (Matson et al., 1966c; Modiano et al., 1972).

The origin and maintenance of genetic variation

The ultimate source of genetic variation is mutation. We have presented some evidence that this rate is not markedly different, if different at all, in the Aymará from that occurring in tropical forest aborigines, despite the fact that Andean populations are exposed to different environmental conditions, including higher cosmic radiation.

We mentioned previously that gene frequencies for variable loci are not correlated with altitude. Restricting our attention to the Chilean Aymará and using chi-square analysis for testing inter-village heterogeneity at each altitude, all four systems vary significantly among the altiplano villages. Furthermore, the HP system showed significant between-village heterogeneity in all three ecogeographic areas. It seems interesting to evaluate the effect of removing the variability caused by the large number of related individuals included in our samples. We used the method described by Chakraborty (1978), in conjunction with genealogical data obtained by interview, to correct the gene counts and gene frequencies for the inclusion of related individuals (see Table 1). After correcting the gene frequencies the between-village heterogeneity observed in the altiplano and the heterogeneity at all altitudes detected for the HP system was no longer significant. This suggests that much of the apparent heterogeneity in gene frequencies is due to non-random sampling.

Next we intended to test between-altitude heterogeneity in an effort to detect the operation of selection. Before doing so, however, two potential sources of error had to be removed – migration between ecogeographic areas and the ethnic heterogeneity of the populations at each altitude. To cope with these problems we used only those individuals who were permanent residents at each altitude and separated the population at each altitude into three categories based on ethnicity as defined previously. This yielded a sample of 1,370 permanent residents made up of 39% Aymará (n = 530), 47% mestizo (n = 650) and 14% Spanish (n = 190). Utilizing only these data, we tested for between-niche variability, again using chi-square analysis. No pattern of significant between-niche heterogeneity was detectable. Thus, there appear to be no systematic changes in gene frequencies nor patterns of heterogeneity that would suggest selection at these particular loci among the Aymará. Parenthetically, O'Rourke and Suarez (1985), in a study of the gene frequencies associated with six polymorphic loci in 70 South American Indian populations, but not including the one of which we write, concluded that 'variables of local ecology do not appear to explain gene frequency distributions in South America.'

The ethnicity code we used conservatively classifies both Aymará and Spanish as mestizo when neither maternal nor paternal patrinyms are available; hence, removing the bias caused by the frequent taking of Spanish names for upward

TABLE 3
Parent-offspring stochastic backward migration matrix for Chilean Aymará villages

Birthplace of progeny	Birthplace of parents 1	2	3	4	5	6	7	8	9	10	11	12	n
Village													
1 Azapa	.035								.107				21
2 Lluta		.040	.122	.102		.020							49
3 Putre			.575	.053		.012	.020			.100	.078		194
4 Socoroma		.029		.417	.045					.088			28
5 Murmuntani			.136	.264	.045					.045	.082		17
6 Chapiquiña						.620					.009	.269	95
7 Belén			.016				.529					.163	49
8 Tignamar							.068	.675				.077	41
9 Visviri									.863				159
10 Caquena		.036	.007				.022		.007	.733	.030	.022	135
11 Parinacota			.027				.071		.061	.127	.479	.014	57
12 Guallatiri												.833	69

n = number of parent-offspring pairs

social mobility. Although between-altitude differences within the three ethnic categories are not significant, there are significant differences between the Aymará and Spanish for all four systems analyzed. Differences between the Aymará and mestizo are significant only for the ESD locus, and the mestizo and Spanish differ only at two loci: ACPI and HP, confirming the expected biological and cultural considerations. In the absence of evidence of selection, it is reasonable to believe that the pattern of genetic variation observed among Aymará villages is the result of an interaction between gene flow and random genetic drift. Consequently, we turn now to an analysis of the migration structure of the Aymará.

Bodmer and Cavalli-Sforza (1968) suggested summarizing migrational data in the form of migration matrices where the birthplaces of parents are given as columns and those of offspring as rows. When father-offspring and mother-offspring migration are different, as is often the case as a consequence of the social structure of the population, both matrices can be averaged. Each scalar of the matrix is divided by the row totals, including the birthplaces of parents located outside of the geographic area considered in the analysis. The resulting 'backward stochastic migrational matrix' can be manipulated algebraically to generate an estimate of the expected Wahlund variance. Table 3 illustrates such a matrix obtained from information provided by 914 parent-offspring pairs. According to this matrix, on the average, 49% of the children are born in the same village as their parents. There is, however, great variation among villages located in the altiplano, the sierra or the lowland valleys. The average percentages for these ecogeographic areas are 73%, 48% and 4%, respectively.

Bodmer and Cavalli-Sforza's (1968) algorithm generated an expected Wahlund variance of 0.0106 which is approximately reached after 12 generations in the Chilean Aymará population. The observed Wahlund variance for the four variable loci is 0.0116. This value is reduced 10%, that is to say to 0.0104, if gene frequencies are adjusted for the inclusion of relatives. Bodmer and Cavalli-Sforza's (1968) drift model assumes basically that (1) the migration structure has remained constant through time, (2) the angular transformation used in the derivation of the formulae makes the variances of the gene frequencies independent of the means, and finally (3) generations are not overlapping. The first two of these assumptions seem justified since village sizes have remained relatively constant over the last 230 years at least (Chapter 4), and Bodmer and Cavalli-Sforza have argued that the angular transformation works well so long as the frequencies are not too near 0 or 1. We tried to cope with the third assumption by using effective population sizes instead of the census sizes of the various villages.

According to these findings the bulk of genetic variation encountered among the Aymará is the result of chance, despite the fact that this population is exposed to contrasting, rigorous environmental conditions. The small number of inhabitants of most villages reduces drastically the probability that all alleles are transmitted from one generation to the next. Given the actual village sizes this process would theoretically lead to the fixation of alleles after approximately 200 generations. In practice the random loss has been compensated for by intervillage migration and gene flow from adjacent areas giving rise probably to a 'steady state'. Although chance is also responsible for most genetic variation in tropical forest Indians the mechanisms originating and maintaining it are somewhat different. Instead of orthodox genetic drift counteracted by intervillage migration, 'founder' and 'lineal' effects are only partially offset by gene flow resulting from village fusions.

Several authors (Ward, 1972; Spielman, 1973; Neel, Rothhammer and Lingoes, 1974) found in Yanomama Indians of southern Venezuela and northern Brazil a good correspondence of among-village biological distances, particularly genetic ones, with geographic locations. It was suggested that 'the tendency of Yanomama villages to progressive fissionings and the recent centrifugal expansion of the tribe may result in unusually large and structural intervillage distances, factors which may play a role in the degree of correspondence observed' (Neel, Rothhammer and Lingoes, 1974). In contrast with these findings, previous reports have failed to detect the same tendency among the Aymará. In fact, Rothhammer and Spielman (1972) found a small, nonsignificant association between erythrocyte antigen markers and geographic distances among six Aymará hamlets. This result is supported by a very low, statistically nonsignificant correlation obtained by us between electrophoretically determined marker genes and geographic distances among the 14 Aymará villages in the present analysis. We presented previously Wahlund variance and heterozygosity estimates based on 24 loci for Aymará villages (Tables 2). On the basis of gene frequencies for the same loci published by Weitkamp et al. (1973), Tanis et al. (1973), and Neel (1978b) we computed similar estimates for 7 Aymará and 7 Yanomama villages as well as for 12 Amerindian tribes (Aymará, Ayoreo,

TABLE 4
Measures of variability among 7 Andean hamlets,
7 tropical forest villages and 12 Amerindian tribes

	Wahlund Variance			Heterozygosity		
Loci	7 Aymará villages	7 Yanomama villages	12 tribes	7 Aymará villages	7 Yanomama villages	12 tribes
ACPI	0.0176	0.0000	0.1174	0.3870	0.0000	0.1282
ESD	0.0293	0.0161	0.1138	0.3782	0.2486	0.3630
PGMI	0.0115	0.0810	0.0587	0.3061	0.0767	0.2126
HP	0.0049	0.0420	0.1071	0.4674	0.2949	0.4487
Total 24 loci	0.0026	0.0058	0.0165	0.0641	0.0258	0.0480

Baniwa, Cayapo, Guaymi, Kraho, Macushi, Makiritare, Panoa, Piaroa, Wapishana and Yanomama) (Table 4). It is noteworthy that despite the fact that the analysis was perforce restricted to 7 villages, because ESD gene frequencies are only available for Yanomama villages 03 U, 03 KP, 03 LMN, 03 T, 03 RS, 03 Q and 03 W, and that the Aymará and Yanomama villages are located in an area of similar dimensions (45,000 km^2), tropical forest aborigines exhibit, on the average, higher Wahlund variances and lower heterozygosity values than Andean Indians. When comparing Wahlund variance estimates with those obtained in 12 Amerindian tribes, it turns out that the seven Yanomama villages are 36% and the Aymará villages 15% as variable as the Central and South American Indians.

This notable difference in the magnitude of the genetic variation encountered between Andean and tropical forest tribes is directly attributable to different migrational patterns, which in turn are a consequence of different social organizations. The constant fissioning of villages (and kinship subgroups) in the tropical forest which is the direct result of social tensions, but more generally the practice of a slash and burn technology results in higher homozygosity and intervillage variation. Andean tribes are sedentary. They found adequate environmental conditions for the practice of agriculture thousands of years ago. Moreover, their migrational patterns reflect zonal complementarity and regional interactions rather than a search for independent cultivating grounds (Lynch, 1981).

We may conclude that although chance is largely responsible for the genetic variation observed in indigenous Andean populations as well as tropical forest tribes, there are observable differences in magnitude between the two groups. Furthermore, the differences seen are the result of different migration patterns which are part of their social structures and represent in each case adaptations to regional environmental conditions.

FRANCISCO ROTHHAMMER

Chapter 15
ETHNOGENESIS AND AFFINITIES TO OTHER SOUTH AMERICAN ABORIGINAL POPULATIONS

The ethnology of South American aborigines has been the object of extensive research. Three decades ago, the application by some anthropologists of a more or less static, anatomic approach to the study of skeletal remains resulted in the creation of different subspecific, immutable categories called 'types' or 'races', such as the Andeans, the Pampeans, the Fueguians or the Lagoa Santans among others. The existence of these different 'types' had then to be explained, and to do so the occurrence of various discrete migrational waves was invoked (Imbelloni, 1938; Rivet, 1958), in a manner similar to the attribution of the existence of different species to independent acts of creation in pre-Darwinian times.

In the late forties, osteotypology was gradually replaced by hemotypology. It was not until twenty years ago that human population geneticists entered the evolutionary field armed with different concepts and methodologies. Subsequently, biological relationships between South American aborigines were explored employing marker genes, anthropometric, dermatoglyphic, dental traits and craniometric distances among other variables (Fitch and Neel, 1969; Ward et al., 1975; Blanco and Chakraborty, 1975; Chakraborty et al., 1976; Palomino et al., 1977; Marcellino et al., 1978; Rothhammer et al., 1979; Spielman et al., 1979; and Rothhammer et al., 1984). Recently, using craniometrical isocline maps and distances based on genetic markers among linguistic groupings, Rothhammer and Silva (1989) tested models of population displacement based on archaeological data.

Available information, including that provided by archaeological findings, osteologic collections, linguistic affinities and genetic markers, is used in what follows to explore the relationships of the Aymará to other South American aboriginal populations, in an effort to establish their geographic origin. Additional objectives are the estimation of the time span they have lived at high altitudes and have existed as a biocultural entity.

Geographic logic

Based heavily on geographic logic and meager archaeological evidence, Bennett and Bird (1964) provided a reconstruction of the principal migrational routes of the first South Americans. According to these authors, the nomadic hunters, fishermen and gatherers, crossed the Isthmus of Panama and entered the northern Andean region by way of the Cauca and Magdalena rivers in Colombia. Some of the nomadic hunters probably migrated eastward into Venezuela and

William J. Schull and Francisco Rothhammer (eds.), The Aymará: Strategies in Human Adaptation to a Rigorous Environment, 203-210. *©1990 by Kluwer Academic Publishers.*

Guyana and others, after adjusting to high altitude, southward into the central and south Andean areas.

Bennett and Bird (1964) also considered an alternative route by way of the chain of Caribbean islands, but believed that despite the development of water travel in Amazonia and southern Chile, there was still little evidence to support the utilization of this transport system by the nomadic hunters who first reached the South American continent. The Amazonian and tropical jungles of the Pacific coast of Colombia and Ecuador, probably offered less favorable conditions for human existence than the highlands, where apparently enough game was available to support nomadic hunters. These small displacements did not alter the main migrational wave which moved southward into northwestern Argentina. Once this area was peopled, one group entered the open park country of the east Brazilian highlands and another one, expanded throughout the Pampas and Patagonia, arriving in Tierra del Fuego as early as 8500 BC. The Chilean archipelago was peopled after water travel developed.

Archaeologic evidence

It is obviously not our purpose to review all archaeologic evidence for paleoindian and archaic cultural periods in South America, but to mention only a few facts that may be relevant to the origin of Andean populations. Absolute chronology suggests that man was hunting now extinct animals in northwestern Venezuela in late Pleistocene times. Four radiocarbon determinations have provided dates between 11,000 and 14,500 BC (Lanning and Patterson, 1967). Near Bogota, Colombia, in Tequendama, Correal and van der Hammen (1977) provided evidence of human occupation before 8000 BC. Some 12,000 years ago, nomadic hunters were already present in the central Andes (MacNeish et al., 1970; Lynch and Kennedy, 1970; Lynch, 1983). Various rock shelters in northern Chile exhibit unequivocal signs of human occupation before 8000 BC (Núñez, 1983). Radiocarbon determinations on the Chilean Pacific coast, at the outlet of the Camarones valley and near Antofagasta, gave antiquities of roughly 5500 BC and 7500 BC, respectively (Niemeyer and Schiapacasse, 1977; Núñez, 1983). Recent archaeological evidence suggests that eastern Brazil was peopled very early (Schmitz, 1985). Doubtlessly, the reviewed data give support to the migration model of Bennett and Bird (1964) based on geographic logic. It seems reasonable to suggest that the tropical forest aborigines descended from the paleoindian bands that settled first in eastern Brazil.

Particularly important for elucidating the origin of Andean peoples and cultures is the work of Donald W. Lathrop. In one of his extensive publications (Lathrop, 1970), he reviews geoecological, technological, linguistic and archaeological information regarding tropical forest inhabitants and postulates that the origin of Andean culture is strongly related to the Tropical Forest Culture, that developed in the upper Amazon area. Lathrop (1970) thinks that the spread of this culture was bound to manioc cultivation, which may have started between 5000 and 7000 BC in the humid lowlands to the east of the

TABLE 1
Localities or tribes, countries of origin and approximate dates of five Andean craniologic collections

Locality or archeologic site	Country	Approximat Chronology
Cerro de Luna	Venezuela	1300 AD
Samabaquies	Brazil	1800 BC
Patallacta	Perú	1400 AD
Paucarcancha	Perú	1400 AD
Torontoy	Perú	1400 AD
Tiwanaku	Bolivia	1000 AD

Andes. On the basis of ecological, archaeological and linguistic considerations he also arrived at a model of Arawakan and Tupian distribution, which assumes that around 3000 BC, speakers of Proto-Arawakan and Tupian were concentrated on the flood plain of the Central Amazon. As a consequence of the development of agriculture, the increased population had to move out, looking for other areas of alluvial bottom land. The population expansion is supposed to have occurred in two directions along available waterways using canoes. The Proto-Arawak speakers moved to the north and southwest, whereas the Proto-Tupi speakers to the southeast. It is highly probable that Andean tribes descended from Arawak speakers that peopled the upper Amazon.

Craniologic evidence

Unfortunately very limited craniometric data are available for the northern and central Andes (Rothhammer and Silva, 1989). Despite the fact that only means and, in a few instances, standard deviations have been published, we have selected six collections for a comparative analysis. Table 1 exhibits the names of the localities or archaeologic sites, countries of origin and approximate chronology. The Cerro de Luna collection (Marcano, 1893) was exhumed in Venezuela close to the Orinoco River. Patallacta, Paucarcancha and Torontoy are located in the Peruvian highlands near Cuzco. The skulls analyzed were recovered from a number of caves and rock shelters mostly along the Urubamba drainage and seriated by Newman (MacCurdy, 1923). The Tiwanaku collection (Posnansky, 1914) is a pooled sample of different sites located close to Lake Titicaca, near Tiwanaku. A Sambaqui sample from the Atlantic coast of Brazil is included for comparison (Mello at Alvin, 1978). According to archaeological evidence (Ponce Sangines, 1978; Rothhammer, this volume) and geographic location, the Tiwanaku collection may, as a first approximation, be considered to represent the ancestors of the historic Aymará.

Seven face measurements, namely, (1) bizygomatic breadth, (2) minimal frontal breadth, (3) nasal height, (4) orbital height, (5) orbital breadth, (6) palatal length and (7) palatal breadth were selected for analysis because previous

TABLE 2
Means of seven craniometric variables
in six prehistoric populations of South America

	Sample Size	Bizygomatic breadth (cm)	Frontal breadth (cm)	Nasal height (cm)	Orbital breadth (cm)	Orbital height (cm)	Palatal length (cm)	Palatal breadth (cm)
Cerro de Luna	65	13.10	9.62	5.01	3.77	3.42	5.25	4.01
Sambaquies	23	13.56	9.73	5.15	3.86	3.41	5.06	3.84
Patallacta	22	13.19	9.24	4.90	3.62	3.45	4.60	3.93
Paucarancha	66	12.81	8.92	4.68	3.56	3.45	4.42	3.94
Torontoy	13	12.81	8.75	4.86	3.60	3.43	4.45	3.89
Tiwanaku	25	12.81	8.44	4.94	3.70	3.61	4.51	4.03

experience has shown that these measurements are relatively unaffected by artificial cranial deformation (Cocilovo, 1975). The means for the seven measurements (Table 2) were obtained averaging both sexes. This procedure seems justified since the two sexes were similarly represented.

Multivariate craniometric distances (Mahalanobis' D^2) among the six samples were computed using a within population variance-covariance matrix. Although we hesitate to assign levels of significance to the distance statistics, they may be used to evaluate the relative biologic proximity of Tiwanaku to any of the other collections. Craniometrically similar groups may either descend one from the other or share a common ancestor. Our previous results (Rothhammer et al., 1982) suggest that the seven craniometric traits included in the analysis exhibit little evolutionary change in a time span of 1,500 years. Therefore chronologic differences among samples should not bias the results importantly.

It is noteworthy that Tiwanaku is closest to Patallacta and Paucarcancha. The three Peruvian samples are separated by relatively small distances. Sambaquies, on the other hand, is surprisingly close to the Venezuelan sample.

Before trying to interpret our findings it should be noted that climatic as well as altitudinal factors may significantly influence growth and development (Mueller et al.; Palomino; this volume). Craniometric distances between high and low altitude populations may include these effects. A partial regression analysis of the craniometric measurements on various climatic variables, as well as latitude, longitude and altitude in a sample of roughly 1,119 skulls belonging to 25 prehistoric populations of South America (Rothhammer and Silva, 1990) demonstrated that, on the average, as much as 11.0% of craniometric variability for facial measurements could be attributed to climate and 7.5% to altitude. This variation is significant and if added to measurement and sampling error, could have distorted our results.

Coming back to the interpretation of distances, we suggest that if the aforementioned factors have not biased our analysis, the Aymará, represented by the Tiwanaku series, and the Quechua, in turn represented by the Patallacta, Torontoy, and Paucarcancha skulls, are biologically related. The proximity of the

TABLE 3
Craniometric distances (Mahalanobis D^2) between six prehistoric populations of South America

	Cerro de Luna	Sambaquies	Patallacta	Paucaranca	Torontoy
Sambaquies	1.985				
Patallacta	5.858	4.393			
Paucarancha	9.259	8.565	0.958		
Torontoy	9.036	7.595	1.140	0.615	
Tiwanaku	12.994	12.812	2.307	4.188	5.000

Brazilian Sambaquies to the Venezuelan sample may indicate the existence of common ancestors. It may be suggested that these ancestors were related to the populations that first settled in eastern Brazil (Rothhammer and Silva, 1989).

Paleoserological evidence

Little is still known about the distribution of marker genes in prehistoric populations of South America and more specifically in highland populations. The early work of Matson (1936) conveyed the impression that blood groups A and B were absent in prehistoric populations of South America. Nevertheless, Boyd and Boyd (1937) found type A and B and Gilbery and Lubran (1952) type A individuals among mummies of Colombia and Perú. More recently Allison et al. (1978) published the results of extensive ABO typing of Peruvian mummies and found the A and B antigens in relatively high frequencies. These authors found the AB genotype to be unexpectedly high and attributed their findings to the existence of a 'primitive' cis ABO haplotype. Although we are skeptical about both the finding and the interpretation, it is possible that the prehistoric populations of South America did, in fact, have the A antigen. Recently, Llop and Rothhammer (1988) reported the finding of one A individual among 54 mummies of the Azapa valley. Allison (personal communication) has also detected the presence of A individuals in northern Chile. The technical difficulties inherent in the typing of mummified tissues promote caution in the acceptance of these findings. If, however, they are verified, many admixture estimates of South American Indians will have to be revised.

Stastny (1974) reported some years ago the successful typing of HLA antigens in mummies using an indirect linfocitotoxicity test. Immunologists reacted skeptically, finding Stastny's efforts 'imaginative' (Amos and Kostyu, 1980). However, Hossaini and Allison (1976), using a modified technique, have reported typing HLA antigens in Chilean and Peruvian mummies and more recently Hansen and Gurtler (1983) in Eskimo bodies from the 15th Century.

Future work will tell us more about the limitations and advantages of paleoserology as a methodological approach for tracing population affinities. Presently, the data are still too scanty to draw conclusions.

Linguistic evidence

Numerous comprehensive attempts to classify the native languages of South American Indians have been published (see for example Mason, 1963; Greenberg, 1959; Loukotka, 1967). Mason (1963) includes Aymará and Quechua in a subphylum which he designates as kechumaran. Greenberg (1959) lists Aymará and Quechua among the languages of the Andean subfamily of the Andean-Equatorial family. Loukotka (1967) includes Aymará in his group of languages of Andean tribes. There is, consequently, general agreement among linguists that the Aymará and Quechua are closely related. We note that our craniometric analysis demonstrated a similar trend. It is of interest to explore the linguistic affinities of the Aymará and Quechua to other Indian tribes. In this respect, Greenberg's (1959) classification is of help. This author includes Arawak and Tupi among the languages of the Equatorial subfamily, which in turn are grouped with the Andean linguistic subfamily in a greater Andean-Equatorial family. Ge, Pano and Carib constitute a different family. Accordingly, if linguistic affinities are also indicators of biological relationships, we should expect that the Aymará are more related to the Arawak and Tupi, than to the Ge, Pano or Carib speaking tribes.

Serological evidence

Thousands of South American Indians have been bled in recent years by investigators driven by an urgency to study their genetic composition before they become extinct or too admixed. Despite this generalized effort it is surprisingly difficult to collect a reasonable amount of marker gene frequencies to compute genetic distances between specific sets of aboriginal populations. As previously mentioned, the results of genetic distance analysis among South American Indian populations have not contributed substantially to the solution of the problem of the origin and evolutionary relationships of these tribal populations. There is no question that the small sample size and the subsequent large standard deviation of many tribal gene frequencies is a major source of bias. To correct this deficiency, we increased sample size constructing weighted linguistic subdivision gene frequency means for Mataco, Ge, Tupi, Arawak and Pano speakers for eight red cell antigen and serum protein systems (ABO, MNS, RH, P, FY, K, DI and HP). Gene frequencies were extracted from the literature recently reviewed by Callagari-Jaques (1985). Nei's (1972) standard genetic distance was computed among linguistic groups and the following Andean tribes: Aymará-Quechua, Uro-Chipaya, Atacameño and Mapuche (Table 4). It is noteworthy that the Arawak are closest to the Ge. Since Ge is, according to Loukotka (1967), a paleoamerican language, this result suggests that the Arawak speakers (and the Tupi) are related to the prehistoric band that peopled eastern Brazil. Furthermore, corroborating Lathrop's (1970) model, the Arawak and Tupi are genetically related. Interestingly too, the Aymará-Quechua exhibit a small distance to the Arawak, indicating that their homeland was probably the

TABLE 4
Nei's genetic distances among various South American Indian linguistic groupings

	Mataco	Ge	Tupi	Arawak	Pano	Aymará-Quechua	Uro-Chipaya	Atacameño
Ge	0.0176							
Tupi	0.0164	0.0201						
Arawak	0.0131	0.0074	0.0105					
Pano	0.0164	0.0196	0.0296	0.0166				
Aymará-Quechua	0.0170	0.0183	0.0367	0.0124	0.0133			
Uro-Chipaya	0.0531	0.0844	0.0753	0.0539	0.0324	0.0371		
Atacameño	0.0384	0.0252	0.0628	0.0271	0.0282	0.0142	0.0545	
Mapuche	0.0477	0.0397	0.0721	0.0378	0.0369	0.0121	0.0641	0.0232

tropical forest. Previously we called attention to the fact that linguists have grouped the Aymará-Quechua together with the Arawak speakers in one Andean Equatorial family (Greenberg, 1959). Moreover, validating linguistic classifications, with the exception of the Uro-Chipaya, the genetic distances among all of the other Andean peoples are small. In passing, we note that the Mapuche are closely related to the Aymará, suggesting that their homeland was the altiplano. Linguistic and craniometric data (Rothhammer et al., 1984) strongly support this hypothesis.

Ferrell et al. (1980) reported the presence among the Chilean Aymará of an unusual PGMI phenotype which is apparently identical to the PGMI 1-10^{MAC} 1 phenotype observed by Neel et al. (1977a) among the Brazilian Macushi, to a PGMI observed by Van der Does et al. (1978) in the northern Chilean village of Socaire, and by Tchen et al. (1978) among the Wayampi of French Guiana. It is not surprising to find the same PGM variant among the Aymará and in Socaire, a village located close to San Pedro in the Atacama desert. This area, populated by Indians designated as the Atacameño in previous reports and gene frequency tabulations (Post et al., 1968), has had extensive contact with southern Bolivia and northwestern Argentina over the last 5,000 years or so.

If we exclude the possibility of an independent origin, the presence of the PGMI variant in northern Brazil and French Guiana suggests that the variant was introduced by migrants from tropical eastern South America. It is interesting to note that among 19 tribes selected for a distance analysis, Neel et al. (1977b) found that the Aymará are closest to the Macushi.

As we have earlier noted, archaeologic evidence suggests that the Andes were first peopled by small bands of nomadic hunters who first crossed the Columbian and Equatorial highlands, and thereafter the Peruvian one some 12,000 years ago. Some groups descended to the lower mountain regions of Perú and Chile, but the main stream moved to eastern Brazil and the Argentinean Pampas. According to archaeological evidence (Schmitz, 1985), the bands that settled in the eastern Brazilian highlands, started a remarkable cultural elaboration that may have given rise to the Tropical Forest Culture. Tropical forest colonists, following the tributaries of the Amazon at the eastern slope of the Andes, probably arrived on the highlands and the Chilean coast around 6000 BC, as judged by radiocarbon dates obtained at the outlet of the Azapa valley (Rivera and Rothhammer, 1986). On the coast they presumably survived, first, through collecting shellfish and then later adapting their technology to the extraction of fish. In the highlands they started early to practice some forms of primitive agriculture (Lynch, 1983) and to domesticate llamas, as early 5000 BC Later, these populations elaborated such cultures as Pucara, Wankarani, Chiripa, Tiwanaku, Mollo and Inca (Chapter 4). Archaeologic and biological evidence indicate furthermore, that the coastal groups did not interrupt their relationships with the tropical forest. In fact, many cultural artifacts, characteristic of tropical South America, were excavated in northern Chile at the outlet of the Azapa and Camarones valleys, in a site that has been dated at 1000 BC (Rivera, 1975).

Linguistic and serologic evidence complement the archaeological and craniometrical findings. The presence of a similar PGMI variant and the relatively small distances of the Aymará-Quechua from the Arawak speakers suggest that the homeland of Andean peoples was the tropical forest.

THE EDITORS

Chapter 16
EPILOGUE

Investigations of the kind that we have described grow progressively more difficult, partly because of their cost, partly because multidisciplinary studies are more tedious to implement than smaller investigations with a narrower range of objectives, and partly because their full return may not be realized for years. If multi-disciplinary studies are to continue, as they should, we must become more efficient in their organization and management, but these efficiencies can only grow out of experience. Rarely, however, are investigators able or encouraged to look at their achievements, or their lack, from the hindsight of years, and venture notions as to how things might have been done differently. We attempt to do this here on the supposition that the lessons we have learned may prove profitable to other investigators either in their selection of a research strategy or in its field conduct. To give structure to our remarks we focus on two areas, namely, (a) the scientific issues our findings have raised, and (b) the practical ones related to the conduct of a study with over a dozen investigators and an ambitious set of objectives.

Scientific issues

As stated at the outset, the aims of this study were, on the one hand, to describe the health problems of the Aymará and the association of these with the environments in which they reside in northern Chile and western Bolivia, and on the other hand, to examine the role of genetic variability in adaptation to an hypoxic environment, and the relationship of the Aymará, a presumably adapted people, to other indigenes of South America. Achievement of the first of these was essentially an exercise in descriptive epidemiology, and the results need no elaboration here, they speak for themselves. However, it is important to note that beyond the immediate commentary these results afford on the association of overt ill-health with the environmental niches under study, they also provide a systematic basis for the planning of health care needs in the sierra and altiplano, and the training of personnel to dispense this care. To the Aymará these are undoubtedly more important considerations than an inquiry into the biology of adaptation.

Generations of students of the indigenous peoples of the Andean highlands have accepted the fact that their body builds, and in particular, their relatively larger chest dimensions are an outgrowth of adaptation to the hypoxia of altitude. Much of this belief, however, rests on a post hoc ergo propter hoc argument, whereas in fact, there is nothing that requires the peculiar morphology of the Andean dweller to be adaptive merely because it is there. To

William J. Schull and Francisco Rothhammer (eds.), The Aymará: Strategies in Human Adaptation to a Rigorous Environment, 211-217. *©1990 by Kluwer Academic Publishers.*

be adaptational, in sensu strictu, implies not only that these traits are heritable, but that they are or have been associated with greater reproductive fitness. Increased fitness could arise either as a result of a greater probability of survival of some phenotypes through the reproductive years without an actual increase in the mean fertility of surviving individuals, or a greater fertility at the individual level without a change in the probability of survival, or both an increase in the survival probability as well as mean fertility. Thus, ideally, studies of adaptation would establish not only the heritability of the presumably adaptive traits but their reproductive fitnesses. Only family studies, taking genetic ancestry into account, can address these issues rigorously. However, ethnicity comparisons within the same environmental niches, although they do not provide heritability estimates, can afford some insight into adaptation since they involve contrasting the average genotype in one population with that in another. It should be borne in mind, of course, that such comparisons will underestimate the role of genetic variation since the latter is invariably greater within populations than it is between populations.

We began our inquiry with the simple, but legitimate notion that adaptation to the rigors of an hypoxic environment might be reflected in the pattern of occurrence or the distribution of genetic variation at a large number of loci. Variability at some of these could be directly assessed, as in the instance of individual genotypes for the erythrocytic enzymes; whereas at others, genetic variability could only be inferred from the continuous distribution of individual measurements and the known segregation of genes within families, for example in the case of the anthropometric or physiological measurements. Thus, in a sense, our approach embraced two traditional methods of studying genetic variability, namely, that of the 'unmeasured' and the 'measured' genotype (sometimes termed the candidate gene).

We turn now to our findings and the following specific questions: Are the chest dimensions and lung function measurements actually heritable? How variable are they? How do they change with migration from an area of lesser to one of greater oxygen stress (or vice versa)? Is there evidence of a differential fertility? Simple, categorical answers to these questions are not presently possible. However, briefly put, we found the following: Ethnicity and altitude effects are separable in the main. Ethnicity, independent of altitude, has its greatest effect on body proportions and a lesser effect on size. Altitude changes in body proportions occur in measurements most probably related to physiological functions, and such changes are more pronounced during growth. Chest measurements are, nonetheless, the major physical correlates of lung function irrespective of altitude, sex, or age, and when these measurements are considered singly, maximum chest circumference provides the greatest amount of physiological information.

We found that heritability estimates of the lung function measurements (adjusted for age, sex, and height) range between 30 and 50%, values somewhat lower than the heritability of height in the individuals studied. However, lung function correlations between like sexed relatives, one or both of whom had migrated to a different altitude, were lower than the correlations between sex matched relatives who had not moved, suggesting either a genotype-environment interaction or an environmental contribution. This did not occur for height. Upward migration was associated with increased chest depth, FVC and FEV_1, but not height nor the other chest measurements. Downward migration had no significant effect on any of the variables. These results suggest that the chest and lung function variables are heritable and concur with the findings of others who have noted the importance of hypoxia in the development of lung function. But they do not fully resolve the issue of whether adaptation in the Darwinian sense exists for at least two reasons. First, the changes observed in chest depth, FVC and FEV_1 with migration to higher altitudes, particularly at younger ages, suggest the existence of considerable developmental plasticity. Whether this plasticity is itself genetically determined is not clear. And it seems unlikely that the role of genetic factors in its origin will be answerable in cross-sectional investigations such as the present one. This argues for a need for longitudinal family studies in which the control is the individual him or herself. Second, there is little or no evidence as yet that a greater reproductive fitness is conferred upon those individuals with lung function measurements that are presumably more advantageous in an hypoxic environment. Without such evidence there are other plausible genetic explanations for the peculiar morphology of the Andean indigenes, such as selective migration or genetic drift.

Insofar as the specific or 'candidate' genetic loci we measured are concerned, we are faced with the conclusion that there is no evidence favoring the adaptational hypothesis in their distribution. But how reasonable is that conclusion? Many of the specific loci studied, and in particular those associated with the pentose pathway, proved uninformative; they were monomorphic. Is this because of the selection of loci since those studied were all involved in the coding of the structure of proteins, and not their regulation? Moreover, the three dozen or so that could be examined at that time represent a very small sampling of one's genetic constitution. What strategies for detecting adaptation at the molecular or cellular level should be adopted in future studies? Would more recently devised techniques, such as the use of restriction fragment length polymorphisms, that have revealed more genetic diversity than has generally been thought to exist, be more informative? Similarly techniques for sequencing DNA, coupled with the amplification of segments of DNA using the polymerase chain reaction, make possible the study of genetic variation in enzymes not easily investigated with conventional one-dimensional electrophoresis. Or would these approaches too fail, for regulation and not structure is the key?

Would more be learned through studies that examine the responsiveness of specific genetic constitutions to hypoxic stress? Much as one can look, for example, at the response of different apolipoprotein genotypes to dietary loading? But what genes would one select as candidates for this approach? Would it be glucose-6-phosphate dehydrogenase, certainly an interesting enzyme itself, given that two chromosomes, the 6th and the X, appear to be involved in its activity? Or would it be 2,3 diphosphoglycerate mutase? Although this genetic locus has appeared to be monomorphic in most but not all populations, the newer techniques might reveal it to be more variable than supposed, and the functional properties of hemoglobin are regulated by this gene product. This gene, as well as the one for G-6-PD, has been cloned. Or would it be still some other enzyme? Should the genetic emphasis be placed upon in-depth studies of a limited number of families rather than the largely ecologic tack that we took? And if so, should these studies focus initially on oxygen transport, or tissue utilization of oxygen?

Would more be gained, initially at least, by focussing on obvious instances of transitory or lasting maladjustment to hypoxia? There is, for example, substantial individual variation in the susceptibility to acute mountain sickness and its severity, although acute mountain sickness is said to affect to some degree about 30 percent of lowland individuals on abrupt exposure to an altitude of 3000 m, and as many as 75 percent to an altitude of 4500 m. Symptoms of this disorder will abate in the majority of persons after three to seven days, but some will pass into a state of chronic illness. Susceptible and nonsusceptible individuals can be distinguished by a variety of physiologic measures both before and after ascent. Among others Johnson and Rock (1988), for example, have called attention to the fact that a diuretic response generally occurs in individuals who remain well at altitude, but water retention is common among those who do not. Little is known, however, about the role of genetic factors in this susceptibility whether it be with respect to acute or chronic illness; at least we can find no published information on familial correspondence in susceptibility. Family studies coupled with what is known about the pathogenesis of acute mountain sickness might provide interesting insights. For example, acetazolamide, one of the two drugs that have been convincingly demonstrated to prevent or ameliorate the symptoms of acute mountain sickness, is an inhibitor of the enzyme carbonic anhydrase and produces a metabolic acidosis which, in turn, stimulates respiratory drive and increases arterial oxygen tension. Although the mechanism of action of acetazolamide is complex, it has been argued that its efficacy rests on increased bicarbonate excretion leading to the metabolic acidosis described, and that the resulting increase in arterial hydrogen ion concentration stimulates the peripheral chemoreceptors, increasing ventilation reflexively. This, in turn, prompts a 'blowing off' of carbon dioxide, a fall in alveolar CO_2 and a rise in partial oxygen pressure (Birmingham Medical Research Expeditionary Society Mountain Sickness Study Group, 1981).

Multiple loci are known to be involved in the coding of tissue specific carbonic anhydrase isozymes, but none of the loci tested appears especially variable on one-dimensional electrophoresis in most populations although the majority of the surveys that have been conducted would not have detected null variants and these are known to occur. Although their significance and frequency have not been rigorously pursued in Andean populations, a mutation apparently in a control gene for CA I has been described in macaque populations which results in almost the total absence of CA I and a marked reduction (60%) in CA II. The effect of this mutation is comparable then to acetazolamide inhibition of carbonic anhydrase. It is tempting to speculate, as Tashian and Osborne (1975) have done, that such a mutation in the human might possibly confer a preadaptive potential for tolerance to low oxygen stress. It is known, although the data are limited, that red cell concentrations of CA I are about 20% lower among Andean indigenes than normal Caucasians or Negroes, and approximate the levels seen in red cells with high fetal hemoglobin levels (Tashian, 1977). Presumably some genetic variability also exists in the metabolism of acetazolamide, or dexamethasone, the other effective drug, and a search for such variability might be informative.

Patently we still cannot answer a central question of biology: Does adaptation in a Darwinian sense actually exist in the human, or is our normal range of physiologic response to extreme environments so broad that genetic adaptation cannot be observed? Has our failure to observe such adaptation stemmed from an overly simplistic attitude toward the environment? As we have tried to show, the ecologic gradient in which we have worked differs more than merely in changes in partial oxygen pressure, there are important differences in water and plant-borne trace metals that impinge on a variety of enzymatic processes.

Practical issues

The success of a multi-dimensional field study often revolves around a series of pragmatic decisions. These involve the choice of the measurements to be made, sample selection and recruitment of participants, and a variety of logistical matters. We describe briefly some of the decisions we had to confront here.

Choice of measurements: Given the organizational difficulties in implementing a study of the nature here described, there is an irresistible urge to measure all that one can possibly measure. This frequently culminates in burdensomely complicated questionnaires, or examinations that are overly long, trying the participant's patience and potentially compromising the individual measurements themselves. These remarks should not be construed as a defense for a simplistic approach, but rather a recognition that each individual measurement should have a clearly defined purpose, one consonant with the overall objectives of the study.

Sample selection and description: Many field studies fail to satisfy the norms of good epidemiology. Most employ opportunistic samples and while the sizes are generally given, it is disconcerting to find no mention of participation rates nor a detailed explanation of the selection and recruitment procedures. The latter can be particularly important when the representativeness of the sample of the population of presumed inference is suspect; moreover, it merits bearing in mind that in the underdeveloped countries of the world participants often seek medical help only to find that this is not one of the aims of the research or the investigator(s) may not be qualified to extend health care. Participation may occur nonetheless out of a sense of intimidation not that such was intentional, and the participant experience a sense of frustration. Obviously there is a need to inform participants fully in a comprehensible manner, and to share those findings that may be of health value. This is best achieved, perhaps, through systematic exit interviews that afford the participant an opportunity to query the investigator about the health implications of particular findings.

One possible means of obtaining depth in selected areas of observation and yet sufficient breadth to permit broader inferences is multiphase sampling. One selects a sample and then a subsample. Certain observations are made upon all elements in the sample and others are made only on the elements within the subsample. The objective is to obtain some experience upon the subsample, to tie this functionally to a more readily obtained observation in the large sample, and thereby to predict some parameter in the population.

Study implementation: Collection of blood and other samples and their transport has been made more difficult by regulations governing the importation of specimens, and the increasing unwillingness of many airlines to transport preservatives, such as liquid nitrogen. It is wise to clear one's proposed procedures with the appropriate authorities before presuming that no problems will arise. But even then, logistic difficulties are common. For example, we carried nitrogen dewars above those necessary to hold the specimens we anticipated collecting on the supposition that liquid nitrogen might be troublesome to obtain locally or to get into and out of the field. This proved wise, but the problems encountered were even greater than we had foreseen. The nearest source of liquid nitrogen proved to be Santiago, and this required dedicating two dewars to an endless circuit to and from this city. It is also worth noting that nitrogen loss at altitude is more rapid, and although we had anticipated this, we had not fully appreciated how rapidly the loss can occur.

Although at the time of these studies the techniques for the preservation of leukocytes were still primitive, it is clear in retrospective that an attempt should have been made to preserve these cells. Their preservation would have provided a means to examine variation among the Aymará at the major histocompatibility locus, to have studied genetic variation in enzymatic systems not represented in the red cell or serum, and possibly most importantly, given recent advances in DNA technology, and in particular the development of the polymerase chain reaction to which we have previously referred, to probe deeper the issue of gene-disease associations and to afford a more comprehensive measure of genetic variability.

We would also urge investigators, wherever practical, to use standardized questionnaires. For example, the health questionnaires we used had embedded within them the Rose-Blackburn assessment of cardiovascular risk factors as well as the London School of Hygiene's evaluation of pulmonary health. These have the merit of facilitating cross-study comparisons, and many of these conventional epidemiological tools have been standardized on a wide variety of populations. Undoubtedly there are other such standard instruments that we could have used, but did not simply because we were unaware of their existence. It would be helpful, therefore, if some sort of clearing-house existed, that made these instruments available to interested investigators. However, not all of one's needs can be met in this manner, and there will inevitably be idiosyncratic elements in every questionnaire. In our own case, for example, it would have been helpful to have pretested and refined the final questionnaires before their actual use in the field. This need was appreciated, and some preliminary testing did occur in Houston, but a more thorough one in Chile could have avoided ambiguities that arose through locally different idiomatic use of Spanish and Aymará, and would have revealed questions that were not eliciting the responses that were being sought. It would also have been helpful if the interviewers had been provided with detailed maps and lists of the names of villages along the border of northern Chile and western Bolivia. Many names occur on both sides, and such maps and lists would have expedited the work of the interviewers who, although Chilean, were not fully familiar with the area. It also soon became obvious that we had not allowed sufficient time for daily checking and quality control of the questionnaires. This is not a matter of moment, perhaps, when there is a single interviewer, but when multiple ones are being used, these procedures are essential if comparability is to be obtained.

Data management: At this juncture in time, it is or should be inconceivable that a field investigation would begin without proper prior thought to the machine management and retrieval of the data that are to be collected. And in this regard, current investigators have options available to them that were denied their predecessors. Small, but powerful battery powered computers now make it practical to begin the establishment of a machine retrievable data base in the field, and the development of an interactive relationship between the investigator(s) and the data collected. For example, screening of the data for errors can occur as the information is actually entered, and this obviously facilitates the identification and resolution of improbably extreme values since the value can be verified while the participant is still available. The importance of a machine retrievable data base resides, however, in more than just the ease of analysis it affords the investigator; multidisciplinary studies are resources and the data should be seen as having continuing value. However, that value is sorely compromised if the data cannot be shared with others or cannot be conveniently plumbed as new research directions emerge.

Lastly, a cautionary note regarding individual responses to the hypoxia of altitude. We, as undoubtedly others who have worked at elevations in excess of 3000 meters, went reasonably well informed on the symptoms associated with oxygen deprivation – such as exhaustion, lack of appetite, a throbbing in the temples, a rapid pounding of the heart on slight exertion, and occasionally even lying down. And we were medically prepared to cope with these developments. We were, however, less well attuned to some of the psychological difficulties – irascibility, pugnacity, and a shortening attention span (see also La Barre, 1948). While these can impair the function of a single investigator, working alone or only with indigenous aides, they become even more important in a group, such as ours, where cooperativeness is essential, and shortness of temper soon pollutes an already harsh working environment. We offer no solution to this problem, but if investigators are aware that even individuals who are normally well tempered can be affected, understanding is wider and umbrage is less likely to be taken.

REFERENCES

Abelson, A. E.
1976 Altitude and fertility. Hum. Biol. 48:83-92.

Abelson, A. E., Baker, T. S. and Baker, P. T.
1974 Altitude, migration and fertility in the Andes. Soc. Biol. 21:12-27.

Abramson, F. D.
1971 Spontaneous fetal death in man: A methodological and analytical evaluation. Doctor of Philosophy Dissertation. Ann Arbor, MI: University of Michigan.

Acosta, J. de
1590 Historia natural y moral de las Indias. Biblioteca de autores españoles desde la formación del lenguaje hasta nuestra días. Tomo LXXIII. Obras del Padre... de al Compañia de Jesús. Estudio preliminar y edición del P. Francisco Mateos de la misma compañia. Madrid, Spain: Ediciones Atlas. 1954, pp. 1-247.

Agostoni, A., Gerli, G. C., Beretta, L., Palazzini, G., Buso, G. P., Xusheng, H. and Moschimi, G.
1983 Erythrocyte antioxidant enzymes and Se serum levels in an Andean population. Clin. Chim. Acta 133:153-157.

Aldunate, C. J., Armesto, J., Castro, V. and Villagrán, C.
1981 Estudio etnobotánico en una comunidad precordillerana de Antofagasta: Toconce. Bol. Mus. Nac. Hist. Nat. 38:183-223.

Allard, C. and Goulet, C.
1973 Serum uric acid: Not a discriminator of coronary heart disease in men and women. Can. Med. Assoc. J. 109:986-988.

Allison, M. J. and Gerszten, E.
1982 Paleopathology in South American Mummies - Application of Modern Techniques. Richmond, VA: Medical College of Virginia, Department of Pathology.

Allison, M. J., Gerszten, E. and Fouant, M.
1983 Paleopathology – Today's laboratory investigates yesterday's diseases. Diagn. Med. Sept/Oct, pp. 28-48.

Allison, M. J., Mendoza, D. and Pezzia, A.
1973 Documentation of a case of tuberculosis in a Pre-Columbian American. Am. Rev. Respir. Dis. 107:985-991.

Allison, M. J., Gerszten, E., Munizaga, J. and Santoro, C.
1980 Metastatic tumor of bone in a Tiahuanaco female. Bull. N. Y. Acad. Med. 56:581-587.

Allison, M. J., Hossaini, A. A., Munizaga, J. and Fung, R.
1978 ABO blood groups in Chilean and Peruvian mummies. Am. J. Phys. Anthropol. 49:139-142.

Allison, M. J., Pezzia, A., Hasegawa, L. and Gerszten, E.
1974 A case of hookworm infestation in a Pre-Columbian American. Am. J. Phys. Anthropol. 41:103-105.

Allison, M. J., Focacci, G., Gerszten, E., Fouant, M., Cebelin, M.
1982 La sifilis una enfermedad Americana? Chungará 9:275-284.

Allison, M. J., Gerszten, E., Shadony, J., Munizaga, J. and González, M.
1979 Paracoccidioidomycosis in a northern Chilean mummy. Bull. N. Y. Acad. Med. 55:670-683.

Amos, D. B. and Kostyu, D. D.
1980 HLA - a central immunological agency of man. *In* Advances in Human Genetics. Vol. 10. H. Harris and K. Hirschhorn, (eds.) pp. 137-208. New York: Plenum Press.

Appleton, F.
1967 Possible influence of altitude on blood pressure. Circulation 36 (Suppl. II):55.

Arias-Stella, J. and Saldana, M.
1963 The terminal portion of the pulmonary arterial tree in people native to high altitude. Circulation 28:915-925.

Arriaza, B., Allison, M. and Gerszten, E.
1988 Maternal mortality in pre-Columbian Indians of Arica, Chile. Am. J. Phys. Anthropol. 77:35-41.

Arteaga, A., Lacassie, Y. and Castro, N.
1968 Estudio de la alimentación y del estado nutritivo de la población indígena de la precordillera de Arica, Chile. Rev. Chil. Pediatr. 39:631-644.

Ashworth, J. T., Allison, M. J., Gerszten, E. and Pezzia, A.
1976 The pubic scars of gestation and parturition in a group of Pre-Columbian and colonial Peruvian mummies. Am. J. Phys. Anthropol. 45:85-89.

Bailit, H. L., Workman, P. L., Niswander, J. D. and MacLean, C. J.
1970 Dental asymmetry as an indicator of genetic and environmental conditions in human populations. Hum. Biol. 42:626-638.

Bailit, H. L.
1975 Dental variation among populations: An anthropologic view. Dent. Clin. North Am. 19(1):125-139.

Baker, P. T.
1978 The adaptive fitness of high-altitude populations. *In* The Biology of High Altitude People. P. T. Baker, (ed.) pp. 317-350. Cambridge, England: Cambridge University Press.

Ballew, C. and Haas, J. D.
1986 Hematologic evidence of fetal hypoxia among newborn infants at high altitude in Bolivia. Am. J. Obstet. Gynecol. 155:166-169.

Bangham, C. R. M. and Hackett, P. H.
1978 Effects of high altitude on endocrine function in the Sherpas of Nepal. J. Endocr. 79:147-148.

Barcroft, J.
1925 The Respiratory Function of the Blood. Part I. Lessons from High Altitudes. p. 194. Cambridge: Cambridge University Press.

Barnett, H. and Einhorn, A. (eds.)
1980 Pediatrics, Edition 17. New York: Appleton-Century-Crofts.

Barr, R. D. and Galbraith, P. R.
1983 Lithium and hematopoiesis. Can. Med. Assoc. J. 128:123-126

Barr, R. D., Koekebakker, M., Brown, E. A., and Falbo, M. C.
1987 Putative role for lithium in human hematopoiesis. J. Lab. Clin. Med. 109:159-163.

Barton, S. A., Lenart, V., Palomino, H., Murillo, F., Weidman, W. and Schull, W. J.
1976 High altitude, indigenous origin and continuous monitoring. Aviat. Space Environ. Med. 47:592-596.

Bass, N. M.
1982 Dentofacial orthopedics in the correction of the skeletal class II malocclusion. *In* Clinical Alterations of the Growing Face. Craniofacial Growth Series Monograph No. 14. J.A. McNamara, K.A. Ribbens, R.P. Howe, (eds.) pp. 193-251. Ann Arbor, MI: University of Michigan.

Bastien, J. W.
1987 Healers of the Andes: The Kallawaya Herbalists and Their Medicinal Plants. Salt Lake City, Utah: University of Utah Press.

Beall, C. M.
1976 The effects of high altitude on growth, morbidity, and mortality of Peruvian infants. Ph.D. Dissertation. University Park, PA: Pennsylvania State University.

Beecher, R. M. and Corruccini, R. S.
1981 Effects of dietary consistency on craniofacial and occlusal development in the rat. Angle Orthod. 51:61-69.

Behm, H.
1983 Final report on the research project on infant and childhood mortality in the Third World. *In* Infant and Child Mortality in the Third World. pp. 9-33. Paris: CICRED-WHO.

Bennett, W. C.
1963 The Andean highlands: An introduction. *In* Handbook of South American Indians. Vol. II. The Andean Civilizations. J.H. Steward, (ed.) pp. 1-60. New York: Cooper Square Publ. Inc.

Bennett, W. C. and Bird, J. B.
1964 Andean Culture History. Garden City, NY: The Natural History Press, p. 257.

Bert, P.
1878 Barometric pressure. Researches in experimental physiology. (Translated by M.A. Hitchock and I.A. Hitchock from French). Columbus, OH: College Book Co., 1943. Reprinted in French, Paris: Centre National de la Recherche Scientifique, 1979.

Bhatia, K. K., Blake, N. M. and Kirk, R. L.
1979 The frequency of private electrophoretic variants in Australian Aborigines and indirect estimates of mutation rate. Am. J. Hum. Genet. 31:731-740.

Bhatia, K. K., Blake, N. M., Serjeantson, S. W. and Kirk, R. L.
1981 Frequency of private electrophoretic variants and indirect estimates of mutation rate in Papua New Guinea. Am. J. Hum. Genet. 33:112-122.

Bibby, B. G.
1970 Inferences from natural occurring variation in caries prevalence. J. Dent. Res. 49:1194-1199.

Bird, J. B.
1963 The cultural sequence of the northern Chilean coast. *In* Handbook of South American Indians. Volume II. The Andean Civilizations. J.H. Steward, (ed.) pp. 587-594. New York: Cooper Square Publ. Inc.

Birmingham Medical Research Expeditionary Society Mountain Sickness Study Group
1981 Acetazolamide in control of acute mountain sickness. Lancet 1:180-183.

Björk, A. and Helm, S.
1961 Need for orthodontic treatment as reflected in the prevalences of malocclusion in various ethnic groups. Acta Socio-Med. Scand. (Suppl. 1).

Blanco, R. and Chakraborty, R.
1975 Genetic distance analysis of twenty-two South American Indian populations. Hum. Hered. 25:177-193.

Bodmer, W. F. and Cavalli-Sforza, L. L.
1968 A migration matrix model for the study of random genetic drift. Genetics 59:565-592.

Boerwinkle, E., Chakraborty, R. and Sing, C. F.
1986 The use of measured genotype information in the analysis of quantitative phenotypes in man I. Models and analytical methods. Ann. Hum. Genet. 50:181-194.

Bonavia, D., León-Velarde, F., Monge C., Sánchez-Griñán, M.I. and Whittembury, J.
1985 Acute mountain sickness: Critical appraisal of the Pariacaca story and on-site study. Respir. Physiol. 62(1):125-134.

Borgoño, J. M., Venturino, H. and Vicent, P.
1980 Estudio clinico epidemiologico de hidroarsenicismo en la II region (1977). Rev. Med. Chile 108:1039-1048.

Bowen, W. J., Velez, H., Aguila, M. Velasquez, H., Sierra, L. I. and Gillespie, G.
1977 The microbiology and biochemistry of plaque, saliva and drinking water from two communities with contrasting levels of caries in Colombia. South Am. J. Dent. Res. (Special Issue C):32-39.

Boyd, W. C. and Boyd, L. G.
1937 Blood grouping tests on 300 mummies with notes on the precipitin test. Immunol. 32:307-319.

Bradshaw, B. S.
1969 Fertility differences in Peru: A reconsideration. Popul. Stud. 23:5-19.

Brewer, G. J.
1967 Genetic and population studies of quantitative levels of adenosine triphosphate in human erythrocytes. Biochem. Genet. 1:25-34.

Browman, D. L.
1985 Cultural primacy of Tiwanaku in the development of later Peruvian states. Díalogo Andino 4:59-72.

Brown, T., Barrett, M. J. and Darroch, J. N.
1965 Craniofacial factors in two ethnic groups. Growth 29:109-123.

Brush, S. B.
1982 The natural and human environment of the central Andes. Mountain Res. Develop. 2:19-38.

Buck, A. A., Sasaki, T. T. and Anderson, R. I.
1968 Health and Disease in Four Peruvian Villages: Contrasts in Epidemiology. Baltimore, MD: Johns Hopkins Press.

Burgos, J. J.
1979 Climatic controls on the South American continent. *In* Ecology of Grasslands and Bamboolands in the World. M. Numata, (ed.) pp. 20-29. The Hague: W. Junk Publishers.

Buskirk, E.
1971 Work and fatigue in high altitude. *In* Physiology of Work Capacity and Fatigue. Springfield, ILL: Charles C. Thomas.

Cabrera, A. L.
1968 Ecología vegetal de la Puna. Colloq. Geographicum 9:91-116.

Cabrera, A. L. and Willink, A.
1973 Biogeografía de America Latina. Serie de Biología, No. 13, Washington, D.C.: Organization of American States, 117 p.

Cabrera, R.
1980 The influence of maternal age, birth order and socioeconomic status on infant mortality in Chile. Am. J. Public Health 70:174-177.

Callagari-Jaques, S. M.
1985 Variabilidade genética e seu significado evolutivo en indios sud-americanos. Thesis. Rio Grande do Sul, Porto Alegre, Brazil: Federal University.

Castillo, B., Solis, F. and Mardones, G.
1983 Influencia del sector salud en los niveles de la mortalidad infantil Chilena. *In* Infant and Child Mortality in the Third World. pp. 49-70. Paris: CICRED-WHO.

Castro, M., Villagrán, C. and Kalin Arroyo, M.
1982 Estudio etnobotánico en la precordillera y altiplano de los Andes del Norte de Chile (18-19° S) *In* El Ambiente Natural y las Poblaciones Humanas de los Andes del Norte Grande de Chile (Arica, Lat. 18° 28' S). Vol II. A. Veloso and E. Bustos, (eds.) pp. 133-205. Montevideo, Uruguay: Oficina Regional de Ciencia y Tecnología de UNESCO para América Latina e el Caribe (ROSTLAC).

Castro, N., Rosales, E., Luengo, N. and Arteaga, A.
1972 Caracteristicas alimentarias y nutricionales de algunas poblaciones indigenas de Chile. Presented IX International Nutrition Congress, Mexico City.

Chakraborty, R.
1978 Number of independent genes examined in family surveys and its effect in gene frequency estimation. Am. J. Hum. Genet. 30:550-552.

Chakraborty, R.
1981 The distribution of the number of heterozygous loci in an individual in natural populations. Genetics 98:461-466.

Chakraborty, R. and Roychoudhury, A. K.
1978 Mutation rates from rare variants of proteins in Indian tribes. Hum. Genet. 43:179-183.

Chakraborty, R., Blanco, R., Rothhammer, F. and Llop, E.
1976 Genetic variability in Chilean Indian populations and its association with geography, language and culture. Soc. Biol. 23:73-82.

Chakraborty, R., Clench, J., Ferrell, R. E., Barton, S. A. and Schull, W. J.
1983 Genetic components of variations of red cell glycolytic intermediates at two altitudes among the South American Aymara. Ann. Hum. Biol. 10:173-184.

Chan, H. S. L., Saunders, E. F., and Freedman, M. H.
1980 Modulation of human hematopoiesis by prostaglandins and lithium. J. Lab. Clin. Med. 95:125-132.

Chaves, A.
1965 Presion arterial en altura. Thesis. Lima, Perú: Universidad Nacional Mayor de San Marcos, Facultad de Medicina.

Christiansen, J. A.
1977 The utilization of bitter potatoes to improve food production in the high altitude of the tropics. Ph.D. Dissertation. New York: Cornell University.

Chow, M., Durand, B., Feldman, M. and Mills, M.
1979 Handbook of Pediatric Primary Care. New York: John Wiley and Sons.

Chung, C. S., Niswander, J. D., Runck, D. W., Bilben, S. E. and Kau, M. C. W.
1971 Genetic and epidemiologic studies of oral characteristics in Hawaii's schoolchildren. II. Malocclusion. Am. J. Hum. Genet. 23:471-495.

Chung, C. S., Runck, D. W., Niswander, J. D., Bilben, S. E. and Kau, M. C. W.
1970 Genetic and epidemiologic studies of oral characteristics in Hawaii's school children. I. Caries and periodontal disease. J. Dent. Res. 49:1374-1385.

Ciswicka-Sznajderman, M., Ignatowska-Switalska, M. H., and Sznajderman, M.
1972 Uric acid level, coronary heart disease and serum lipids. Pol. Med. J. 11:233-237.

Clarke, W. B., Webber, C. E., Koekebakker, M., and Barr, R. D.
1987 Lithium and boron in human blood. J. Lab. Clin. Med. 109:155-158.

Clegg, E. J.
1978 Fertility and early growth. *In* The Biology of High Altitude Peoples. P.T. Baker, (ed.) pp. 65-116. Cambridge, MA: Cambridge University Press.

Clegg, E. J. and Harrison, G. A.
1971 Reproduction in human high altitude populations. Hormones 2:13-25.

Clench, J., Ferrell, R. E. and Schull, W. J.
1982 Effect of chronic altitude hypoxia on hematologic and glycolytic parameters. Am. J. Physiol. 242 (Regulatory Integrative Comp. Physiol. 11): R447-451.

Clench, J., Ferrell, R. E., Schull, W. J. and Barton, S. A.
1981 Hematocrit and hemoglobin, ATP and DPG concentrations in Andean man: The interaction of altitude and trace metals with glycolytic and hematologic parameters in man. *In* The Red Cell: Fifth Ann Arbor Conference. G.J. Brewer, (ed.) pp. 747-762. New York: Alan R. Liss.

Cobo, B.
1891-92 Historia del nuevo mundo. Vol. 2-3. Sevilla, Spain: Imp. de E. Rasco, Bustos Tavera.

Cocilovo, J. A.
1975 Estudio de dos factores que influencian la morfología craneana en una colección Andina: El sexo y la deformación artificial. Rev. Inst. Antropol. 2:197-212.

Comstock, G.
1957 An epidemiologic study of blood pressure levels in a biracial community in the Southern United States. Am. J. Hygiene 65:271-315.

Cornoni-Huntley, J., Harlan, W. and Leaverton, P.
1979 Blood pressure in adolescence. The U. S. Health Examination Survey. Hypertension 1:566-571.

Correal, G. and van der Hammen, T.
1977 Investigaciones Arqueológicas en los Abrigos Rocosos del Tequendama. Vol. 1. Bogota: Biblioteca Banco Popular, 194 p.

Corruccini, R. S., Potter, R. H. Y. and Dahlberg, A.
1983 Changing occlusal variation in Pima Amerindians. Am. J. Phys. Anthropol. 62:317-324.

Cosio, G. Z.
1973 Hematic and cardiopulmonary characteristics of the Andean miner. Bull. Pan. Am. Health Organ. 7(1):26-33.

Cracraft, J.
1982 A nonequilibrium theory for the rate-control of speciation and extinction and the origin of macroevolutionary patterns. Syst. Zool. 31:348-365.

Cruz-Coke, R., Cristoffanini, A. P., Aspillaga, M. and Biancani, F.
1966 Evolutionary forces in human populations in an environmental gradient in Arica, Chile. Hum. Biol. 38:421-438.

Cruz-Coke, R.
1977 The genetic description of high-altitude populations. *In* The Biology of High-Altitude Peoples. P.T. Baker, (ed.) pp. 47-63. Cambridge, MA: Cambridge University Press.

Cuneo Vidal, R.
1919 El cacicazgo de Tacna. Revista Histórica. Tomo 6, Lima, Perú.

Dauelsberg, P.
1983 Tojotojone: Un paradero de cazadores arcaicos. Características y secuencias. Chungará 11:11-31.

Davis, H.
1965 The ISO zero-reference level for audiometers. Arch. Otolaryng. 81:145-149.

Dawber, T. R.
1963 Coronary heart disease. Bibl. Cardiol. (Basel) 13:9-24.

Dempster, W. L., Adams, W. J. and Dubbles, R. A.
1963 Arrangement in the jaws of the roots of teeth. J. Am. Dent. Assoc. 67:779-797.

Department of Health Education and Welfare (DHEW)
1978 Cardiovascular profile of 15,000 children of school age in three communities. 1971-1975. Washington, D. C.: DHEW Publication No. (NIH) 78-1472.

Díaz, B., Gallegos, D., Murillo, F., Covarrubias, E., Covarrubias, T., Rona, R., Weidman, W., Rothhammer, F. and Schull, W. J.
1978 The multinational Andean genetic and health program. II. Disease and disability among the Aymara. Bull. Pan. Am. Health Organ. 12:219-235.

Donayre, J.
1966 Population growth and fertility at high altitude. *In* Life at High Altitude. pp. 74-79. Washington, D. C.: Pan American Health Organization Publ. No. 140.

Dorus, E., Pandey, G. N. and Davis, J. M.
1975 Genetic determinant of lithium ion distribution. II. An in vitro and in vivo monozygotic-dizygotic twin study. Arch. Gen. Psychiatry 32:1097-1102.

Dorus, E., Pandey, G. N., Frazer, A. and Mendels, J.
1974 Genetic determinant of lithium ion distribution. I. An in vitro monozygotic-dizygotic twin study. Arch. Gen. Psychiatry 31:463-465.

Douglas, J. W. B.
1966 The age of reaching puberty: Some associated factors and some educational implications. Scientific Basis Med. Annual Rev. 91-105.

Douglas, J. W. B. and Simpson, H. R.
1964 Height in relation to puberty, family size and social class. A longitudinal study. Millbank Memorial Fund Q. 42:20-35.

Duellman, W. E.
1979 The Herpetofauna of the Andes: Patterns of distribution, origin, differentiation and present communities. *In* The South American Herpetofauna: Its Origin, Evolution and Dispersal. Monograph 7. W. E. Duellman, (ed.) pp. 371-460. Lawrence, KS: Museum of Natural History, The University of Kansas.

Duke-Elder, S
1941 Diseases of the Inner Eye. Vol. 3 of Textbook of Ophthalmology. St. Louis, MO: C.V. Mosby Co.

Duke-Elder, S., and Dobree, J. H.
1967 Diseases of the Retina. Vol. 10 of Systems of Ophthalmology. St. Louis, MO: C.V. Mosby Co.

Ebbing, J. E.
1965 Gramatica y Diccionario Aimará. La Paz, Bolivia: Editorial Don Bosco.

Eisenberg, J. F. and Redfond, K. F.
1982 Comparative niche structure and evolution of mammals of the Neartic and Southern South America. *In* Mammalian Biology in South America. Special Publication Series Vol. 16. N.A. Mares and H.H. Genoways, (eds.) pp. 77-84. Pittsburgh, PA: Pymatuning Laboratory of Ecology, University of Pittsburgh.

Erf, L. A.
1956 Radioactive phosphorus in the treatment of primary polycythemia (Vera). *In* Progress in Hematology. L. M. Tocantins, (ed.). New York: Grune and Stratton.

Esquef, L.
1972 Dietary habits of the peasant of the Bolivian highlands. Nutritional Newsletter (FAO) 10:16-20.

Ferrell, R. E., Bertin, T. and Schull, W. J.
1981 Electrophoretic study of glycolytic enzymes in a human population living at high altitude: The Aymara of Northern Chile and Western Bolivia. Hum. Genet. 56:397-399.

Ferrell, R. E., Bertin, T., Barton, S. A., Rothhammer, F. and Schull, W. J.
1980 A multinational Andean genetic and health program. IX. Gene frequencies of 20 serum protein and erythrocyte enzyme systems in the Aymara of Chile. Am. J. Hum. Genet. 32:92-102.

Ferrell, R. E., Bertin, T., Young, R., Barton, S. A., Murillo, F. and Schull, W. J.
1978 The Aymara of Western Bolivia. IV. Gene frequencies of eight blood groups and 19 protein and erythrocyte enzyme systems. Am. J. Hum. Genet. 30:539-549.

Figueroa, L., Razmilíc, B., Allison, M. and González, M.
1987 Quebrada Camarones, habitat arsenical: La vida humana, animal y vegetal en esta área del norte Chileno tiene extremas y hasta dramáticase características debido al alto contenido de arsénico del agua y del suelo. CRECES 4 (Vol. 8):5-8.

Fitch, W. M. and Neel, J. V.
1969 The phylogenetic relationships of some Indian tribes of Central and South America. Am. J. Hum. Genet. 21:384-397.

Flatz, G.
1989 The genetic polymorphism of intestinal lactase activity in adult humans. *In* The Metabolic Basis of Inherited Disease. C.R. Scriver, A.L. Beaudet, W.S. Sly and D. Valle, (eds.) pp. 2999-3006. New York: McGraw-Hill Information Services Co.

Forbes, D.
1870 On the Aymara Indians of Bolivia and Peru. J. Ethnological Soc. Lond. II:193-305.

Fouant, M., Allison, M. J., Gerszten, E. and Focacci, G.
1982 Parasitos intestinales entre los indigenas pre-Colombinos. Chungará 9: 285-300.

Franklin, W. L.
1982 Biology, ecology and relationship to man of the South American camelids. *In* Mammalian Biology in South America. Special Publication Series, Vol. 6. M. A. Mares and H. H. Genoways, (eds.) pp. 457-489. Pittsburgh, PA: Pymatuning Laboratory of Ecology, University of Pittsburgh.

Frayser, R., Houston, C. S., Gray, G. W., Bryan, A. C. and Rennie, I. D.
1971 The response of the retinal circulation to altitude. Arch. Intern. Med. 128:708-711.

Freij, L. and Wall, S.
1977 Exploring child health and its ecology. The Kirkos study in Addis Ababa. Acta Paediatr. Scand. (Suppl.) No. 267, pp. 1-180.

Freij, L. and Wall, S.
1979 Quantity and variation in morbidity: THAID-Analysis of the occurrence of gastroenteritis among Ethiopian children. Int. J. Epidemiol. 8:313-325.

Frere, M., Rijks, J. Q. and Rea, J.
1978 Estudio agroclimatológico de la zona Andina. Geneva: World Meteorological Organization, Technical Notes No. 161, 297 pp.

Frisancho, A. R.
1975 Functional adaptation to high altitude hypoxia. Science 187:313-319.

Frisancho, A. R.
1978 Human growth and development among high-altitude populations. *In* The Biology of High-Altitude Peoples. P.T. Baker, (ed.) pp 117-171. Cambridge, MA: Cambridge University Press.

Frisancho, A. R.
1988 Origins of differences in hemoglobin concentration between Himalayan and Andean populations. Respir. Physiol. 72:13-18.

Frisancho, A. R. and Baker, P. T.
1970 Altitude and growth: A study of the patterns of physical growth of a high altitude Peruvian Quechua population. Am. J. Phys. Anthropol. 32:279-292.

Frisancho, A. R., Borkan, G. A. and Klayman, J. E.
1975 Pattern of growth of lowland and highland Peruvian Quechua of similar genetic composition. Hum. Biol. 47:233-243.

Frisancho, R. and Greksa, L. P.
1989 Developmental responses in the acquisition of functional adaptation to high altitude. *In* Human Population Biology: A Transdisciplinary Science. M.A. Little and J.D. Haas, (eds.) pp. 203-221. New York: Oxford University Press.

Galofre, F.
1979 Pobreza y los primeros años de la ninez. Situacion en America Latina y el Caribe. Santiago, Chile: CEPAL/Proyecto 1/3.

Geerdink, R. A., Bartstra, H. A., and Van Veen, J. M. S.
1974 Serum proteins and red cell enzymes in Trio and Wajana Indians from Surinam. Am. J. Hum. Genet. 26:581-587.

Gilbery, B. E. and Lubran, M.
1952 Blood groups of South American Indian mummies. Man 52:115-117.

Gilmore, R. M.
1950 Fauna and ethnozoology of South America. *In* Handbook of South American Indians. Vol VI. J.H. Steward, (ed.) pp. 345-464. New York: Cooper Square Publ. Inc.
Gilroy, T. E., Brewer, G. J. and Sing, C. F.
1978 Quantitative genetics of human erythrocyte intermediate concentrations. *In* The Red Cell. G.J. Brewer, (ed.) pp. 363. New York: Alan R. Liss.
Glass, R. L.
1982 Secular changes in caries prevalence in two Massachusetts towns. J. Dent. Res. 61:1352-1355.
Glorig, A. and Nixon, J.
1962 Hearing loss as a function of age. Laryngoscope 72:1596-1610.
Goldsmith, R. I., Rothhammer, F. and Schull, W. J.
1977 Mydriasis and heredity. Clin. Genet. 12:128-133.
Goldsmith, R. I., Rothhammer, F. and Schull, W. J.
1979 The multinational Andean genetic and health program. III. Ophthalmic disease and disability among the Aymara. Bull. Pan Am. Health Organ. 13(1):58-65.
González, F. O.
1974 Arica. Nevados de Payachata. International Symposium on Vulcanology, pp. 1-34.
Graber, T. M.
1972 Orthodontics Principles and Practice. pp. 204-210. Philadelphia, PA: W.B. Saunders.
Greenberg, M.
1959 Linguistic classification of South America. *In* Native Peoples of South America. J. H. Steward and L. C. Faron, (eds.). New York: McGraw-Hill.
Greene, J. C. and Vermillion, J. R.
1964 The simplified oral hygiene index. J. Am. Dent. Assoc. 68:7-31.
Guerra-Garcia, R., Velasquez, A. and Whittembury, J.
1965 Urinary testosterone in high altitude natives. Steroids 6:351-355.
Haas, J. D.
1976 Prenatal and infant growth and development. *In* Man in the Andes. P.T. Baker and M.A. Little, (eds.) pp. 161-179. Stroudsburg, PA: Dowden, Hutchinson and Ross, Inc.
Haas, J. D.
1981 Maternal-fetal responses to pregnancy as indicators of human adaptability at high altitude. *In* Environmental and Human Population Problems at High Altitude. C. Jest, (ed.) pp. 81-85. Paris: Centre National de la Recherche Scientífigue.
Haas, J. D., Frongillo, E. A., Stepick, C. D., Beard, J. L. and Hurtado G. L.
1980 Altitude, ethnic and sex difference in birth weight and length in Bolivia. Hum. Biol. 52:459-477.
Hall, A. P.
1965 Correlations among hyperuricemia, hypercholesterolemia, coronary disease and hypertension. Arthritis Rheum. 8:846-852.
Hammond, N.
1976 The early history of American agriculture: Recent research and current controversy. Proc. Trans. R. Soc. Lond. B 275:120-127.
Hansen, H. E. and Gurtler, H.
1983 HLA types in mummified Eskimo bodies from the 15th Century. Am. J. Phys. Anthropol. 61:441-452.
Harris, R. D., Phillips, R. L., Williams, P. M., Kuzma, J. W. and Fraser, G. E.
1981 The child-adolescent blood pressure study: 1. Distribution of blood pressure levels in Seventh-Day Adventist and non-Seventh-Day Adventist children. Am. J. Public Health 71(12):1342-1349.
Heath, D., Smith, P., Rios Dalenz, J., Williams, D. and Harris, P.
1981a Small pulmonary arteries in some natives of La Paz, Bolivia. Thorax 36:599-604.
Heath, D. and Williams, D. R.
1981 Man at High Altitude. Edinburgh: Churchill Livingstone.
Heath, D., Williams, D., Harrist, P., Smith, P., Kruger, H. and Ramirez, A.
1981b The pulmonary vasculature of the mountain-viscacha (*Lagidium peruanum*). The concept of adapted and acclimatized vascular smooth muscle. J. Comp. Pathol. 91:293-301.

Heer, D. M.
1964 Fertility differences between Indian and Spanish-speaking parts of Andean countries. Popul. Stud. 18:71-84.
Heiser, C. B. Jr. and Nelson, D. C.
1974 On the origin of the cultivated chenopods (*Chenopodium*). Genetics 78:503-505.
Heiser, C. H.
1979 Origins of some cultivated New World plants. Ann. Rev. Ecol. Syst. 10:309-326.
Hellegers, A., Metcalfe, J., Huckabee, W. E., Prystowsky, H., Meschia, G. and Barron, D. H.
1961 Alveolar PCO_2 and PO_2 in pregnant and nonpregnant women at high altitude. Am. J. Obstet. Gynecol. 82:241-245.
Heloe, L. A. and Hangejorden, O.
1981 The rise and fall of dental caries. Some global aspects of dental caries epidemiology. Community Dent. Oral Epidemiol. 9:251-301.
Hernández, S.
1970 Geografía de Plantas y Animales de Chile. Santiago, Chile: Editorial Universitaria, S.A.
Hershkovitz, P.
1972 The recent mammals of the neotropical region: A zoogeographic and ecological review. *In* Evolution, Mammals and Southern Continents. A. Keast, F. Erk, B. Glass, (eds.) pp. 311-431. Albany, NY: State University of New York Press.
Hertig, A. T., Rock, J. and Adams, E. C.
1956 A description of 34 human ova within the first 17 days of development. Am. J. Anat. 98:435-494.
Heyden, S. L., Walker, L., Hames, C. G., and Tyroler, H. A.
1971 Decrease of serum cholesterol level and blood pressure in the community: Seven to nine years of observations in the Evans County study. Arch. Intern. Med. 128:982-986.
Hidalgo, J.
1972 Culturas protohistóricas del Norte de Chile. Santiago, Chile: Departamento de História, Facultad de Filosofía y Educación, Universidad de Chile.
Hidalgo, J.
1978 Revisita a los altos de Arica en 1750. Arica, Chile: Departamento de Antropologia, Universidad del Norte.
Hinchcliffe, R.
1962 Aging and sensory thresholds. J. Gerontol. 17:45-60.
Hossaini, A. A. and Allison, M. J.
1976 Paleoserologic studies: ABO and histocompatibility antigens in mummified American Indians. MCV Quarterly 12:67-73.
Hudson, E. H.
1965 Treponematosis in perspective. Bull. WHO 32:735-748.
Hurtado, A.
1937 Aspectos fisiológicos y patológicos de la vida en la altura. Lima, Perú: Imprenta Rimac.
Hurtado, A.
1944 Relación de los estudios de altura con la clínica y la fisiología en general. Gaceta Médica (Lima, Perú) 1:57-59.
Hurtado, A.
1964 Acclimization to high altitudes. *In* The Physiological Effects of High Altitude. W.H. Weihe, (ed.) pp. 1-17. Oxford, England: Pergamon Press.
Imbelloni, J.
1938 Tabla clasificatoria de los Indios. Regiones biológicas y grupos spaciales humanos de America. Physio. 12:229-249.
Interdepartmental Committee on Nutrition for National Defense (ICNND)
1961 Chile Nutrition Survey: 1960, A Report by the Interdepartmental Committee on Nutrition for National Defense. Washington, D.C.: U.S. Government Printing Office.
International Classification of Diseases (ICDA)
1968 U.S. Department of Health, Education and Welfare. Public Health Service. National Center for Health Statistics. Eighth Revision. Washington, D.C.: U.S. Government Printing Office.
International Demographic Tapes: Chile
1980 Houston, TX: The University of Texas Health Science Center at Houston, School of Public Health, Computer Room.

Iyengar, V.
1988 Biological trace element research: A multidisciplinary science. Sci. Total Environ. 71:1-5.

Iyengar, G. V. and Gopal-Ayengar, A. R.
1988 Human health and trace elements including effects on high-altitude populations. AMBIO 17:(1):31-35.

Jackson, M. R., Meyhew, T. M. and Haas, J. D.
1987 The volumetric composition of human term placentae: Altitudinal, ethnic and sex differences in Bolivia. J. Anat. 152:173-187, 1987.

Jacobs, D.
1972 Hyperuricaemia and myocardial infarction. S. Afr. Med. J. 46:367-369.

Jefferson, J. W. and Griest, J. H.
1977 Primer of Lithium Therapy. Baltimore, MD: The Williams and Wilkins Co.

Jinks, J. L. and Mather, J.
1955 Stability in development of heterozygotes and homozygotes. Proc. R. Soc. Lond. B 143:561-578.

Johnson, J. D., Kretchmer, N. and Simmons, F. J.
1974 Lactose malabsorption: Its biology and history. Adv. Pediatr. 21:197-237.

Johnson, T. S. and Rock, P. B.
1988 Current concepts: Acute mountain sickness. N. Engl. Med. J. 319:841-845.

Juberg, R. C.
1966 Selection in the ABO, Rhesus and MNSs blood group polymorphisms in an Amish isolate of Northern Indiana. Ph.D. Dissertation. Ann Arbor, MI: University of Michigan.

Kalin Arroyo, M., Villagrán, C., Marticorena, C. and Armesto, J.
1982 Flora y relaciones biogeográficas en los Andes del Norte de Chile. *In* El Ambiente Natural y las Poblaciones Humanas de los Andes del Norte Grande de Chile (Arica, Lat. 18° 28' S). Vol. I. A. Veloso and E. Bustos, (eds.) pp. 71-92. Montevideo, Uruguay: Oficina Regional de Ciencia y Tecnología de la UNESCO para América Latina y el Caribe (ROSTLAC).

Kaplan, L., Lynch, T. and Thomas, C. E.
1973 Early cultivated beans (*Phaseolus vulgaris*) from an intermontane Peruvian valley. Science 179:5.

Kashiwazaki, H., Suzuki, T., and Takemoto, T.
1988 Altitude and reproduction of the Japanese in Bolivia. Hum. Biol. 60:831-845.

Keast, A.
1972 Comparisons of contemporary mammal faunas of Southern Continents. *In* Evolution, Mammals and Southern Continents. A. Keast, F.C. Erk, B. Glass, (eds.) pp. 433-501. Albany, NY: University of New York Press.

Keller, C.
1946 El Departamento de Arica, Republica de Chile Censo Economico Nacional. Vol 1. Santiago, Chile: Zig-Zag.

Kelley, M. A.
1979 Parturition and pelvic changes. Am. J. Phys. Anthropol. 51:541-546.

Kelly, J. E.
1979 Basic data on dental examination findings of persons 1-74 years, United States, 1971-1974. Vital and Health Statistics: Series 11, Data from the National Health Survey, No. 214. DHEW Publ., PHS 79-1662.

Kempe, H., Silver, H. and O'Brien, D.
1982 Current Pediatric Diagnosis and Treatment. 7th Ed. Los Altos, CA: Lange Medical Publishers.

Kimura, M. and Ohta, T.
1969 The average number of generations until extinction of an individual mutant gene in a finite population. Genetics 63:701-709.

King, D. L.
1983 Etiology of malocclusion. Birth Defects Original Article Series 19:83-94.

Kirk, R. L., McDermid, E. M., Blake, N. M., Gajdusek, D. C., Leyshon, W. C. and MacLennan, R.
1974 Blood group, serum protein and red cell enzyme groups of Amerindian populations in Colombia. Am. J. Phys. Anthropol. 41:301-316.

Klein, R., Klein, B. E., Cornoni, M. C., Maready, J., Cassell, J. C. and Tyroler, H. A.
1973 Serum uric acid: Its relationship to coronary heart disease risk factors and cardiovascular disease, Evans County, Georgia. Arch. Intern. Med. 132:401-410.

Kolbrick, J. L.
1970 Effects of hypoxia and acetazolamide on color sensitivity zones in the visual field. J. Appl. Physiol. 28:741-747.

Koning, H. W.
1987 Setting Environmental Standards: Guidelines for Decision-Making. Geneva: World Health Organization.

Krogman, W. M.
1960 Oral structures genetically and anthropologically considered. Ann. N.Y. Acad. Sci. 85:17-41.

Kruger, H. and Arias-Stella, J.
1970 The placenta and the newborn infant at high altitudes. Am. J. Obstet. Gynecol. 106:586-591.

La Barre, W.
1948 The Aymara Indians of the Lake Titicaca Plateau, Bolivia. Am. Anthropologist 50:1-250.

Lanning, E. P. and Patterson, T. C.
1967 Early man in South America. Sci. Am. 217:44-50.

Lathrop, D. W.
1970 The Upper Amazon. Southampton: Thames and Hudson, 256 p.

Lavelle, C. L. B., Forster, T. D. and Flinn, R. M.
1971 Dental arches in various ethnic groups. Angle Orthod. 41:293-297.

Lazarus, J. H.
1986 Endocrine and Metabolic Effects of Lithium. New York: Plenum Medical Book Co.

Leistol, K.
1982 Social conditions and menarcheal age: The importance of early years of life. Ann. Hum. Biol. 9:521-537.

Leon, J. A.
1939 Algunas consideraciones sobre los Camelidos de los Andes. Boletin del Museo de Historia Natural Javier Prado 11:95-105.

Leonard, W. R.
1989 Nutritional determinants of high-altitude growth in Nuñoa, Peru. Am. J. Phys. Anthropol. 80:341-352.

Leonard, W. R. and Thomas, R. B.
1989 Biosocial responses to seasonal food stress in highland Peru. Hum. Biol. 61:65-85.

Lerner, I. M.
1954 Genetic Homeostasis. London: Oliver and Boyd, 134 p.

Lewis, J. G. and Gardner, J. E.
1960 The relation of serum uric acid to haemoglobin level in patients with cardiac and respiratory disease. J. Clin. Pathol. 13:502-505.

Lichty, J. A., Ting, R. Y., Bruns, P. D. and Dyar, R.
1957 Studies of babies born at high altitude. I. Relation of altitude to birth weight. J. Dis. Childh. 93:666-678.

Livingstone, F. B.
1984 The Duffy blood groups, vivax malaria and malaria selection in human populations: A review. Hum. Biol. 56:413-425.

Livshits, G. and Kobylianski, E.
1984 Biochemical heterozygosity as a predictor of developmental homeostasis in man. Ann. of Hum. Genet. 48:173-184.

Liu, K.
1977 Dental condition of two tribes of Taiwan aborigenes-Ami and Atayal. J. Dent. Res. 56:117-127

Llerena, L. A.
1973 Determinacion de hormona luteinizante por radioinmunoensayo. Variaciones fisiologicas y por efecto de la altura. Doctoral Thesis. Lima, Perú: Universidad Peruana Cayetano Heredia, Instituto de Investigaciones de Altura.

Llop, E. and Rothhammer, F.
1988 A note on the presence of blood groups A and B in Pre-Columbian South America. Am. J. Phys. Anthropol. 75:107-112.

Loe, H., Theilade, E. and Jensen, S. B.
1965 Experimental gingivitis in man. J. Periodontol. 36:177-187.

Loukotka, C.
1967 Classification of South American Indian Languages. Los Angeles: University of California, Los Angeles Press.

Lynch, T. F.
1981 Zonal complementarity in the Andes. A history of the concept. *In* Networks of the Past-regional Interaction in Archaeology. P.D. Francis, F.J. Kerise, P.G. Duke, (eds.) Proceedings of the Twelfth Annual Conference, The Archaeological Association of the University of Calgary.

Lynch, T. F.
1983 The Paleo-Indians. *In* Ancient South Americans. J.D. Jennings, (ed.) pp. 87-137. San Francisco: W.P. Freeman.

Lynch, T. F. and Kennedy, K. A. R.
1970 Early human cultural and skeletal remains from Guitarrero Cave, Northern Peru. Science 169:1307-1309.

MacCurdy, G. G.
1923 Human skeletal remains from the highlands of Peru. Am. J. Phys. Anthropol. 6:217-329.

MacNeish, R. S., Berger, R. and Protsch, R.
1970 Megafauna and man from Ayacucho, highland Peru. Science 168:975-977.

Makela, M., Weidman, W., Barton, S. A., Rothhammer, F. and Schull, W. J.
1978 The multinational Andean genetic and health program. IV. Altitude and the blood pressure of the Aymara. J. Chron. Dis. 31:587-603.

Malecot, G.
1969 The Mathematics of Heredity. Revised Edition. San Francisco, CA: Freeman Publishers.

Marcano, G.
1893 Ethnographic precolombine du Venezuela. Mem. South Am. Anthropol. Paris 5:1-86.

Marcellino, A. J., Da Rocha, F. and Salzano, F.
1978 Size and shape differences among six South American Indian tribes. Ann. Hum. Biol. 5:69-74.

Marckwardt, A. M.
1973 Evaluation of an experimental short interview form designed to collect fertility data: The case of Peru. Demography 10:639-657.

Marek, K. and Kujawska, A.
1973 L'influence des lesions pneumaconiotiques precoces sur la fonction respiratoire. Bull. Physio-Path. Resp. 9:1173-1187.

Mares, M. A. and Ojeda, R. A.
1982 Patterns of diversity and adaptation in South American hystricognath rodents. *In* Mammalian Biology in South America. M.A. Mares and H.H. Genoways, (eds.) pp. 393-432. Pittsburgh, PA: Pymatuning Laboratory of Ecology, University of Pittsburgh, Special Publication Series Vol 6.

Mares, M. A., Ojeda, R. A. and Kosco, M. P.
1979 Observations on the distribution and ecology of the mammals of Salta Province, Argentina. Ann. Carnegie Mus. 50:151-206.

Marienfeld, C. J., Robins, M., Sandridge, R. P. and Findlan, C.
1964 Rheumatic fever and rheumatic heart disease among U.S. college freshmen, 1956-1960. Public Health Rep. 79:789-811.

Marquez, S.
1967 Patrullajes en el Altiplano de Chile. Santiago: Editorial Orbe.

Marticorena, E., Peñaloza, D., Severino, J., and Hellriegel, K.
1962 Frequency of patent ductus arteriosus at high altitude. Fourth World Congress of Cardiology, Mexico.

Marticorena, E., Severino, J. and Chaves, A.
1967 Presion arterial sistemica en el nativo de altura. Arch. Inst. Biol. Andina 2:18.

Mason, J. A.
1963 The language of South American Indians. *In* Handbook of South American Indians. Vol. VI. J.H. Steward, (ed.) pp. 157-318. New York: Cooper Square Publ. Inc.

Matson, G. A.
1936 A procedure for the serological determination of blood-relationship of ancient and modern peoples with special reference to the American Indian. J. Immunol. 30:459-470.

Matson, G. A., Swanson, J. and Robinson, A.
1966a Distribution of hereditary blood groups among Indians in South America. III. In Bolivia. Am. J. Phys. Anthropol. 25:13-34.
Matson, G. A., Sutton, H. E., Swanson, J. and Robinson, A.
1966b Distribution of hereditary blood groups among Indians in South America. II. In Peru. Am. J. Phys. Anthropol. 24:325-350.
Matson, G. A., Sutton, H. E., Swanson, J., Robinson, A. R. and Santiana, A.
1966c Distribution of hereditary blood groups among Indians in South America. I. In Ecuador. Am. J. Phys. Anthropol. 24:51-70.
Maurer, J. F. and Rupp, R. R.
1979 Hearing and Aging: Tactics for Intervention. New York: Grune and Stratton.
May, J. M. and McLellan, D. L. (eds.)
1974 The Ecology of Malnutrition in Western South America: Columbia, Ecuador, Peru, Bolivia and Chile. New York: Hafner Press.
Mazess, R. B.
1965 Neonatal mortality and altitude in Peru. Am. J. Phys. Anthropol. 23:209-213.
Mazess, R. B. and Baker, P. T.
1964 Diet of Quechua Indians living at high altitude: Nuñoa, Peru. Am. J. Clin. Nutr. 15:341-351.
McClung, J.
1969 Effects of High Altitude on Human Birth. Cambridge, MA: Harvard University Press.
McEwin, R., McEwin, K and Loudon, B.
1974 Raised serum uric acid levels with myocardial infarction. Med. J. Aust. 1:530-532.
McFarland, R. A.
1937a Psycho-physiological studies of high altitudes in the Andes: (I) The effects of rapid ascents by airplane and train. J. Comp. Psychol. 23:191-225.
McFarland, R. A.
1937b Psycho-physiological studies of high altitudes in the Andes: (II) Sensory and motor responses during acclimatization. J. Comp. Psychol. 23:227-240.
McFarland, R. A.
1937c Psycho-physiological studies of high altitudes in the Andes: (IV) Sensory and circulatory response of the Andean residents at 17,500 feet. J. Comp. Psychol. 24:189-220.
McFarland, R. A.
1969 The effects of altitude on pilot performance. *In* Aviation and Space Medicine. Oslo: Universitetsforlaget.
McFarland, R. A.
1972 Psychophysiological implications of life at altitude and including the role of oxygen in the process of aging. *In* Physiological Adaptations: Desert and mountains. New York: Academic Press.
McFarlane, R. W.
1975a Northern Chile. *In* Flamingos. J. Kear, N. Duplaix-Hall, (eds.) pp. 84-90. Berkhamsted, England: T. & A. D. Poyser Ltd.
McFarlane, R. W.
1975b The status of certain birds in Northern Chile. Bull. of the International Council for Bird Preservation No. XII. pp. 300-309.
Meggers, B. J.
1971 Amazonia: Man and Culture in a Counterfeit Paradise. Chicago: Aldine Atherton, Inc.
Mello at Alvin, M. C.
1978 Caracterizacao da morfologia craniana des populacoes pre-históricas do litoral meridional brasíleiro (Paraná e Santa Catarina) Arq. Antropol. Anat. 3:293-318.
Melnick, M., Shields, E. D. and Bixler, D.
1976 Periodontosis: A phenotypic and genetic analysis. Oral Surg. 42:32-41.
Mendlewicz, J., Fieve, R. R., Stallone, F. and Fleiss, J. L.
1972 Genetic history as a predictor of lithium response in manic-depressive illness. Lancet I:599-600.
Merck Index: An Encyclopedia of Chemicals and Drugs.
1976 Rahway, N.J.: Merck & Co., Inc. p. 173.
Mestriner, M. A., Salzano, F. M., Neel, J. V. and Ayres, M.
1976 Esterase D in South American Indians. Am. J. Hum. Genet. 28:257-261.

Mew, J. R. C.
1981 Factors influencing maxillary growth. Proceedings of Symposium Anatomischam Institute. Rostock.

Miller, G. R.
1979 An introduction to the ethnoarcheology of the Andean camelids. Ph.D. Thesis. Berkeley, CA: University of California.

Mills, L. F.
1966 Epidemiological studies of occlusion. IV. The prevalence of malocclusion in a population of 1,455 school children. J. Dent. Res. 45:332-336.

Mitton, J. B.
1978 Relationship between heterozygosity for enzyme loci and variation of morphological characters in natural populations. Nature 273:661-662.

Modiano, G., Bernini, L., Carter, N. D., Benerecetti, S. A. S., Detter, J. C., Bauer, E. W. et al.
1972 A survey of several red cell and serum genetic markers in a Peruvian population. Am. J. Hum. Genet. 24:111-123.

Molina, E. G. and Little, A. V.
1981 Geoecology of the Andes: The natural science basis for research planning. Mountain Res. Develop. 1:115-144.

Molina, S. and Piñera, S.
1979 La pobreza en Americana Latina: Situacion, evolucion y orientaciones de Politicas. Santiago, Chile: CEPAL/Proyecto 1/1.

Moncloa, F.
1966 Physiological patterns: Endocrine factors. *In* Life at High Altitude. pp. 36-39. Washington, D. C.: Pan American Health Organization Publ. No 140.

Monge, M. C.
1948 Acclimatization in the Andes. Baltimore, MD: Johns Hopkins Press.

Monge M., C. and Monge C., C.
1966 High Altitude Disease: Mechanism and Management. Springfield, ILL: Charles C. Thomas.

Monge, C., León-Velarde, F. and Arregui, A.
1989 Increasing prevalence of excessive erythrocytosis with age among healthy high-altitude miners. N. Engl. J. Med. 321:1271.

Moore, L. G., Hershey, D. W., Jahnigen, D. and Bowes, W.
1982a The incidence of pregnancy-induced hypertension is increased among Colorado residents at high altitude. Am. J. Obstet. Gynecol. 144:423-428.

Moore, L. G., Jahnigen, D., Rounds, S. S., Reeves, J. T. and Grover, R. F.
1982b Maternal hyperventilation helps preserve arterial oxygenation during high-altitude pregnancy. J. Appl. Physiol. (Respirat. Environ. Exercise Physiol.) 52:690-694.

Moore, L. G., Rounds, S. S., Jahnigen, D., Grover, R. F. and Reeves, J. T.
1982c Infant birth weight is related to maternal arterial oxygenation at high altitude. J. Appl. Physiol. (Respirat. Environ. Exercise Physiol.) 52:695-699.

Moore, L. G., Brodeur, P., Chumbe, O., D'Brot, J., Hofmeister, S. and Monge, C.
1986 Maternal hypoxic ventilatory response, ventilation, and infant birth weight at 4,300 m. J. Appl. Physiol. 60:1401-1406.

Morgan, W. K. C., Lapp, N. L. and Seaton, A.
1972a Respiratory impairment in simple coal workers' pneumoconiosis. J. Occup. Med. 14:839-844.

Morgan, W. K. C., Reger, R., Burgess, D. B. and Shoub, E.
1972b A comparison of the prevalence of coal workers' pneumoconiosis and respiratory impairment in Pennsylvania bituminous and anthracite miners. Ann. NY Acad. Sci. 200:252-259.

Mueller, W. H.
1979 Fertility and physique in a malnourished population. Hum. Biol. 51:153-166.

Mueller, W. H.
1983 The genetics of human fatness. Yearbook Phys. Anthropol. 26:215-230.

Mueller, W. H.
1986 The genetics of size and shape in children and adults. *In* Human Growth, A Comprehensive Treatise, 2nd Edition. F. Falkner and J.M. Tanner, (eds.) pp. 145-168. New York: Plenum Publ. Corp.

Mueller, W. H. and Reid, R. M.
1979 A multivariate analysis of fatness and relative fat patterning. Am. J. Phys. Anthropol. 50:199-208.

Mueller, W. H., Lasker, G. W. and Evans, F. G.
1981a Anthropometric measurements and Darwinian fitness. J. Biosoc. Sci. 13:309-316.

Mueller, W. H., Schull, W. J. and Rothhammer, F.
1981b Studies of the Aymara of highland, intermontane and coastal Chile. *In* Health in the Andes. J.W. Bastein and J.M. Donahue, (eds.) pp. 69-81. Washington, D.C.: American Anthropological Assn.

Mueller, W. H., Yen, F. I., Rothhammer, F. and Schull, W. J.
1978b The multinational Andean genetic and health program. VI. Physiological measurements of lung function in an hypoxic environment. Hum. Biol. 50(4):489-513.

Mueller, W. H., Yen, F. I., Rothhammer, F. and Schull, W. J.
1978c The multinational Andean genetic and health program. VII. Lung function and physical growth: Multivariate analysis in high and low altitude populations. Aviat., Space and Environ. Med. 49:1188-1196.

Mueller, W. H., Chakraborty, R., Barton, S. A., Rothhammer, F. and Schull, W. J.
1980a Genes and epidemiology in anthropological adaptation studies. Familial correlations in lung function in populations residing at different altitudes in Chile. Med. Anthropol. 4:366-384.

Mueller, W. H., Soto, P., Schull, V., Rothhammer, F. and Schull, W. J.
1978a The multinational Andean genetic and health program. V. Growth and development in an hypoxic environment. Ann. Hum. Biol. 5:329-352.

Mueller, W. H., Murillo, F., Palomino, H., Badzioch, M., Chakraborty, R., Fuerst, P. E. and Schull, W. J.
1980b The Aymara of Western Bolivia. V. Growth and development in an hypoxic environment. Hum. Biol. 52:529-546.

Munizaga, J., Allison, M. J. and Paredes, C.
1978 Cholelithiasis and cholecystitis in pre-Columbian Chileans. Am. J. Phys. Anthropol. 48:209-212.

Muñoz, I. and Focacci, G.
1983 Asentamientos aldeanos en los valles costeros de Arica. Documento de trabajo No. 3. Arica, Chile: Universidad de Tarapaca, 124 p.

Murillo, F., Barton, S. A., Palomino, H., Lenart, V. and Schull, W. J.
1980 The Aymara of Western Bolivia: Health and disease. Bull. Pan Am. Health Organ. 14:52-64.

Murphy, R. M.
1976 Mammalia Americae Australe: A table of taxonomic and vernacular names. Ciencia Interamericana 17(1):16-32, 17(2):18-30 and 17(3):26-35.

Murra, J. V.
1960 Rite and crop in the Inca state. *In* Culture in History: Essays in Honor of Paul Radin. S. Diamond, (ed.) New York: Columbia University Press, 207.

Murra, J. V.
1968 Aymara kingdom in 1567. Ethnohistory 15:115-151.

Murra, J. V.
1972 El 'control vertical' de un máximo de pisos ecológicos en la economía de las sociedades Andinas. Visita de la Provincia de León de Huanaco (1562). I. Ortíz de Zuñiga, (ed.) Huanaco, Perú: Universidad Nacional Hernilio Valdizar.

Murra, J. V.
1975 Control vertical de pisos ecológicos en la economía de las sociedades Andinas. *In* Formaciones Económicas y Políticas del Mundo Andino. Lima, Perú: Instituto de Estudios Peruanos.

Nadas, A., Ellison, R. and Weidman, W. (Eds.)
1977 Report from the Joint Study of the Natural History of Congenital Heart Defects. Circulation 56 (Suppl. 1):1-87.

Nano, H. M., Gavarini, O. and Perez, H. A.
1960 RO 1-7683/15: A new and effective mydriatic. Am. J. Ophthalmol. 49:958-967.

Neel, J. V.
1973 Private genetic variants and the frequency of mutation among South American Indians. Proc. Natl. Acad. Sci. 70:3311-3315.

Neel, J. V.
1978a The population structure of an Amerindian tribe, the Yanomama. Ann. Rev. Genet. 12:365-413.

Neel, J. V.
1978b Rare variants, private polymorphisms, and locus heterozygosity in Amerindian populations. Am. J. Hum. Genet. 30:465-490.

Neel, J. V. and Rothman, E. D.
1978 Indirect estimates of mutation rates in tribal Amerindians. Proc. Natl. Acad. Sci. USA, 75:5585-5588.

Neel, J. V. and Schull, W. J.
1968 On some trends in understanding the genetics of man. Perspect. Biol. Med. 11:565-602.

Neel, J. V., Rothhammer, F. and Lingoes, J. C.
1974 The genetic structure of a tribal population, the Yanomama Indians. X. Agreement between representations of village distances based on different sets of characteristics. Am. J. Hum. Genet. 26:281-303.

Neel, J. V., Tanis, R. J., Migliazza, E. C., Spielman, R. S., Salzano, F., Oliver, W. J. et al.
1977a Genetic studies of the Macushi and Wapishana Indians. I. Rare genetic variants and a 'private polymorphism' of esterase A. Hum. Genet. 36:81-107.

Neel, J. V., Gershowitz, H., Spielman, R. S., Migliazza, E. C., Salzano, F. M. and Oliver, W. J.
1977b Genetic studies of the Macushi and Wapishana Indians. II. Data on 12 genetic polymorphisms of red cell and serum proteins. Gene flow between the tribes. Hum. Genet. 37:207-219.

Nei, M.
1972 Genetic distance between populations. Am. Natur. 106:283-292.

Nei, M.
1977 Estimation of mutation rates from rare protein variants. Am. J. Hum. Genet. 29:225-232.

Nie, N., Hall, C., Jenkins, J., Steinbrenner, K. and Bent, D.
1975 Statistical Package for the Social Sciences. Ed. 2. New York: McGraw-Hill Co.

Niemeyer, H. and Schiapacasse, V.
1977 Investigaciones de un sitio temprano de cazadores-recolectores arcaicos en la desembocadura del Valle Camarones. Actas del VII Congr. de Arq. Chil. Altos de Vilches. 1:115-118.

Niswander, J. D.
1967 Further studies on the Xavante Indians: VII. The oral status of the Xavantes of Simoes Lopes. Am. J. Hum. Genet. 19:543-553.

Niswander, J. D.
1975 Genetics of common dental disorders. Dent. Clin. North Am. 19:197-206.

Núñez, L.
1974 La Agricultura Prehistoria en los Andes Meridionales. Santiago: Editorial Orbe, Universidad del Norte, pp. 96-116.

Núñez, L.
1983 Paleoindian and archaic cultural periods in the arid and semi-arid regions of northern Chile. Adv. World Archaeol. 2:161-203.

Ohlbaum, M. K.
1969 The effects of hypoxia on certain aspects of visual performance. Am. J. Optom. 46:235-249.

Olmsted, R. W., Alvarez, M. C., Moroney, J. D. and Eversden, M.
1964 The pattern of hearing following acute otitis media. J. Pediatr. 65:252-255.

Omran, A. R., McEwen, W. J., and Zaki, M. H.
1967 Epidemiological Studies in Bolivia. RISM Bolivia Project. New York: Research Institute for the Study of Man.

O'Rourke, D. H. and Suarez, B. K.
1985 Patterns and correlates of genetic variation in South Amerindians. Ann. Hum. Biol. 13:13-31.

Ortíz de Zuñiga, I.
1972 Visita de la Provincia de Leon de Huánaco en 1562. Huánaco, Perú: Universidad Nacional Hermilio Valdizan.

Page, L. B., Damon, A., and Moellering, R. C.
1974 Antecedents of cardiovascular disease in six Solomon Islands Societies. Circulation 49:1132-1146.

Palomino, H.
1978 The Aymará of Western Bolivia: III. Occlusion, pathology and characteristics of the dentition. J. Dent. Res. 57:459-467.

Palomino, H. and Pereira, G.
1971 Genetica oral en Mapuches. I. Estudio de diferencias etnicas intrapoblacionales. Rev. Med. Chil 99:132-138.

Palomino, H., Chakraborty, R. and Rothhammer, F.
1977 Dental morphology and population diversity. Hum. Biol. 49:61-70.

Palomino, H., Mueller, W. H. and Schull, W. J.
1979 Altitude, heredity and body proportions in northern Chile. Am. J. Phys. Anthropol. 50:39-50.

Palomino, H., Barton, S. A., Murillo, F. and Schull, W. J.
1978 The Aymara of Western Bolivia: II. Maxillofacial and dental arch variation. Am. J. Phys. Anthropol. 49:157-166.

Pandey, G. N., Ostrow, D. G., Haas, M., Dorus, E., Casper, R. C., Davis, J. M. and Toteson, D. C.
1977 Abnormal lithium and sodium transport in erythrocytes of a manic patient and some members of his family. Proc. Nat. Acad. Sci. 74:3607-3611.

Patterson, B. and Pascual, R.
1972 The fossil mammal fauna of South America. *In* Evolution, Mammals and Southern Continents. A. Keast, F.C. Erk and B. Glass, B., (eds.) pp. 247-309. Albany, NY: State University of New York Press.

Pearson, O. P.
1951 Mammals in the highlands of Southern Peru. Bull. Mus. Comp. Zool. 106:117-174.

Pearson, O. P.
1958 A taxonomic revision of the rodent genus *Phyllotis*. Univ. of California Publ. in Zool. 56:391-496.

Pearson, O. P.
1982 Distribución de pequeños mamíferos en el Altiplano y los desiertos del Perú. *In* Zoología Neotropical. Actas del VIII Congreso Latinoamericano de Zoología. P. Salinas, (ed.) p. 263-284. Mérida, Venezuela.

Pearson, O. P. and Patton, J. L.
1976 Relationships among South American phyllotine rodents based on chromosome analysis. J. Mamm. 57:339-350.

Pearson, O. P. and Ralph, C. P.
1978 The diversity and abundance of vertebrates along an altitudinal gradient in Peru. Lima, Peru: Memorias Museo de Historia Natural Javier Prado, No. 18, 97 pp.

Peñaloza, D., Gamboa, R., Dyer, J., Echevarria, M. and Marticorena, E.
1959 The influence of high altitudes on the electrical activity of the heart. 1. Electrocardiographic and vectorcardiographic observations in the newborn, infants and children. Am. Heart J. 59:111-128.

Peñaloza, D., Gamboa, R., Marticorena, E., Echevarria, M., Dyer, J. and Gutierrez, E.
1961 The influence of high altitudes on the electrical activity of the heart. 2. Electrocardiographic and vectorcardiographic observations in adolescence and adulthood. Am. Heart J. 61:101-115.

Peñaloza, D., Sime, F., Banchero, N., Gamboa, R., Cruz, J. and Marticorena, E.
1963 Pulmonary hypertension in healthy men born and living at high altitudes. Am. J. Cardiol. 11:150-157.

Peñaloza, J. B.
1971 Crecimiento y desarollo sexual del adolescente Andino. Doctoral Thesis. Lima, Perú: Universidad Nacional de San Marcos.

Penso, G.
1978 Back to nature. World Health p. 28-31, July.

Perrin, E. B. and Sheps, M. C.
1964 Human reproduction: A stochastic process. Biometrics 20:28-45.

Picón-Reátegui, E.
1978 The food and nutrition of high-altitude populations. *In* The Biology of High-Altitude Peoples. P.T. Baker, (ed.) pp. 219-249. Cambridge: Cambridge University Press.

Piñera, S.
1979 Definicion, medicion y analisis de la pobreza: Aspectos conceptualies y metodologicos. Santiago, Chile: CEPAL/Proyecto 1/3.

Pizzimenti, J. and de Salle, R.
1980 Dietary and morphometric variation in some Peruvian rodent communities: The effect of feeding strategy on evolution. Biol. J. Linnean Soc. 13:263-285.

Plank, S. J. and Milanesi, M. L.
1973 Fertility in rural Chile. Soc. Biol. 20:151-159.

Pollitt, E.
1980 Child poverty in South America: Reflections on its magnitude, and the basic-need developmental approach: A retrospect on the International Year of the Child. (Paper presented at the meeting of the American Association for the Advancement of Science. San Francisco, CA).

Ponce Sangines, C.
1978 Bolivian Precolumbian Cultures. La Paz, Bolivia: Confirmado.

Posnansky, A.
1914 Una metrópoli prehistórica en la América del Sud. *In* Südamerika. D. Reiner, (ed.) Berlin: Ernst Vohsen.

Post, R. H., Neel, J. V. and Schull, W. J.
1968 Tabulations of phenotype and gene frequencies for 11 different genetic systems studied in the American Indian. *In* Biomedical Challenges Presented by the American Indian. pp.141-185. Washington, D. C.: Pan American Health Organization. Publication No. 165.

Potter, R. G.
1963 Birth intervals: Structure and change. Popul. Stud. 17:155-166.

Puffer, R. and Serrano, C.
1975 Patterns of mortality in childhood. Washington, D. C.: Pan American Health Organization. Publication No. 262.

Purchas, S.
1905 Hakluytus Posthumus or Purchas His Pilgrimes. 20 Volumes. See Vol. XV. pp. 27-29. Glasgow: James MacLehose and Sons.

Quilici, J. C.
1973 Applicaciones de la hemotipologia el estudio de grupos Neoamericanos de los Andes: Los altiplanidos. Définition et Analyse Biologique des Populations Amérindennes. J.C. Quilici, (ed.) pp. 247-261. Toulouse, France: Centre d'Hémotypologie.

Raffo, E.
1934 Observations oto-rhino-laryngologiques chez les habitants des hauts plateaux, a 4000 metres. Rev. Suc. Am. Med. Chir. 5:91.

Ramfjord, S. P.
1959 Indices for prevalence and incidence of periodontal disease. J. Periodont. 39:27-35.

Ramos, V. A.
1989 The birth of Southern South America. Am. Sci. 77:444-450.

Rao, S. and Tewani, S. V.
1968 Prevalence of periodontosis among Indians. J. Periodont. 39:27-35.

Razmilíc, B., Figueroa, L., and González, M.
1989 Arsenic concentations in the waters, sediments, soils and some foods of three watersheds in Northern Chile: A survey.

Reeves, A. L.
1976 The toxicology of arsenic-noncarcinogenic effects. *In* Health Effects of Occupational Lead and Arsenic Exposure: A Symposium. B.W. Carnow, (ed.) pp. 237-246. HEW Publ. No. (NIOSH) 76-134. Washington, D.C.: Superintendent of Documents.

Reig, O. A.
1983 Distribution patterns and evolutionary history of High Andean rodents. Unpublished manuscript, 40 pp.

Rennie, D. and Morrissey, J.
1975 Retinal changes in Himalayan climbers. Arch. Ophthalmol. 93:295-300.

Report of the 2nd Task Force on Blood Pressure Control in Children - 1987
1987 Task force on blood pressure control in children. Pediatrics 79(1):1-25.

Rivera, M.
1975 Una hipotesis sobre movimientos poblaciones altiplanicos y transaltiplanicos a las costas norte de Chile. Chungará 5:7-32.

Rivera, M. and Rothhammer, F.
1986 Evaluacion biológica y cultural de poblaciones Chinchorro: Nuevos elementos para la hipótesis de contactos trans altiplanicos cuenca Amazonas-Costa Pacifico. Chungará 16-17:295-306.

Rivet, P.
1958 As origens do Homen America. Sao Paulo: Auharubia.

Roberts, S. S.
1989 Molecular archaeology: PCR amplifies the pace of discovery. J. NIH Res. 1:129-133.

Rose, G. A. and Blackburn, H.
1968 Cardiovascular Survey Methods. WHO Monograph Series 56. Geneva: World Health Organization.

Rothhammer, F. and Rosales, P.
1990 Microevolution of the maxillodental system in pre-Columbian populations of northern Chile. Homo 39:148-153.

Rothhammer, F. and Schull, W. J.
1980 Adaptacion genetica de poblaciones Andinas. Actas IV Congr. Latinoam. Genet. 2:357-368.

Rothhammer, F. and Silva, C.
1989 Peopling Andean South America. Am. J. Phys. Anthropol. 78:403-410.

Rothhammer, F. and Silva, C.
1990 Cranimetrical variation among South American prehistoric populations: Climatical, altitudinal, chronological and geographic contributions. Am. J. Phys. Anthropol. 82:9-17.

Rothhammer, F. and Spielman, R. S.
1972 Anthropometric variation in the Aymara: Genetic, geographic and topographic contributions. Am. J. Hum. Genet. 24:371-380.

Rothhammer, F., Allison, M. J., Núñez, L., Standen, V. and Arriaza, B.
1985 Chagas disease in pre-Columbian South America. Am. J. Phys. Anthropol. 68:495-498.

Rothhammer, F., Chakraborty, R. and Llop, E.
1979 Dermatoglyphic variation among South American tribal populations and its association with marker gene, linguistic and geographic distances. *In* Dermatoglyphics – 50 Years Later. W. Wertelecki and C. Plato, (eds.) pp. 269-278. Birth Defects Original Article Series 15 (6).

Rothhammer, F., Cocilovo, J. A. and Quevedo, S.
1984 El poblamiento temprano de Sud America. Chungará 13:99-108.

Rothhammer, F., Cocilovo, J. A., Quevedo, S. and Llop, E.
1982 Microevolution in prehistoric Andean populations. I. Chronologic craniometric variation. Am. J. Phys. Anthropol. 58:391-396.

Rotta, A. and López, A.
1958 Electrocardiographic patterns in man at high altitudes. Circulation 19:719.

Rowe, J. H.
1963 Inca culture at the time of the Spanish conquest. *In* Handbook of South American Indians. Vol. II. J.H. Steward, (ed.) pp. 183-330. New York: Cooper Square Publ. Inc.

Roychoudhury, A. K. and Nei, M.
1988 Human Polymorphic Genes World Distribution. New York: Oxford Univeristy Press.

Ruedi, L., von
1944 Gehoruntersuchungen an ohrgesunden und ohrkranken ver suchspersonen auf dem Jungfrau-Joch n (3460 m). Acto Oto-Laryngol. 32:176-188.

Ruiz, L. and Peñaloza, D.
1977 Altitude and hypertension. Mayo Clinic Proc. 52:442-445.

Russell, A. L.
1956 A system of classification and scoring for prevalence surveys of periodontal status. J. Dent. Res. 35:350-359.

Sacro-Pollitt, C.
1981 Birth in the Peruvian Andes: Physical and behavioral consequences in the neonate. Child. Dev. 52:839-846.

Salas, R., Kast, R. F., Montecinos,F. and Salas, I.
1966 Geología y recursos minerales del departamento de Arica. Provincia de Tarapacá. Instituto de Investigaciones Geológicas Chile en colaboración con la Junta de Adelanto de Arica. Boletín No. 21.

Salzano, F. M., Neel, J. V., Weitkamp, L. R. and Woodall, J. P.
1972 Serum proteins, hemoglobins and erythrocyte enzymes in Brazilian Cayapo Indians. Hum. Biol. 44:443-458.

Santolaya, R., Donoso, H., Apud, E. and Sanudo, M. C.
1973 Electrocardiograma y capacidad aerobica en nativos residentes de altura del altiplano chileno, como indice de aclimatacion. Rev. Med. Chil. 101:433-448.

Santoro, C. and Chacama, J.
1982 Secuencia cultural de las tierras altas del área centro sur Andina. Chungará 9:22-45.

Sarmiento, G.
1975 The dry plant formations of South America and their floristic connections. J. Biogeog. 2:233-255.

Sauer, C. O.
1963 Cultivated plants of South and Central America. *In* Handbook of South American Indians Vol. VI. J.H. Steward, (ed.) pp. 487-543. New York: Cooper Square Publ. Inc.

Sawyer, D., Allison, M. J., Elzay, R. P. and Pezzia, A.
1978a A study of dental caries, missing teeth, attrition, osteitis, calculus and bone loss. MCV Quart. 14:181-188.

Sawyer, D., Allison, M. J., Elzay, R. P., Page, D. G. and Pezzia, A.
1978b Maxillary and mandibular jaw-size in Pre-Columbian Peru. MCV Quart. 14:101-108.

Saxen, L.
1980 Heredity of juvenile periodontitis. J. Clin. Periodontal 7:276-288.

Schiappacasse, V. and Niemeyer, H.
1984 Descripción y análisis interpretativo de un sitio arcaico temprano en la Quebrada de Camarones. Museo Nacional de Historia Natural Publ. No. 41.

Schless, A. P., Frazer, A., Mendels, J., Pandey, G. N. and Theodorides, V. J.
1975 Genetic determinant of lithium ion metabolism. II. An in vivo study of lithium ion distribution across erythrocyte membranes. Arch. Gen. Psychiat. 32:337-340.

Schmitz, P. I.
1985 Cacadores e Colectores de Pre-historia do Brazil. Sao Leopoldo, Brazil: UNISINOS. 63 p.

Schulhof, R. J.
1978 Consideration of airway in orthodontics. J. Clin. Orthod. 12:440-444.

Schull, W. J. and Neel, J. V.
1965 The Effects of Inbreeding on Japanese Children. New York: Harper and Row.

Schull, W. J. and Rothhammer, F.
1977 A multinational Andean genetic and health program: A study of adaptation to the hypoxia of altitude. *In* Physiological Variation and its Genetic Basis. Society for the Study of Human Biology Vol. 17. J.S. Weiner, (ed.) pp. 139-169. London: Taylor and Francis.

Schull, W. J., Ferrell, R. E. and Rothhammer, F.
1978 Genes, enzymes and hypoxia. *In* Ecological Genetics. P. Brussard, (ed.) pp. 73-90. New York: Springer-Verlag.

Selowsky, M.
1978 The economic dimension of malnutrition in young children. A World Bank Working Paper. No. 294. The World Bank.

Shults, W. T. and Swan, K. C.
1975 High-altitude retinopathy in mountain climbers. Arch. Ophthalmol. 93:404-408.

Sime, F., Banchero, N., Peñaloza, D., Gamboa, R., Cruz, J. and Marticorena, E.
1963 Pulmonary hypertension in children born and living at high altitudes. Am. J. Cardiol. 11:143-149.

Simonson, E.
1961 Differentiation Between Normal and Abnormal in Electrocardiography. St. Louis, MO: Mosby.

Simpson, B. B.
1975 Pleistocene changes in the flora of the high tropical Andes. Paleobiology 1:273-294.

Simpson, B. B.
1979 Quaternary biogeography of the high montane regions of South America. *In* The South American Herpetofauna: Its Origin, Evolution and Dispersal. Monograph 7. W.I. Duellman, (ed.) pp. 157-188. Lawrence, KS: Museum of Natural History, The University of Kansas.

Singh, D., Kochar, R. C. and Kacker, S. K.
1976 Effects of high altitude on inner ear function. J. Laryngol. Otol. 90:1113-1120.

Singh, S. M. and Zouros, E.
1978 Genetic variation associated with growth rate in the American oyster (*Crossostrea virginica*). Evolution 32:342-353.

Slots, J. and Genco, R. J.
1984 Black-pigmented bacteroides species, capnocytophaga species, and actinobacillus actinomycetemcomitans in human periodontal disease: Virulence factors in colonization, survival and tissue destruction. J. Dent. Res. 63:412-421.

Smouse, P.
1984 Genetic architecture of swidden agricultural tribes from the lowland rain forests of South America. *In* Current Developments in Anthropological Genetics. Vol. 2: Ecology and Population Structure. M. Crawford and J. Mielke, (eds.) pp. 139-178. New York: Plenum Press.

Snedecor, G. and Irwin, M. R.
1933 On the chi-square test for homogeneity. Iowa State College J. Sci. 8:75-81.

Sobrevilla, L. A., Romero, I., Moncloa, F., Donayre, J. and Guerra-Garcia, R.
1967 Endocrine studies at high altitude. III. Urinary gonadotropins in subjects native to and living at 14,000 feet and during acute exposure of man living at sea level to high altitudes. Acta Endocrin. 56:369-375.

Sofaer, J. A., Niswander, J. D., MacLean, C. J. and Workman, P. L.
1972 Population studies on southwestern Indian tribes. V. Tooth morphology as an indicator of biological distance. Am. J. Phys. Anthrop. 37:357-366.

Solares, A.
1941 Kerato-conjunctival lesions observed at high altitudes in Bolivia. Am. J. Ophthalmol. 24:900-914.

Solimano, G. and Hakim, P.
1978 Development, Reform and Malnutrition in Chile. Cambridge, MA: MIT Press.

Solimano, G. and Vine, M.
1980 Undernutrition, infection and infant mortality. Seminar on Biological and Social Aspects of Mortality and the Length of Life. International Union for the Scientific Study on Population. Fiuggi Terme, Italy, May 13-16th, 1980.

Soule, M. E.
1979 Heterozygosity and developmental stability: Another look. Evolution 33:396-401.

Spielman, R. S.
1973 Differences among Yanomama Indian villages: Does the pattern of allele frequency, anthropometrics and map locations correspond? Am. J. Phys. Anthropol. 39:461-479.

Spielman, R. S., Migliazza, E. C., Neel, J. V., Gershowitz, H. and Torres de Arauz, R.
1979 The evolutionary relationships of two populations: A study of the Guaymi and the Yanomama. Current Anthropol. 20:377-388.

Spotorno, A. E.
1982 Conservation of South American mammals – Round Table. *In* Mammalian Biology in South America. M.A. Mares and H.H. Genoways, (eds.) pp. 527-528. Pittsburgh, PA: Special Publication Series, Pymatuning Laboratory of Ecology, University of Pittsburgh, Vol 6.

Squier, E. G.
1878 Peru: Incidents of Travel and Exploration in the Land of the Incas. London: Macmillan and Co.

Stastny, P.
1974 HLA antigens in mummified pre-Columbian tissues. Science 183:864-866.

Steinbock, T.
1976 Paleopathological Diagnosis and Interpretation: Bone diseases in Ancient Human Populations. Springfield, ILL: C.C. Thomas.

Stinson, S.
1980 The physical growth of high altitude Bolivian Aymara children. Am. J. Phys. Anthropol. 52:377-385.
Stinson, S.
1982 The effect of high altitude on the growth of children of high socioeconomic status in Bolivia. Am. J. Phys. Anthropol. 59:61-71.
Stinson, S.
1985 Chest dimensions of European and Aymara children at high altitude. Ann. Hum. Biol. 12:333-338.
Stockard, C. R.
1941 The Genetic and Endocrine Basis for Differences in Form and Behavior as Elucidated by Studies of Contrasted Pure-line Dog Breeds and Their Hybrids. Philadelphia, PA: Wistar Institute.
Stycos, J. M.
1963 Culture and differential fertility in Peru. Popul. Stud. 16:257-270.
Suomi, J. D.
1978 Occurrence of dental caries among children and youths in the United States. J. Prev. Dent. 5:20-23.
Tanis, R. J., Neel, J. V., Dovey, H. and Morrow, M.
1973 The genetic structure of a tribal population, the Yanomama Indians. IX. Gene frequencies for 18 serum protein and erythrocyte enzyme systems in the Yanomama and five neighboring tribes: Nine new variants. Am. J. Hum. Genet. 25:655-676.
Tashian, R. E.
1977 Evolution and regulation of the carbonic anhydrase isozymes. Isozymes: Curr. Top. Biol. Med. Res. 2:21-62.
Tashian, R. E. and Osborne, W. R. A.
1975 Some genetic and molecular aspects of enzyme adaptations. *In* Physiological Adaptation to the Environment. F. J. Vernberg, (ed.) pp. 37-49. New York: Intext Educational Publ.
Tchen, P., Seger, J., Bois, E., Grenand, F., Fribourg-Blanc, A. and Feingold, N.
1978 A genetic study of two French Guiana Amerindian populations. II. Rare electrophoretic variants. Hum. Genet. 45:317-326.
Thomas, O.
1900 New Peruvian species of *Conepatus*, *Phyllotis* and *Akodon*. Ann. Mag. Nat. Hist. (7), 6:466-469.
Tichauer, R.
1963 The Aymara children of Bolivia. Pediatrics 62:399-412.
Tietze, C.
1957 Reproductive span and rate of reproduction among Hutterite women. Fertil. Steril. 8:89-97.
Tschopik, H.
1963 The Aymara. *In* Handbook of South American. Indians Vol. II. J.H. Steward, (ed.) pp. 501-575. New York: Cooper Square Publ. Inc.
Tschudi, J. J., von
1847 Travels in Peru during the Years 1838-1842. On the Coast, in the Sierra, across the Cordillera and the Andes, into the Primeval Forests. First English Edition. London: David Bogue.
Tucker, A., McMurty, I. F., Reeves, J. T., Alexander, A. F., Will, D. H. and Grover, R. F.
1975 Lung vascular smooth muscle as a determinant of pulmonary hypertension at high altitude. Am. J. Physiol. 228:762-767.
Uhle, M.
1919 La arqueología de Arica y Tacna. Bol. de la Soc. Ecuat. de Est. Hist. Am. Quito Vol. III:1-48.
UNICEF/CEPAL
1979 Indicators on the situation of children in Latin America and the Caribbean. No 49. 318. Santiago, Chile.
United States A. I. D.
1975 Bolivia Health Sector Assessment. Mission to Bolivia. La Paz, Bolivia.
Urzua Urzua, L.
1969 Arica, Puerta Nueva. Santiago, Chile: Editorial Andres Bello.

USPHS

1970 U.S. Public Health Service: Community Water Supply Study: Analysis of National Survey Findings. Washington, D.C.: U.S. Department of Health, Education, and Welfare.

Vahter, M.

1983 Metabolism of arsenic. *In* Biological and Environmental Effects of Arsenic. Vol. 6 Topics in Environmental Health. B.A. Fowler, (ed.) pp. 171-198. Amsterdam: Elsevier Science Publishers B.V.

Valsik, J. A.

1965 The seasonal rhythm of menarche: A review. Hum. Biol. 37:74-90.

Van Der Does, J. A., Rubinstein, P. and Khan, P. M.

1978 A rare PGM_1 variant in Chilean Aymara Indians. Hum. Genet. 34:327-329.

Van Liere, E. J. and Stickney, J. C.

1963 Hypoxia. Chicago: University of Chicago Press

Veloso, A., Salaberry, M., Navarro, J., Iturra, P., Valencia, J., Penna, M. and Díaz, N.

1982 Contribución sistemática al conocimiento de la Herpetofauna del extremo Norte de Chile. *In* El Ambiente Natural y las Poblaciones Humanas de los Andes del Norte Grande de Chile (Arica, Lat. 18° 28'S) Vol. II. A. Veloso and E. Bustos, (ed.) pp. 135-268. Montevideo, Uruguay: Oficina Regional de Ciencia y Tecnología de UNESCO para América Latina y el Caribe (ROSTLAC).

Villagrán, C., Kalin Arroyo, M. and Armesto, J.

1982 La vegetación de un transecto altitudinal en los Andes del Norte de Chile (18-19° S). *In* El Ambiente Natural y la Poblaciones Humanas de los Andes del Norte Grande de Chile (Arica, Lat. 18°28' S). Vol I. A. Veloso and E. Bustos, (eds.) pp. 13-70. Montevideo, Uruguay: Oficina Regional de Ciencia y Tecnología de UNESCO para América Latina y el Caribe (ROSTLAC).

Villagrán, C., Kalin Arroyo, M. and Marticorena, C.

1983 Efectos de la desertización en la distribución de la flora Andina de Chile. Rev. Chil. Natural 56:137-157.

Vogel, J., Pryor, R. and Blount, S.

1964 The cardiovascular system in children from high altitude. J. Pediatr. 64:315-322.

Vogel, J., Weaver, W., Rose, R. et al.

1962 Pulmonary hypertension on exertion in normal man living at 10,150 feet. Med. Thorac. 19:461-477.

Vuilleumier, B. S.

1971 Pleistocene changes in the fauna and flora of South America. Science 173:771-780.

Vuilleumier, F. and Simberloff, D.

1980 Ecology versus history as determinants of patchy and insular distributions in high Andean birds. Evolutionary Biol. 2:235-379.

Waddington, C. H.

1942 Canalization of development and the inheritance of acquired characters. Nature 150:563-565.

Waerhang, J.

1966 Epidemiology of periodontal disease. *In* Workshop in Periodontics. S.P. Ramfjord, D.A. Kerr, M.M. Ash, (eds.) pp. 179-211. Ann Arbor, MI.

Wagenvoort, C. and Wagenvoort, N.

1973 Hypoxic pulmonary vascular lesions in man at high altitude and in patients with chronic respiratory disease. Pathologia et Microbiologia 39(3):276-282.

Walker, E. P.

1975 The Mammals of the World. Baltimore, MD: Johns Hopkins University Press.

Ward, R. H.

1972 The genetic structure of a tribal population, the Yanomama Indians. V. Comparison of a series of genetic networks. Ann. Hum. Genet. 36:21-43.

Ward, R. H., Gershowitz, H., Layrisse, M. and Neel, J. V.

1975 The genetic structure of a tribal population, the Yanomama Indians. VI. Gene frequencies for 10 blood groups and the AGH-Le secretor traits in the Yanomama and their neighbors; the uniqueness of the tribe. Am. J. Hum. Genet. 27:1-30.

Webb, D.

1978 A history of savanna vertebrates in the New World. Part II. South America and the Great Interchange. Ann. Rev. Ecol. System. 9:393-426.

Weidman, M.
1975 High-altitude retinal hemorrhage. Arch. Ophthalmol. 93:401-403.
Weir, E. K., Tucker, A., Reeves, J. T., Will, D. H. and Grover, R. F.
1974 The genetic factor influencing pulmonary hypertension in cattle at high altitude. Cardiovasc. Res. 8:745-749.
Weitkamp, L. R., Franglen, G., Rokala, D. A., Polesky, H. F., Simpson, N. E., Sunderman, F. W. et al.
1969 An electrophoretic comparison of human serum albumin variants: Eight distinguishable types. Hum. Hered. 19:159-169.
Weitkamp, L. R., McDermid, E. M., Neel, J. V., Fine, J. M., Petrini, C., Bonazzi, L. et al.
1973 Additional data on the population distribution of human serum albumin genes: Three new variants. Ann. Hum. Genet. 37:219-226.
Weiss, K. M., Ferrell, R. E., and Hanis, C. L.
1984 A new world syndrome of metabolic diseases with a genetic and evolutionary basis. Yearbook Phys. Anthropol. 27:153-178.
Wheeler Pires-Ferreira, J., Pires-Ferreira, E. and Kaulicke, P.
1976 Preceramic animal utilization in the Central Peruvian Andes. Science 194:483-490.
Whitehead, L.
1968 Altitude, fertility and mortality in Andean countries. Popul. Stud. 22:335-346.
Wilcox, A. J., Weinberg, C. R., O'Connor, J. F. and Baird, D. D.
1988 Incidence of early loss of pregnancy. N. Engl. J. Med. 319:189-194.
Winterhalder, B. P. and Thomas, R. B.
1978 Geoecology of Southern Highland Peru. A human adaptation perspective. Institute of Arctic and Alpine Research, University of Colorado, Occas. Paper No. 27, pp 1-91.
Wolpoff, M.
1969 The effect of mutations under conditions of reduced selection. Soc. Biol. 16:11-23.
Wormald Cruz, A.
1968 Frontera Norte. Santiago, Chile: Editorial Orbe.
Wormald Cruz, A.
1969 El Mestizo en el Departamento de Arica. Santiago, Chile: Ediciones Rafaga.
Wright, A. C. S., Astudillo, J., Meléndez, E. and Alcayaga, B.
1961 Notes on soils, natural vegetation, and land use in the Department of Arica, Province of Tarapacá, Chile. Supplement to the 1st Quarterly Report of the Assessor in Soils F.A.O.-Chile.
Wright, A. C. S. and Meléndez, E.
1963 Environment, soil and land use in the Department of Arica, Province of Tarapacá, Northern Chile. Supplement to the Quarterly Report of the Assessor in Soils F.A.O.-Chile.
Wright, S.
1965 The interpretation of population structure by F-statistics with special regard to systems of mating. Evolution 19:395-420.
Wu, M., Kuo, T., Hwang, Y., and Chen, C.
1989 Dose-response relation between arsenic concentration in well water and mortality from cancers and vascular diseases. Am. J. Epidemiol. 130:1123-1132
Yabek, S.
1989 Research and practice in pediatric cardiology. Progress in Cardiology Nov. pp. 14-15.
Yen, F. I.
1972 Polimorfismo a nivel molecular de los genes due determinan la fosfatasa ácida del erithrocito en poblaciones humanas del altiplano Peruano. Arch. Inst. Biol. Andina 5:1-12.
Zaldivar, R.
1980 Gradientes geograficas en concentraciones de litio en aguas superficiales y de consumo y en plasma sanguineo de subjetos expuestos. Rev. Med. Chile. 108:822-824.
Ziegler, R.
1951 Electrocardiographic Studies in Normal Infants and Children. Springfield, IL: Charles C. Thomas.

MULTINATIONAL ANDEAN GENETIC AND HEALTH PROGRAM PUBLICATIONS

Bailey, J. K.
1984 Hearing and hypoxia in the Aymara Indians of Chile. Master of Science Thesis. Houston, TX: The University of Texas Health Science Center at Houston, Graduate School of Biomedical Sciences.

Barton, S. A., Lenart, V., Palomino, H., Murillo, F., Weidman, W. and Schull, W. J.
1976 High altitude, indigenous origin and continuous monitoring. Aviat. Space Environ. Med. 47:592-596.

Chakraborty, R.
1976 Cultural, language and geographical correlates of genetic variability in Andean highland Indians. Nature 264:350-352.

Chakraborty, R., Barton, S. A., Ferrell, R. E. and Schull, W. J.
1989 Ethnicity determination by names among the Aymara of Chile and Bolivia. Hum. Biol. 61(2): 159-177.

Chakraborty, R., Ferrell, R. E., Barton, S. A. and Schull, W. J.
1985 Ethnicity determination by names: A case study of validity and reliability in admixed groups in Chile and Bolivia. Am. J. Phys. Anthropol. 66:154 (abstract).

Chakraborty, R., Ferrell, R. E., Barton, S. A. and Schull, W. J.
1986 Genetic polymorphism and fertility parameters in the Aymara of Chile and Bolivia. Ann. Hum. Genet. 50:69-82.

Chakraborty, R., Barton, S. A., Schull, W. J., Hanis, C. and Weidman, W.
1982 Familial component of blood pressure variation in an hypoxic environment. Am. J. Phys. Anthropol. 57:175 (Abstract).

Chakraborty, R., Clench, J., Ferrell, R. E., Barton, S. A. and Schull, W. J.
1983 Genetic components of variations of red cell glycolytic intermediates at two altitudes among the South American Aymara. Ann. Hum. Biol. 10:173-184.

Chakraborty, R., Gershowitz, H., Ferrell, R. E., Barton, S. A. and Schull, W. J.
1985 Immunoglobulin (Gm and Km) allotypes in the Aymara of Chile and Bolivia. Ann. Hum. Biol. 12:533-544.

Clench, J. M. Rigaud
1980 Hematocrit and hemoglobin, ATP and DPG concentrations in Andean man: Variability by sex, age, village, altitude, weight, smoking habits and genetic constitution. Ph.D. Dissertation. Houston, TX: The University of Texas Health Science at Houston, School of Public Health.

Clench, J., Ferrell, R. E. and Schull, W. J.
1982 Effect of chronic altitude hypoxia on hematologic and glycolytic parameters. Am. J. Physiol. 242 (Regulatory Integrative Comp. Physiol.) 11: R447-451.

Clench, J., Ferrell, R. E., Schull, W. J. and Barton, S. A.
1981 Hematocrit and hemoglobin, ATP and DPG concentrations in Andean man: The interaction of altitude and trace metals with glycolytic and hematologic parameters in man. *In* The Red Cell: Fifth Ann Arbor Conference. G.J. Brewer, (ed.) pp. 747-762. New York: Alan R. Liss.

Clench, J., Barton, S. A., Lenart, V., Murillo, F. and Schull, W. J.
1980 Circadian heart rhythmicity in natives living a high altitude. Chronobiologia 7:265-267.

Díaz, B., Gallegos, D., Murillo, F., Covarrubias, E., Covarrubias, T., Rona, R., Weidman, W., Rothhammer, F. and Schull, W. J.
1978 The multinational Andean genetic and health program. II. Disease and disability among the Aymara. Bull. Pan. Am. Health Organ. 12:219-235. (El programa multinacional Andino de genetica y salud: II. Enfermedades e invalideces entre los Aimaras. Bol. Of. Sanit. Panam. 86(1):20-39).

William J. Schull and Francisco Rothhammer (eds.), The Aymará: Strategies in Human Adaptation to a Rigorous Environment, 243-247. *©1990 by Kluwer Academic Publishers.*

Ferrell, R. E., Schull, W. J. and Barton, S. A.
1985 Adenosine triphosphate, diphosphoglyceric acid, and their relationship to reproductivity at altitude. *In* Human Adaptation to Environment. Proceedings of the Symposium on Human Adaptation to Environment: Relative Impacts of Physical, Environmental and Sociocultural Factors. A. Basu and B. Mukhopadhyay, (eds.) Calcutta, India: The Indian Anthropological Society, pp. 43-54.
Ferrell, R. E., Bertin, T. and Schull, W. J.
1981 An electrophoretic study of glycolytic enzymes in a human population living at high altitude: The Aymara of Northern Chile and Western Bolivia. Hum. Genet. 56:397-399.
Ferrell, R. E., Bertin, T., Barton, S. A., Rothhammer, F. and Schull, W. J.
1980 A multinational Andean genetic and health program. IX. Gene frequencies and rare variants of 20 serum proteins and erythrocyte enzymes in the Aymara of Chile. Am. J. Hum. Genet. 32:92-102.
Ferrell, R. E., Bertin, T., Young, R., Barton, S. A., Murillo, F. and Schull, W. J.
1978 The Aymara of Western Bolivia. IV. Gene frequencies for eight blood groups and 19 protein and erythrocyte enzyme systems. Am. J. Hum. Genet. 30:539-549.
Ferrell, R. E., Chakraborty, R., Barton, S. A. and Schull, W. J.
1985 Genetic polymorphisms and fertility parameters in the Aymara of Chile and Bolivia. Am. J. Phys. Anthropol. 66:167 (Abstract).
Goldsmith, R. I., Rothhammer, F. and Schull, W. J.
1977 Mydriasis and heredity. Clin. Genet. 12:128-133.
Goldsmith, R. I., Rothhammer, F. and Schull, W. J.
1979 The multinational Andean genetic and health program. III. Ophthalmic disease and disability among the Aymara. Bull. PAHO 13(1):58-65. (El progama multinacional Andino de genetica y salud: III. Enfermedades e invalideces oftalmicas entre los Aimaras. Bol. Of. Sanit. Panam. 87(3):191-199).
Makela, M., Weidman, W., Barton, S. A., Rothhammer, F. and Schull, W. J.
1978 The multinational Andean genetic and health program. IV. Altitude and the blood pressure of the Aymara. J. Chron. Dis. 31:587-603.
Marcks, S., Barton, S. A., Ferrell, R., and Howell, R. R.
1980 Effects of nontherapeutic environmental exposure to lithium. Am. J. Hum. Genetics 32:147A (abstract)
McFarlane, J. M.
1982 Infection: Its ecological determinants among children in northern Chile. Doctor of Public Health Dissertation. Houston, TX: The University of Texas Health Science Center at Houston, School of Public Health.
Mueller, W. H., Schull, W. J. and Rothhammer, F.
1981 Studies of the Aymara of highland, intermontane and coastal Chile. *In* Health in the Andes. J.W. Bastien and J.M. Donahue, (eds.) pp. 69-91. Washington, D.C.: American Anthropological Assn.
Mueller, W. H., Yen, F. I., Rothhammer, F. and Schull, W. J.
1978 The multinational Andean genetic and health program. VI. Physiological measurements of lung function in an hypoxic environment. Hum. Biol. 50(4):489-513.
Mueller, W. H., Yen, F. I., Rothhammer, F. and Schull, W. J.
1978 The multinational Andean genetic and health program. VII. Lung function and physical growth: Multivariate analysis in high and low altitude populations. Aviat. Space Environ. Med. 49:1188-1196.
Mueller, W. H., Chakraborty, R., Barton, S. A., Rothhammer, F. and Schull, W.J.
1980 Genes and epidemiology in anthropological adaptation studies: Familial correlations in lung function in populations residing at different altitudes in Chile. Med. Anthropol. 4:366-384.
Mueller, W. H., Soto, P., Schull, V., Rothhammer, F. and Schull, W. J.
1978 The multinational Andean genetic and health program. V. Growth and development in an hypoxic environment. Ann. Hum. Biol. 5:329-352.
Mueller, W. H., Ferrell, R. E., Bertin, T., Barton, S. A., Rothhammer, F., and Schull, W.J.
1981 Genetic flexibility and morphological variation in populations residing at different altitudes in Chile. Am. J. Phys. Anthropol. 54:257 (abstract).
Mueller, W. H., Yen, F. I., Soto, P., Schull, V., Rothhammer, F. and Schull, W. J.
1979 The multinational Andean genetic and health program. VIII. Lung function, altitude and migration. Am. J. Phys. Anthropol. 51:183-196.

Mueller, W. H., Murillo, F., Palomino, H., Badzioch, M., Chakraborty, R., Fuerst, P. E. and Schull, W. J.
1980 The Aymara of Western Bolivia. V. Growth and development in an hypoxic environment. Hum. Biol. 52:529-546.
Murillo, F., Barton, S. A., Palomino, H., Lenart, V. and Schull, W. J.
1980 The Aymara of Western Bolivia: Health and disease. Bull. PAHO 14:52-64. (Los Aimaras del Oeste de Bolivia: Salud y enfermedad. Bol. Of. Sanit. Panam. 89(5):415-428).
Palomino, H.
1978 The Aymara of Western Bolivia: III. Occlusion, pathology, and characteristics of the dentition. J. Dent. Res. 57:459-467.
Palomino, H., Mueller, W. H. and Schull, W. J.
1979 Altitude, heredity and body proportions in Northern Chile. Am. J. Phys. Anthropol. 50:39-50.
Palomino, H., Barton, S. A., Murillo, F. and Schull, W. J.
1978 The Aymara of Western Bolivia: II. Maxillofacial and dental arch variation. Am. J. Phys. Anthrop. 49:157-166.
Rothhammer, F.
1977 Microdiferenciación genética de una población indígena de habla Aymará de la provincia de Arica. Ph.D. Dissertation. Santiago, Chile: Faculty of Science, University of Chile.
Rothhammer, F. and Schull, W. J.
1980 Adaptacion genetica de poblaciones Andinas. Actas IV Congr. Latinoam. Genet. 2:357-368.
Rothhammer, F. and Schull, W.J.
1982 Adaptación genética a la altura de una población de habla Aymará de las provincias de Parinacota y Arica, Chile. *In* El Ambiente Natural y las Poblaciones Humanas de los Andes del Norte Grande de Chile (Arica, Lat. 18° 28'S). Vol I. A. Veloso and E. Bustos, (eds.) pp. 1-12. Montevideo, Uruguay: Oficina Regional de Ciencia y Tecnología de la UNESCO para América Latina y el Caribe (ROSTLAC).
Rothhammer, F. and Llop, E.
1982 Estimacion indirecta de tasas de mutacion a partir de variantes electroforeticas en unma poblacion Altiplanica. *In* El Ambiente Natural y las Poblaciones Humanas de los Andes del Norte Grande de Chile (Arica, Lat. 18° 28'S). Vol I. A. Veloso and E. Bustos, (eds.) pp. 13-16. Montevideo, Uruguay: Oficina Regional de Ciencia y Tecnología de la UNESCO para América Latina y el Caribe (ROSTLAC).
Rothhammer, F., Castillo, S. and Schull, W. J.
1985 Risk to disease of Andean populations inhabiting contrasting ecogeographic areas. *In* Diseases of Complex Etiology in Small Populations: Ethnic Differences and Research Approaches. R. Chakraborty and E.J.E. Szathmary, (eds.) pp. 325-344. New York: Alan R. Liss.
Schull, W. J.
1973 Mankind, past and future. Bulletin of The University of Texas Institutions at Houston, 3rd Quarter, pp. 20-26.
Schull, W. J.
1980 Food, water and genes. Fukuoka Acta Medica 71(2):47-60.
Schull, W. J. and Rothhammer, F.
1977 A multinational Andean genetic and health program: A study of adaptation to the hypoxia of altitude. *In* Physiological Variation and its Genetic Basis. Society for the Study of Human Biology Vol. 17. J.S. Weiner, (ed.) pp. 139-169. London: Taylor and Francis.
Schull, W. J. and Rothhammer, F.
1979 Analytical methods for genetic and adaptational studies. *In* The First Americans: Origins, Affinities and Adaptations. W. S. Laughlin and A. Harper, (eds.) pp. 241-255. New York: Gustav Fischer.
Schull, W.J. and Rothhammer, F.
1981 The multinational Andean genetic and health program: A brief description. *In* Environmental and Human Population Problems at High Altitude. C. Jest and P. Baker (eds.) pp. 55-60. Paris, France: Centre National de la Recherche Scientifique.

Schull, W. J., Ferrell, R. E. and Rothhammer, F.
1978 Genes, enzymes and hypoxia. *In* Ecological Genetics. Proc. in the Life Sciences. P. Brussard, (ed.) pp. 73-90. New York: Springer-Verlag.

Schull, W. J., Goldsmith, R. I.,Clench, J., Ferrell, R. E., Barton, S. A. and Rothhammer, F.
1981 2,3-diphosphoglycerate and night vision. Aviat. Space Environ. Med. 52:41-44.

Schull, W. J., Hanis, C., Ferrell, R. E., Clench-Aas, J. and Rothhammer, F.
1983 Psychomotor performance, hypoxia and the Aymara. *In* Proceedings of the Indian Statistical Institute Golden Jubilee International Conference on Human Genetics and Adaptation, Vol. 2. A. Basu and K.C. Malhotra, (eds.) pp. 85-99. Calcutta, India: Indian Statistical Institute.

Weidman, W., Barton, S. A., Lenart, V. and Schull, W. J.
1984-85 Effect of high altitude on age related changes in the pulmonary vascular bed seen in coastal populations. Commemorative Volume Dr. Carlos Monge Sr. 100th Birthday. E. Picon-Reategui, (ed.) Lima, Peru: Arch. Inst. Biol. Andina 13:95-110.

GLOSSARY

alpaca	camel family, domestic Andean animal, sheared for wool
altiplano	*in Chile:* high plateau between two principal Andean mountain chains; east of Cordillera Central mountains in Chile and west of Bolivia, elevation 4000 m or more. *in Bolivia:* high plateau around Lake Titicaca and north-western Bolivia; the high plateau or intermountain basin of Bolivia that lies between the two main cordilleras of the Andes, elevation about 3000 to 4200 m; the high basin area of western Bolivia in which the population is concentrated
Atacama	northern Chilean desert stretching from Arica to Caldera, a distance of about 960 kms.
Atacameños	Literally, 'people of the land', a distinctive Indian language and culture once common to the northern Chilean provinces of Tacna, Arica, Tarapacá, Antofagasta, and Atacama and northwestern provinces of Argentina, Los Andes, Salta and Jujuy. Culturally and linguistically they have been absorbed by the Aymará or Spanish.
ayllu	association of families united by community, territorial, and genealogical links; Indian land tenure unit, a communal kinship group or clan; lineage, through male descent, of an Inca emperor
Aymará (Aimará)	language spoken by Indians of southern Perú, northern Chile, western Bolivia; chiefly in the altiplano
bofedal	green peat bogs, marshy area
callahuayas	traveling herbalists, who dispense medical services consisting of folk knowledge, witchcraft, and herb cures
camanchaca	heavy winter mist on coast
cañihua (qanahua)	(*Chenopodium pallidicaule*) cereal grain

campesino	rural dweller, a peasant
caserio	a cluster of a few houses
charqui	jerky, dried meat, usually llama
chenopodi-aceae	a family of plants occuring in temperate regions of the world to which cañihua and quinoa belong
chicha	fermented drink, usually made from corn
choclo	corn on the cob
cholo	person of mixed Indian and European background, a member of an intermediate social class in Bolivia; generally of mixed racial composition
chuño	freeze dried potatoes, prepared by Aymará and Quechua Indians
coca	(*Erythroxylon coca*) a boxwood-like bush from which cocaine is derived; the leaf is chewed
cóndor	(*Vultur gryphus*) large American vulture which makes its habitat in the high altitudes of the Andes
cordillera (montaña)	mountains
CORFO	Corporación de Fomento de Producción (Chilean Development Corporation)
costa (coast)	coastal plain, western slope of Andes Mountains to Pacific Ocean
criollo	a person born in the New World colonies, of Spanish parents
cuy	guinea pig
departamento	governmental division analogous to state
2,3-DPG	2,3-diphosphoglyceric acid, a glycolytic intermediate in the red cell that binds to hemoglobin to decrease its O_2 affinity
ECG (EKG)	electrocardiogram

ENDESA	Empresa Nacional de Electricidad (National Electricity Enterprise)
fava	see haba
FEV_1	forced expiratory volume in 1 second, a measurement of pulmonary function. Forced expiratory volume is usually reduced in chronic obstructive pulmonary disease.
guanaco	(*Lama guanicoe*) camel family, nondomesticated, superfine wool
haba (hava)	(*Vicia faba*) broad beans, larger than lima beans
hematocrit	fraction of blood that is red cells (%)
hemoglobin	concentraction of hemoglobin in the blood, gm/deciliter
Guallatiri (Huallatiri or Quallatire)	small village in northern Chilean altiplano
ichu	Andean bunch grass
Inca	Quechua-speaking group around Cuzco, Perú and the empire it ruled; ethnic group
JAA	Junta de Adelanto de Arica
junta	a municipal or provincial council
latifundia	large, entailed, private estates; large feudalistic agricultural estate in pre-1952 Bolivia
llama	camel family, domesticated animal, wool producing, beast of burden
llareta	(*Laretia compacta*) cauliflower-like woody plant
MCH	mean corpuscular hemoglobin: hemoglobin (gm/liter)/red blood cell count (millions/mm^3)
MCHC	mean corpuscular hemoglobin concentration: hemoglobin (gm/100 ml × 100/hematocrit (ml/100 ml)

MCV	mean corpuscular volume: hematocrit (ml/1000 ml)/red blood cell (millions/mm^3)
mestizo	person of mixed race, usually European (Spanish) and Indian descent
mitmas	settlers transplanted to colonize part of empire; the class of colonists used by the Inca to consolidate their political territory
mote	hominy
Nandú	(*Pterocnemia pennata*) South American rhea
Norte Grande	northern desert, from border of Perú south to Copiapó River
oca (oqa)	(*Oxalis tuberosa*) carrot-like tuber
paja brava	high altitude tough bunch grass, used to make roofs on houses
pampa	grassy plain
parina	(*Phoenicoparrus andinus*) flamingo
parroquia	parish
perdiz	(*Tinamotis pentlandii*) partridge-like bird
polycythemia vera	(polycythemia rubra vera) A condition of overproduction of red blood cells in the bone marrow. Apparently production is autonomous because the rate is not related to hypoxia or the levels of erythropoietin, as it is in other states of increased red cell production.
portazuela	mountain pass
practicante	untrained person practicing medicine; in Chile medically trained military person providing medical attention, first-aid in mountains
pucará	fort
puna	mountain sickness a high altitude zone of the Andes, above timberline, and suitable only for pasture of llamas and alpacas

quebrada	canyon
Quechua	an Indian who speaks Quechua; Indian language of Bolivia predominant in the valleys; official language of Incas and modern Andean Indians. the most numerous Indian group in western South America; the dominant Indian language
queñoa (queñua)	(*Polylepis incana*) twisted small bush
quinoa (quinua or hupa)	(*Chenopodium quinoa*) high Andes edible small grain cereal with spinach-like leaves; seeds ground for food
SNS	Servicio Nacional de Salud (National Health Service)
sierra	3000 to 3500 meters
solanaceae	a family of tropical and semi-tropical herbaceous plants, including the potato, nightshade, and tobacco
soroche	mountain sickness; also called mareo or veta or puna
surumpe	inflammation of the eyes
Tarapacá	province in northern Chile
Tignamar (Ticnamar)	sierran village in northern Chile
Tiwanaku (Tiwanacu or Tiahuanaco)	a culture of the altiplano of Perú, Bolivia and contiguous areas, deriving its name from the western Bolivian community Tiwanaku; it extended from about 100 BC to 900 AD
tunta	frozen, crushed, dehydrated, washed and redried potatoes
vicuña	(*Vicugna vicugna*) undomesticated Andean animal, finer grade of wool than llama
viscacha	(*Lagidium viscacia*) rabbit-like rodent
Uro-Chipaya	cultural group who lived around Lake Titicaca, western Bolivia, southern Perú coast and northern Chile coast; language unrelated to Quechua or Aymará

INDEX

Studies in Human Biology

1. N. M. Durham and C. C. Plato (eds.): *Trends in Dermatologlyphic Research.* 1990 ISBN 0-7923-0963-4
2. W. J. Schull and F. Rothhammer (eds.): *The Aymara.* Strategies in Human Adaptation to a Rigorous Environment. 1990 ISBN 0-7923-0969-3

KLUWER ACADEMIC PUBLISHERS – DORDRECHT / BOSTON / LONDON